Optical Methods in Sensing and Imaging for Medical and Biological Applications

Optical Methods in Sensing and Imaging for Medical and Biological Applications

Special Issue Editors

Dragan Indjin
Željka Cvejić
Małgorzata Jędrzejewska-Szczerska

MDPI • Basel • Beijing • Wuhan • Barcelona • Belgrade

MDPI

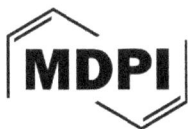

Special Issue Editors

Dragan Indjin
University of Leeds
UK

Željka Cvejić
University of Novi
Sad Serbia

Malgorzata Jedrzejewska-Szczerska
Gdańsk University of Technology
Poland

Editorial Office
MDPI
St. Alban-Anlage 66
4052 Basel, Switzerland

This is a reprint of articles from the Special Issue published online in the open access journal *Sensors* (ISSN 1424-8220) from 2016 to 2018 (available at: https://www.mdpi.com/journal/sensors/special_issues/optical_methods_sensing_imaging)

For citation purposes, cite each article independently as indicated on the article page online and as indicated below:

LastName, A.A.; LastName, B.B.; LastName, C.C. Article Title. *Journal Name* **Year**, *Article Number, Page Range.*

ISBN 978-3-03897-370-6 (Pbk)
ISBN 978-3-03897-371-3 (PDF)

Contents

About the Special Issue Editors

Dragan Indjin joined the School of Electronic and Electrical Engineering, University of Leeds, Leeds, UK in 2001. He currently holds the title of Reader in Optoelectronics and Nanoscale Electronics. His research interests include electronic structures, optical and transport properties, optimization and design of quantum wells, quantum-cascade lasers, and quantum well infrared photodetectors from near- to far-infrared and terahertz spectral ranges. He is currently focused on exploiting quantum-cascade lasers and interband cascade lasers for sensing and imaging applications from security and defense to in vivo biomedical imaging. Dr. Indjin was a recipient of the prestigious Academic Fellowship from the Research Councils UK and University of Leeds, in 2005. He has published more than 150 journal papers (current h-index: 25) and has delivered a number of invited talks and seminars at leading conferences. He has also served as coordinator and project director of major international projects on infrared and terahertz imaging for skin cancer detection and terahertz sensing for security applications.

Željka Cvejić is a Professor at the Faculty of Sciences, University of Novi Sad, Serbia. She obtained an M.Sc. degree from the University of Belgrade, Serbia, and a Ph.D. from the University of Novi Sad. Her goal is to understand how structure and microstructure affect physical and chemical properties of materials. Her main research focus is the design and optimization of electrical, optical, and magnetic properties of nanomaterials. Other fields of interest include crystallography, X-ray diffraction, spectroscopy, scattering, and structure modeling. Her lab is currently developing an ambitious research program concerning the difference of angular distribution for scattered radiation on biological tissue. Also, she aims to address the growing need to identify key spectral peaks and their correct assignment to a chemical structure for the different statuses of biological tissue. Prof Željka Cvejić has published a great number of research articles, with over 240 total citations (h-index: 8) according to Google Scholar.

Małgorzata Jędrzejewska-Szczerska is an Associate Professor in the Department of Metrology and Optoelectronics of Gdańsk University of Technology, where she leads the research group in the area of biophotonics and fiber-optic sensors. She received a Ph.D. in 2008 and a D.Sc. in 2016 from Gdańsk University of Technology. Her main area of research is biophotonics and she focuses on the use of low-coherence interferometry, fiber-optic technology, and the application of optical measurements in biomedicine. Apart from her main research subject, she also deals with research in the areas of: using low-coherence interferometry in metrology, constructing an electronic system supporting behavioral therapy for children with autism, and investigating the biocompatibility of new optoelectronic materials. She has supervised seven doctoral theses and has published more than 60 research articles and review papers. She has served as a leader of many scientific projects and has been awarded by the first edition of the INTER competition, organized by the Foundation for Polish Science for the implementation of interdisciplinary research (2013–2014). She was the winner of the first edition of the eNgage competition of the Foundation for Polish Science for the implementation of the work of disseminating research results (2014–2015). She is the author and co-author of 10 patent applications. Several technical achievements, of which she was a co-founder, were presented at exhibitions of inventions and won medals. For a number of years she has been involved in activities related to the popularization of science among people from outside of the university. She is the co-organizer of a series of actions popularizing science, organized at Gdańsk University of Technology, as well as in schools and kindergartens in the Pomerania region. Since 2013 she has been an Advisor of the Optical Society of American Student Chapter and BioPhoton Students Science Club at Gdańsk University of Technology. From 2016 she has also been an OSA Traveling Lecturer.

Preface to "Optical Methods in Sensing and Imaging for Medical and Biological Applications"

The recent advances in optical sources and detectors have opened up new opportunities for sensing and imaging techniques which can be successfully used in biomedical and healthcare applications. This book, entitled *Optical Methods in Sensing and Imaging for Medical and Biological Applications*, focuses on all aspects of the research and development related to these areas.

With 19 works and a review paper, this book covers different areas of the most advantageous biomedical sensing and imaging applications. These include novel imaging modalities that are efficient tools for the improvement of healthcare quality. The review paper describes multispectral, fluorescent, and photoplethysmographic imaging technologies which ensure patient-friendly remote skin assessment. It relates not only to diagnostics in dermatology, e.g., the identification of skin cancers, but also to the monitoring of patient condition during surgeries (distant control of anesthesia efficiency) and in longer periods of time (development/healing of skin malformations, post-operative follow-up, etc.).

Another interesting example presented in the book is a work on an extended near-infrared multispectral imaging system based on an InGaAs sensor used to improve the diagnosis of skin cancer with respect to that offered by silicon sensors. While the new system provides similar values of sensitivity, it also offers significantly better specificity.

There is still a need for low-cost measuring devices for biology and medicine which can be fulfilled by the fiber-optic sensors. Fiber-optic sensors are insensitive to electric and magnetic field interferences as well as ionizing radiation. This class of sensors is characterized by small size, which allows for nearly pointwise measurements. Moreover, while analyzing signals in the frequency domain, changes in the intensity of the optical signal do not affect the transmitted information. On the other hand, the development in nanotechnology and techniques of depositing thin films open new opportunities for tuning the optical parameters of such sensors. One of the key paper describes the possibility of improving the reflectivity of a fiber-optic Fabry-Pérot cavity by the use of a dielectric film: titanium dioxide (TiO_2). A thin film was deposited on the tip of single-mode fiber-optic via the atomic layer deposition (ALD) technique. The deposition of TiO_2 allows for measurements of samples characterized by a similar refractive index to the silica glass fiber, which are impossible to perform without the film. Another advantage is that TiO_2 introduces better resistance to aggressive chemicals and biocompatibility. This expands the measurement abilities of the sensor; biomedical measurements can be performed as was proven in the article by the successful measurement of the refractive index of glucose and hemoglobin. Another good example is the application of an indium tin oxide (ITO) in an optical fiber sensor for the real-time optical monitoring of the electrochemical deposition of ketoprofen during its anodic oxidation.

The papers contributed to this book also address issues of high relevance for practical applications; for example, in one paper the authors describe the use of in-vivo OCT (optical coherent tomography) imaging for perfusion evaluation in patients with esophageal cancer undergoing gastric tube surgery. The incidence of esophageal cancer is rising and post-operative complications, because of impaired perfusion, account for a high morbidity and even mortality. Described intra-operative perfusion imaging with OCT using speckle contrast percentage is a non-invasive, real-time technique to help the surgeon in decision-making for the desirable anastomosis placement. The widespread and growing amount of human and veterinary prescriptions of pain-killers needs to be followed by the development of novel sensing techniques allowing for the detection of their traces in various biofluids or sludge water. The direct or indirect contamination of the environment by, e.g., ketoprofen (KP) enhances the bacterial resistance against these drugs and has a negative effect on non-targeted organisms, even at very low environmental concentrations. Thus, KP and other pain-killer drugs have been recognized as emerging contaminants. To overcome the aforementioned issues, the authors of one featured paper propose a novel approach for KP detection where an electrochemical method and an indium tin oxide (ITO)-coated optical fiber sensor is used. The described solution offers reliability and accuracy, enabling the development of simple, rapid, and cost-effective approaches for the detection of electroactive compounds like ketoprofen.

One can also find in this book a comprehensive set of results and studies on novel optical techniques and methods in ophthalmology. One of the papers describes the results showing that excimer laser surgery with an advanced eye tracker system achieves much better results of astigmatism refractive error correction. Furthermore, the analyses of biomechanical corneal effects using the dynamic of pterygium disease progression combined with an adequate mathematical model leads to a better prediction of further corneal changes. That gives us a good platform to simulate corneal surgery with a better clinical prediction and potentially a more successful clinical outcome. Another study presented in the book showed that the femtosecond laser gives us the possibility to perform customized surgery with higher precision, that is repeatable and minimally invasive. Supracor is a customized PresyLASIK procedure which is proven to give good refractive results for far, intermediate, and near visual acuity with improvement of contrast vision.

We strongly believe that this book will be a valuable source of information presenting the recent advances in optical methods and techniques, in addition to their applications in the field of biomedicine and healthcare, to anyone interested in this subject.

Dragan Indjin, Željka Cvejić, Małgorzata Jędrzejewska-Szczerska
Special Issue Editors

sensors

MDPI

Review

Multispectral, Fluorescent and Photoplethysmographic Imaging for Remote Skin Assessment

Janis Spigulis

Biophotonics Laboratory, Institute of Atomic Physics and Spectroscopy, University of Latvia, Riga, LV-1586, Latvia; janis.spigulis@lu.lv; Tel.: +371-2948-5347

Academic Editors: Dragan Indjin, Željka Cvejić and Małgorzata Jędrzejewska-Szczerska
Received: 12 April 2017; Accepted: 17 May 2017; Published: 19 May 2017

Abstract: Optical tissue imaging has several advantages over the routine clinical imaging methods, including non-invasiveness (it does not change the structure of tissues), remote operation (it avoids infections) and the ability to quantify the tissue condition by means of specific image parameters. Dermatologists and other skin experts need compact (preferably pocket-size), self-sustaining and easy-to-use imaging devices. The operational principles and designs of ten portable in-vivo skin imaging prototypes developed at the Biophotonics Laboratory of Institute of Atomic Physics and Spectroscopy, University of Latvia during the recent five years are presented in this paper. Four groups of imaging devices are considered. Multi-spectral imagers offer possibilities for distant mapping of specific skin parameters, thus facilitating better diagnostics of skin malformations. Autofluorescence intensity and photobleaching rate imagers show a promising potential for skin tumor identification and margin delineation. Photoplethysmography video-imagers ensure remote detection of cutaneous blood pulsations and can provide real-time information on cardiovascular parameters and anesthesia efficiency. Multimodal skin imagers perform several of the abovementioned functions by taking a number of spectral and video images with the same image sensor. Design details of the developed prototypes and results of clinical tests illustrating their functionality are presented and discussed.

Keywords: multispectral skin imaging; skin autofluorescence and photobleaching; photoplethysmography imaging

1. Introduction

Biomedical imaging has become a powerful tool for diagnostics and monitoring of human health condition. Apart from routine clinical imaging modalities (e.g., x-ray, ultrasound, endoscopy, computed tomography, magnetic resonance imaging), a number of advanced "open air" optical imaging methods and technologies have been introduced recently. Their main advantages are remote operation (avoids infection) and non-invasiveness (does not change the structure of tissues). Besides, digital imaging ensures quantitative documentation on the skin condition and its changes.

There are several commercially available skin diagnostic imaging devices for dermatologists (e.g., *SIAscope* [1], *MelaFind* [2], confocal microscopes [3], multi-photon tomographs [4]), but most of them are bulky, cable-connected to computers and also too expensive for GPs or small clinics. With a perspective on personalized medicine, new more compact and less expensive self-sustaining designs for skin imaging are preferable. The recently commercialized pocket-size digital dermatoscopes [5], video-microscopes [6] and smartphone-based solutions [7] have shown promising potential for primary skin diagnostics. Further developments of portable skin imaging technologies would facilitate their wider and more efficient implementation in hospitals and clinics. They may also prove useful for home monitoring of skin condition, follow-up after skin therapies and for some forensic applications, e.g., for age estimation of bruises [8].

This review paper (which follows a previous review [9]) presents the operational principles, designs and clinical test results of ten portable in-vivo skin imaging prototypes developed over the last five years at the Biophotonics Laboratory of the University of Latvia. Four groups of imaging devices are presented. Multi-spectral imagers offer possibilities for distant mapping of specific skin parameters (e.g., distribution of skin chromophore concentrations) so facilitating better diagnostics of skin malformations. Autofluorescence photobleaching rate imagers show a promising potential for skin tumor identification and margin delineation. Photoplethysmography video-imagers ensure remote detection of cutaneous blood pulsations and can provide real-time information on cardiovascular parameters and anesthesia efficiency. Finally, multimodal skin imagers perform several of the abovementioned functions by taking a number of spectral and video images with the same image sensor. All devices are portable and most of them wireless; original software solutions (not discussed here) provide fast data processing for obtaining clinically significant tissue parameters.

2. Materials and Methods

2.1. Prototype Devices for Multispectral Skin Imaging

Multispectral imaging is a method based on acquisition of a limited number (typically three to 10) of images within relatively narrow non-overlapping spectral bands—so-called spectral images [10]. The captured spectral images of skin can be further converted into parametric images, e.g., 2-D maps that specify distribution of skin chromophore concentrations [11,12]. In the visible spectral range, a relatively simple 3-chromophore skin model can be applied for obtaining chromophore distribution maps over the imaged area [13]. The hardware implementing this approach should ensure easy capture of three narrowband spectral images of skin as fast as possible. One option for that is subsequent narrowband illumination by means of different color LEDs and capturing one spectral image under each illumination mode [11]. This approach was examined earlier by a compact research grade RGB camera-LED illumination ring system [14]. As the next steps, three prototype devices comprising commercial consumer cameras and spectrally specific illuminators were developed.

2.1.1. RGB-LED Add-On Illumination System for Smartphones

Thanks to the rapid development of communication technologies, a number of smartphone camera-based health assessment software applications are available, both in ambient light and under white LED illumination from the same phone [15,16]. Such applications may provide, for instance, information about the potential malignancy of skin lesions [7]. To extend the smartphone applications for skin evaluation, we developed a technique for mapping the main skin chromophores using a RGB light source specially designed as add-on for various smartphone models.

The system design scheme is presented at Figure 1. The smartphone is fixed on a flat sticky surface with a window for its rear camera [17], which is surrounded from bottom by a ring of LEDs mounted within cylindrical screening spacers (6 cm between the skin and camera). The ring includes four types of LEDs, with four diodes of each type: white—to find and adjust location of the skin malformation, and colored—with emission in blue (maximum at 460 nm), green (maximum at 535 nm), and red (maximum at 663 nm) spectral bands (Figure 1b) which are suitable for mapping of three skin chromophores. LEDs are operated in continuous mode and switched on and off manually or automatically by a special software using a Bluetooth connection between the smartphone and the illumination system. Illumination and image detection are performed normally to the skin surface. Two orthogonally oriented polarizers are used in front of the LEDs and smartphone camera, respectively, to reduce detection of skin specular reflection. Five AA 2800 mAh rechargeable battery blocks provide the system power supply.

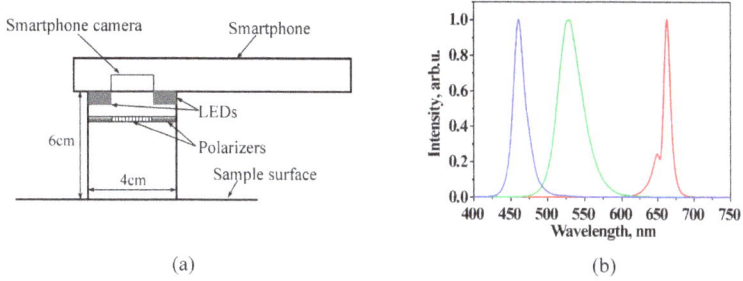

Figure 1. Design scheme of smartphone RGB illuminator (**a**) and normalized emission spectra of the used color LEDs (**b**) [18].

Figure 2a provides more design details of the prototype. A driver placed in the compartment 10 ensures Bluetooth wireless connection between the smartphone and illumination unit and enables automatic sequential on-off switching of the color LEDs within less than 1 s (one image for each illumination band) by command from the smartphone touchscreen. Specially developed software transmits the obtained spectral images via mobile network to a remote server that converts them into distribution maps of the three main skin chromophores (melanin, oxy- and deoxy-hemoglobin) and then transmits the maps back for displaying on the smartphone touchscreen. More details on the RGB-LED smartphone add-on prototype and its tests are provided in [17,18].

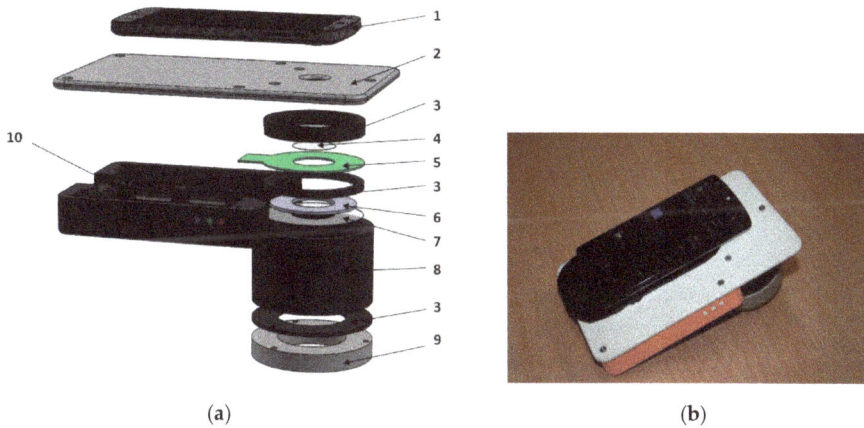

Figure 2. Design details of the smartphone-LED prototype device (**a**) and its outlook with a smartphone on it (**b**): 1—smartphone, 2—sticky fixing platform with a camera window, 3—holding ring, 4—polarizer of the detected light, 5—LED ring comprising four sets of LEDs, 6—light diffuser, 7—illumination polarizer (oriented orthogonally to the polarizer 4), 8—screening spacer, 9—silicone skin contact ring, 10—compartment for batteries and electronic components [17].

2.1.2. Modified Multispectral Video-Microscope

A number of digital microscopes nowadays are small handheld devices connected to a PC via a USB cable; they can be applied also for visual skin assessment [19]. A typical digital microscope consists of a webcam with a high-powered macro-lens and a built-in LED light source. Advantages of such microscopes are their compactness, low power consumption and relatively low price, typically a few hundreds of USD. Most of the digital microscopes have white illumination source(s) and some of them–also ultraviolet illuminators [20]. These devices, however, cannot be used for detailed spectral analysis of skin. To overcome this drawback, we adapted a standard digital microscope (model *DinoLite* AD413, series AM-4013) for multispectral imaging by replacing the built-in LEDs with specifically selected color LEDs and by developing the LED management software.

Figure 3 presents the block diagram of the custom-modified microscope. A standard white/UV LED illuminator ring has been removed and replaced by a lab-designed illuminator ring comprising sixteen LEDs combined in four groups: (1) four infrared 940 nm LEDs; (2) four red 660 nm LEDs; (3) four green 545 nm LEDs; and (4) four blue 450 nm LEDs. To each group of LEDs a current of 80 mA is fed by LED drivers that are controlled by a FTDI USB controller. The two-port USB hub provides control over the LEDs and the original CMOS image sensor of the microscope. The power support, LED switching and CMOS control are executed through the USB interface.

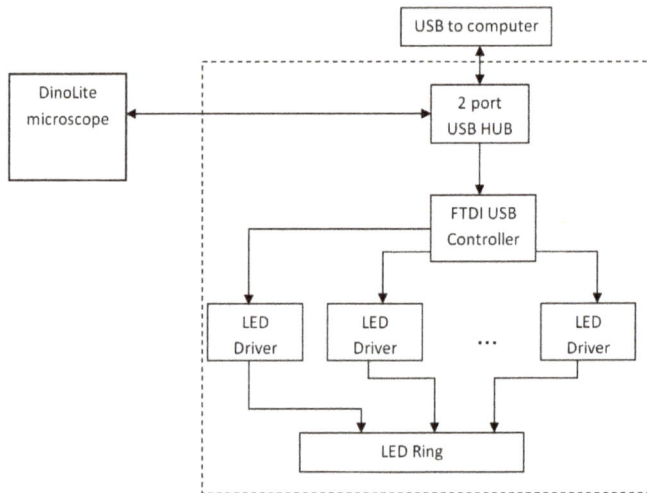

Figure 3. Block diagram of the modified video-microscope [21].

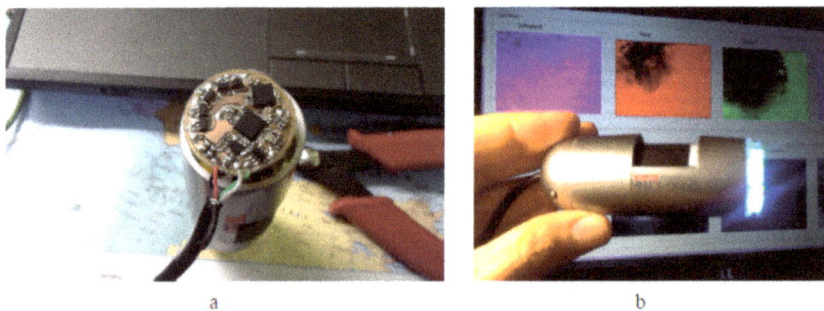

a

b

Figure 4. The developed LED control unit (**a**) and the modified video-microscope with replaced illumination unit (**b**) [21].

The custom-designed control unit module is installed on the rear side of microscope as shown on Figure 4a. The lab-made 16-LED ring is mounted on the front side (Figure 4b); it is even more compact than the original 8-LED *DinoLite* ring. For better homogeneity of skin illumination, a diffuser film is attached to the new LED-ring. To avoid detection of the directly reflected radiation from the skin surface (thus distinguishing the diffusely reflected radiation from the upper layers of skin), a pair of orthogonally-oriented polarizing filters are added: one of them directly after the diffuser, and the other-in front of the camera sensor matrix. The microscope is computer-controlled. The custom-developed program written in MatLab with a standard FTDI USB driver and a custom LED driver (written in C programming language) performs the control over LEDs and the acquisition of images. The software provides two image processing modes: (1) the preview mode, for focusing the microscope to the skin object, and (2) the video acquisition/processing mode, where the software performs sequential switching of LEDs and triggering of the video sensor. Each single measurement includes capturing of four frames (taken within the four wavelength bands). After recording, the images are stored in a 4-image matrix and saved as a data file for further processing. The image processing software allowed mapping of three above-mentioned skin chromophores, erythema index and the melanoma/nevus differentiation parameter [22]. More details on the modified video-microscope and its tests are available in [21,23,24].

2.1.3. Prototypes for Smartphone Monochromatic Spectral Imaging of Skin at Multi-Laser Illumination

If skin is evenly illuminated by several laser sources, monochromatic spectral images can be extracted from a single RGB image file [25], thus making it possible to map several chromophores in a single snapshot. Such an approach speeds-up the image processing and excludes image artefacts caused by the tissue movements. First demonstration of skin hemoglobin snapshot RGB mapping under double-wavelength laser illumination was reported at [26]. Later mapping of three main skin chromophores under triple-wavelength laser illumination was demonstrated with laboratory [27] and smartphone-based [28] setups.

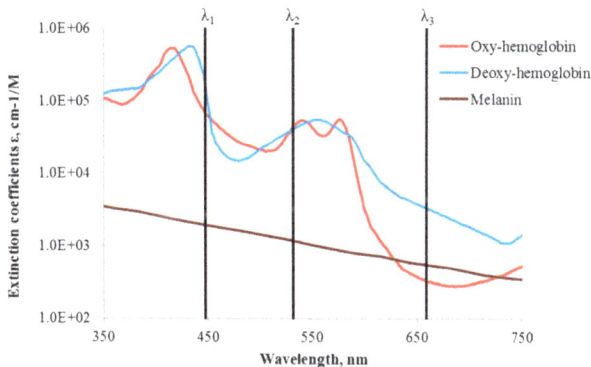

Figure 5. Absorption of three main skin chromophores [29,30] at three fixed wavelengths [28].

The general concept of snapshot skin chromophore mapping at fixed wavelengths is illustrated at Figure 5. Let us suppose that an RGB color image of skin is captured under illumination that comprises only three equal intensity spectral lines at wavelengths λ_1, λ_2 and λ_3 (the vertical lines in Figure 5). With respect to the spectral sensitivity of RGB image sensor and the cross-talk between its detection bands at the fixed wavelengths, three monochromatic spectral images can be extracted from the color image data set by the technique described in [25,31]. If the skin surface reflection is suppressed (e.g., by means of two crossed polarizers), variations in chromophore composition induce changes of the diffusely reflected light intensities at each of the fixed wavelengths. Such variations in the pathology region relatively to the healthy skin can be estimated by measuring reflected light intensities from equally sized regions of interest in the pathology (I_j) and the adjacent healthy skin (I_{oj}). The ratios I_j/I_{jo} at each pixel or pixel's group of three monochromatic spectral images contain information on the concentration increase or decrease of all three regarded chromophores, which can be further mapped over the whole image area [28].

A compact smartphone-compatible three wavelength illuminator has been designed, assembled and tested in the laboratory and clinics. Figure 6 shows the design details (left) and outlook of operating prototype with smartphone on it (right). Flat ring-shaped laser diffuser [17] ensures uniform three wavelength illumination of the round target area with diameter 40 mm. The illumination wavelengths 448 nm, 532 nm and 659 nm are emitted by three pairs of compact 20 mW power laser modules (models *PGL-DF-450nm-20mW-15011564, PGL-VI-1-532nm-20mW-15030443* and *PGL-DF-655nm-20mW-150302232* from Changchun New Industries Optoelectronics Tech. Co., Ltd., Changchun, China). Laser modules (1, Figure 6a—showing three out of six) of each equal-wavelength pair are mounted at opposite sides on the internal wall of a hollow 3D-printed plastic shielding cylinder 2; the round bottom opening of this cylinder is in contact with skin and forms the field of view for the smartphone camera, situated 80 mm apart. All six coaxial laser beams are pointed to the 45-degree conical reflecting edge of a Plexiglass transparent disc 3 (beam collector); after reflections they are turned radial towards the internal ring-shaped flat milky-Plexiglas diffuser 4. In result, the flat diffuser 4 evenly illuminates the 65 mm distant skin target area simultaneously by the three laser wavelengths.

a   b

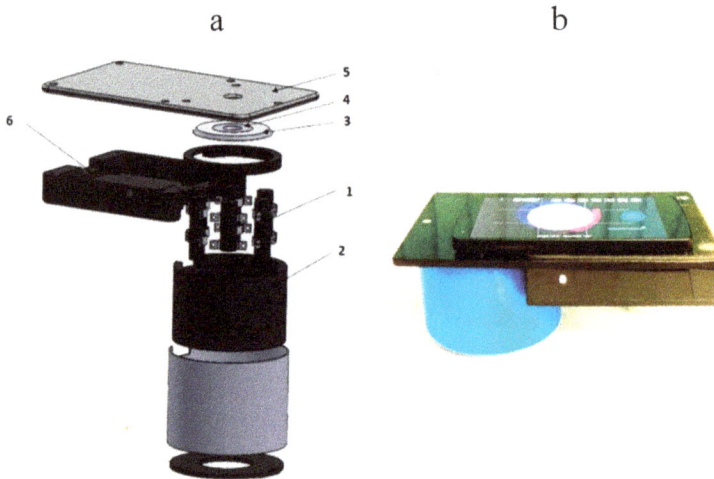

Figure 6. Design scheme of the 3-wavelength laser add-on illuminator (**a**) and the mobile prototype with smartphone on it (**b**): 1—laser modules (3 pairs, 448-532-659nm), 2—shielding cylinder, 3—collector of laser beams, 4—flat ring-shaped diffuser of laser light, 5—sticky platform for the smartphone, 6—electronics compartment [28].

The smartphone is placed on flat sticky platform 5 (Figure 6a) with a round window for the smartphone rear camera, co-aligned with the internal opening of the diffuser 4. The round camera window is covered by a film polarizer; another film with orthogonal direction of polarization covers the diffuser 4 from bottom, so avoiding detection of skin surface-reflected light by the smartphone camera. We used a model *Google Nexus5* smartphone comprising an 8Mpx *SONY IMX179* image sensor with known RGB-sensitivities; spatial resolution of the imaging system was better than 0.1 mm.

The single-snapshot RGB technique is not applicable for express-mapping of more than three skin chromophores. The double-snapshot approach [32] for obtaining four monochromatic images has been implemented in a model device comprising switchable four laser illuminator and a smartphone. Figure 7 shows the design scheme and outlook of a smartphone add-on illuminator intended for mapping of four skin chromophores, e.g., melanin, oxy-hemoglobin, deoxy-hemoglobin and bilirubin. Two of the laser modules can be manually switched on and off, so providing two sets of 3-wavelengths illumination (405, 532, 650 nm and 450, 532, 650 nm). Four rechargeable AA-type batteries are used for power supply. Relatively uniform illumination of round skin spot (dia. 18 mm) is provided by an advanced optical design which also reduces laser speckle artefacts [33]. More details on the multi-laser smartphone add-on prototypes and their test results can be found in [17,28,34].

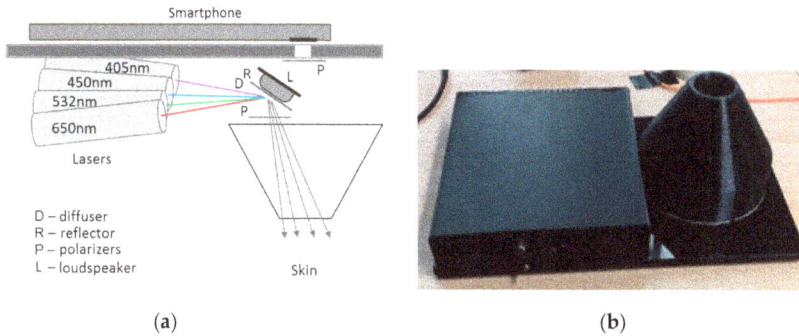

Figure 7. Design scheme (**a**) and outlook (**b**) of the prototype device for switchable 4-wavelengths skin illumination [33,34].

2.2. Prototype Device for Skin Fluorescence Imaging With a Smartphone

If the light is absorbed in skin, it can be further re-emitted at longer wavelengths as autofluorescence (AF), i.e., self-fluorescence without any specific additives on or inside the skin. There is a number of fluorescing compounds called fluorophores in the upper skin, each with its specific emission spectrum. Even if excited by a narrow laser line, several emission spectra overlap and skin autofluorescence spectrum usually is bell-shaped, without a pronounced structure. Besides, a phenomenon called autofluorescence photobleaching (AFPB) normally takes place: the in-vivo skin emitted intensity decreases during continuous optical excitation and does not fully recover after interruptions of the excitation (Figure 8). AFPB causes some interesting effects like low power radiation induced "fingerprints" on in-vivo skin [35].

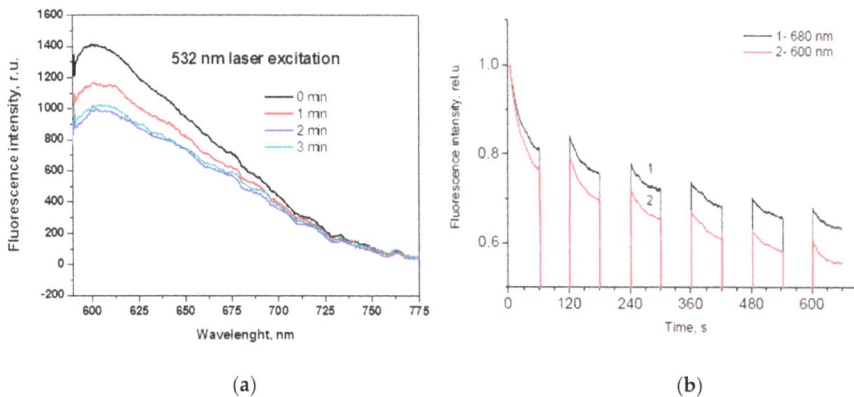

Figure 8. Skin autofluorescence photobleaching at continuous 532nm laser irradiation (~85 mW/cm^2): (**a**)—temporal changes of the emission spectrum [36]; (**b**)—partial recovery of the autofluorescence intensity at two wavelengths after interrupted excitation [37].

The decrease of skin autofluorescence intensity during the laser exposure in most cases can be approximated by a double-exponential expression:

$$I(t) = a \exp(-t/\tau_1) + b \exp(-t/\tau_2) + A \tag{1}$$

where *I*—autofluorescence intensity at a fixed wavelength band, *t*—time, *a* and *b*—weighting coefficients, *A*—the "bottomline" constant, and τ_1, τ_2—the "fast" and "slow" AFPB rate coefficients, respectively. The "fast" AFPB (when sharp intensity decrease is observed) usually takes place during the first 5–15 s of the irradiation, while the "slow" AFPB continues up to several min.

Our first set-up for skin AFPB imaging comprised laser illuminator and consumer photo camera equipped with a band-pass filter in front of the objective; it was operating at a slow video-mode (~2 frames/s) [38]. After the image processing, distribution of τ-values over the imaged skin area was mapped and analyzed. This study showed that the τ-values are sensitive to skin structural changes—e.g., AFPB rates detected from melanin-pigmented nevi were always slower than those detected from healthy skin. Thus, the AFPB rate measurements and spatial mapping may have a potential for skin diagnostics and recovery monitoring, as well as for better skin tumor margin delineation.

As the next step, a smartphone-compatible technique for acquisition and analysis of violet LED excited skin fluorescence intensity and AFPB rate distribution images has been developed and clinically tested [39]. Design of the prototype device is illustrated on Figure 9. For parametric mapping of skin AF intensity decrease rates, a sequence of AF images under continuous 405 nm LED (model LED Engin LZ1-00UA00-U8, spectral band half-width 30 nm) excitation at a power density of ~20 mW/cm² with framerate 0.5 fr/s is recorded for 20 s. Four battery-powered violet LEDs placed within a cylindrical light-shielding wall (which also ensures a fixed 60 mm distance between the smartphone camera and skin) evenly irradiate a 40 mm round spot of the examined skin tissue. A long pass filter (>515 nm) is placed in front of the smartphone camera to prevent detection of the exciting LED emission. The battery/electronics compartment comprises a set of rechargeable batteries and a Bluetooth Low Energy (BLE) module with a driver for communications between the smartphone and illumination unit.

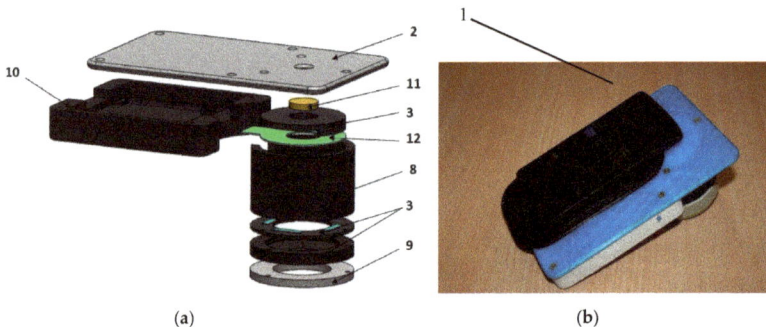

(a)   (b)

Figure 9. Design scheme (**a**) and outlook (**b**) of the prototype device for skin fluorescence imaging with a smartphone: 1—smartphone, 2—sticky fixing plate with camera window, 3—mounting rings, 8—cylindrical screening spacer, 9—silicone skin-contact ring, 10—battery/electronics compartment, 11—long-pass filter, 12—LED ring [17].

The recorded RGB fluorescence images were further separated to exploit the R- and G-images for imaging of skin autofluorescence in the red and green spectral bands, respectively. Due to spectral cut-off by the 515 nm long pass filter, the B band images served only for reference. A *Samsung Galaxy Note 3* smartphone comprising integrated CMOS RGB image sensor with resolution of 13 MP was used for image acquisition. All images were taken at the following settings: ISO-100, white balance—daylight, focus—manual, exposure time—fixed 200 ms. More details on the skin fluorescence imager design and its test results are provided in [17,39].

2.3. Photoplethysmography Video-Imaging Prototypes

The incident cw light can be reflected from the skin surface and also may enter its epidermal and dermal layers where light can be absorbed and/or scattered. A part of back-scattered photons have been travelled via the skin dermal layer where arterial blood volume periodically changes with each heartbeat. As a consequence, also total blood absorption changes with each heartbeat and the back-scattered light intensity is modulated—the detected so-called remission photo-plethysmography (PPG) signal comprises a relatively stable DC component, determined by absorption of the "static" skin structures, and a pulsatile AC component caused by the periodically changing blood absorption [40]. The pulsatile remission PPG signals can be detected not only by specially designed skin contact probes [41], but also distantly, e.g., by video-imaging of skin with subsequent signal processing [42]. This technique is called PPG-imaging (PPGI) or remote PPG (rPPG). The captured video-signals consist of a number of image frames taken at a definite frame rate, e.g., 20 frames per second. Consequently, during one heart activity cycle (~1 s) 20 skin images are obtained, each at different phase of the sub-cutaneous pulse wave. If consecutive frames are compared, the skin-remitted light intensity detected from a fixed area increases and decreases with time, forming the periodic PPGI signal. Specific software [43] allows extracting the arterial pulsations from the video-signal over the whole imaged skin area. The amplitude of PPG peaks may differ between the image pixels due to different blood perfusion of the skin tissues—especially if there is a burn or other dermal skin damage. After the image processing, parametric maps of the PPG signal amplitude distribution (or blood perfusion maps) can be constructed [44].

2.3.1. PPGI Prototype for Palm Anesthesia Monitoring

Figure 10 illustrates the recently designed PPGI prototype device for distant monitoring of anesthesia efficiency during the palm surgeries. The system was intended for recording signals from the curved surface of the hand (dorsal or ventral aspect). The illuminator comprised four bispectral light sources, each consisting of two high-power LED emitters (Roithner LaserTechnik GmbH, Vienna, Austria; green: $\lambda = 530$ nm, 3 W and infrared: $\lambda = 810$ nm, 1 W). To achieve uniform illumination of skin surface, adjustable LED intensity control was introduced via PC based custom developed software. The two wavelengths of illumination were chosen in order to control blood pulsations at two different vascular depths in real time [45].

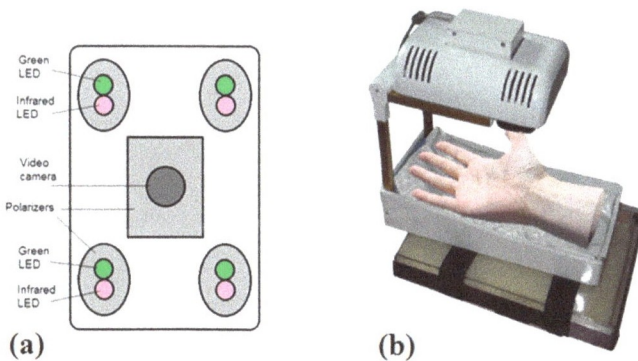

(a)   **(b)**

Figure 10. Dual wavelength photoplethysmography imaging device: bottom view of the imaging system-camera and light sources (**a**) and the whole device with vacuum pillow supporting the palm (**b**) [46].

The microcontroller board (Arduino Nano, Arduino, New York, NY, USA) provided sequential switching of green and IR LEDs and triggering of the captured video frames. The camera control was performed by *uEye* software using manual trigger mode, fixed exposure time, 2 × 2 pixels binning and triggered at 60 frames/s. The monochromatic camera (8 bit CMOS *IDS-uEye UI-1221LE*) was equipped with an *S-mount* 1/2 inch F = 4 mm low distortion, wide-field lens (Lensagon, Lensation GmbH, Karlsruhe, Germany). The camera lens was placed at 15 cm distance from the skin surface so ensuring full view of adult palm (20 cm × 15 cm field of view). In order to reduce skin specular reflectance, orthogonally oriented polarizers were placed behind the camera and all four light sources, respectively. The plastic parts were produced by a 3D printer (*Prusa i3*, custom made, Latvia). The device comprised a plastic enclosure filled with an adjustable vacuum pillow (40 × 20 AB Germa, Kristianstad, Sweden) as the palm support.

2.3.2. Universal Compact PPPGI Prototypes

Another, much smaller PPGI prototype device (Figure 11) for more universal applications related to skin microcirculation control has been developed, as well. It involves near-infrared LED illuminator and a video camera, both placed in custom designed 3D-printed case (4 cm × 4 cm × 4 cm). The illuminator comprises a ring of twelve circularly oriented near-infrared LEDs (peak wavelength 760 nm, current 20 mA each), connected in parallel; stabilized illumination is provided by LED driver (cat4104). Video acquisition is performed by a board-level CMOS video camera (*IDS uEye UI-1221LE*), resolution 752 × 480 pixels, maximum framerate 87 fps., 8-bit monochrome). The camera is equipped with low-distortion S-mount 4 mm lens (Lensagon). In order to reduce skin specular reflectance, cross-oriented polarizers are placed behind the light sources and in front of the camera, respectively. The infrared cut-off filter KC-15 (>700 nm) also is placed in the front of the camera, in order to minimize the influence of ambient illumination. USB-2 cable connection to PC ensures both video-signal processing and the power supply.

For real clinical applications, it is a good choice to use surgical lamp as a light source. A simple and convenient PPGI system for contactless monitoring of anesthesia effectiveness before and during surgical procedures has been developed (Figure 12). The system involves compact lightweight camera (CMOSIS, ADC-8/10/12-bits, resolution 640 × 480 pixels, 502 frames/s, Ximea-xiQ, Cubert GmbH, Ulm, Germany) with a low-distortion lens (3.5 mm f/2.4, Edmund Optics, Barrington, NJ, USA) and green band-pass filter (half-bandwidth 520–580 nm). Both are placed in a custom designed 3D-printed case, adapted for handle attachment to the warm-white-light surgical lamp (Prismalix PRX800, ALM, Soma Technology Inc., Bloomfield, CT, USA), see Figure 12b. The camera is connected via USB-3 cable to a laptop computer which also serves as the power supply of camera. Video acquisition frame rate is 100 Hz (equal to the lamp blinking frequency), so temporal variations of the lamp intensity do not affect the PPGI signal, filtered in the frequency range 0.7–3.0 Hz. More details on the developed PPGI prototype devices and their software can be found in [42–44,46,47].

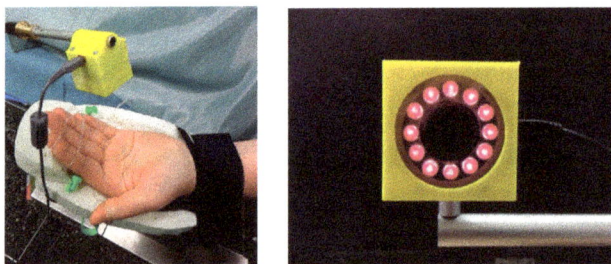

Figure 11. The compact PPGI prototype device in operation (**left**) and the front view of the device (**right**).

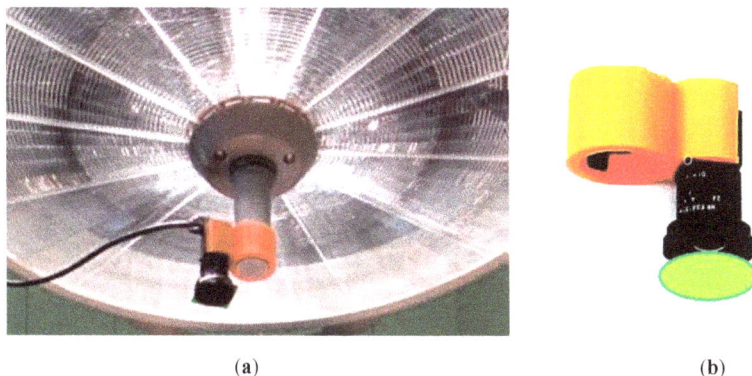

(a)   (b)

Figure 12. The PPGI device attached to a surgical lamp (**a**) and the design of its holder (**b**) [47].

2.4. Multimodal Skin Imagers

2.4.1. SkImager—A Concept Device for Multimodal Skin Imaging

A proof-of-concept prototype device based on inexpensive components and smart software was developed for compact and handy wireless skin diagnostics and monitoring. The multimodal imaging includes capturing by a single camera a number of spectral and video-images from the skin pathology area, with subsequent extraction of clinically significant information. The device captures four consecutive imaging series: (i) RGB image of skin at white polarized LED illumination, helping to reveal hidden subcutaneous structures; (ii) four spectral images at narrowband LED illumination for mapping of the main skin chromophores; (iii) video-images under green LED illumination for mapping of skin blood perfusion; (iv) autofluorescence video-images under UV LED irradiation for mapping of the skin fluorophores. Polarized LED light is used for illumination, and round skin spot of diameter 34 mm is imaged by a CMOS sensor via cross-oriented polarizing filter. To improve the reliability of diagnostics, manipulation with maps of different parameters (i.e., extraction, summing, and division of images) is proposed, as well. Our first prototype version was described earlier [48].

A more advanced prototype device with the preliminary brand-name *SkImager* [49] has been developed (Figure 13). It is a battery-powered fully self-contained wireless device. Its main building blocks are CMOS image sensor, LED illumination system, on-chip microcomputer, touchscreen, memory card and rechargeable battery. The functional diagram of the device is presented at Figure 13c. A *Tegra 2 T20* (Nvidia, Santa Clara, CA, USA) system on chip (SoC) module with a dual-core *Cortex-A9* processor (clock frequency 1 GHz, ARM Inc., San Jose, CA, USA) is used as a central processing unit. It provides smooth operation of all components of the device. A 3 Mpix RGB CMOS matrix with 3.2 micron pixel size (MT9T031) serves as the image sensor; it is connected to the central processor via 10-bit parallel line. Removable SD memory card stores the image information that can be transferred to external processor, e.g., PC. It can be done also via Mini-USB connector which also ensures software installations and updates from outside. On-board and off-board calculations can be performed to extract parametric maps of the examined skin area. The main information input-output device is the built-in 4.3 inch/480 × 272 pixels touchscreen. It displays the operation mode and state of the device (battery charge level, clock, state of the memory card). Power switch button is placed on the side above the slot of memory card (Figure 13b). The device has its holder with integrated contacts for battery charging (Figure 13a). The Li-ion battery (3.6 V, 4.6 Ah) ensures up to 15 h of operation, providing about 100 full measurement cycles. The power consumption under the maximum load (display switched-on, spectral and video image recording and processing) is 3 Watts, or 1 Watt in the waiting mode. Dimensions of the device are 121 mm × 205 mm × 101 mm, weight about 440 g.

(a) (b)

(c)

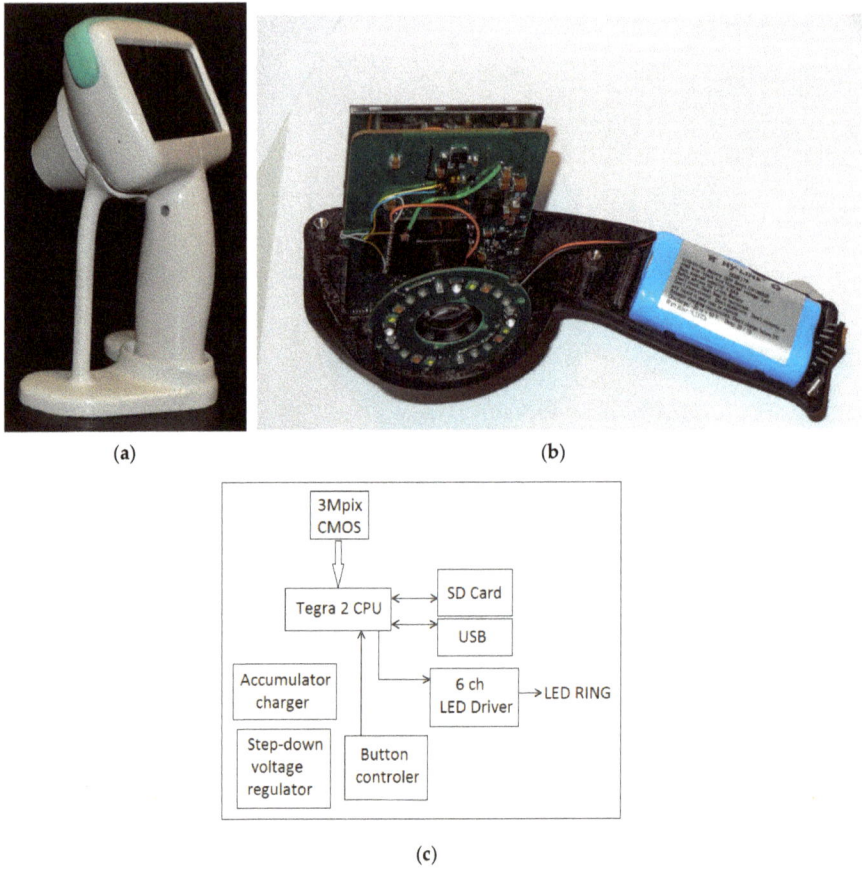

Figure 13. The *SkImager* prototype device in its battery-charging holder (**a**); internal design details (**b**) and functional scheme (**c**) [49].

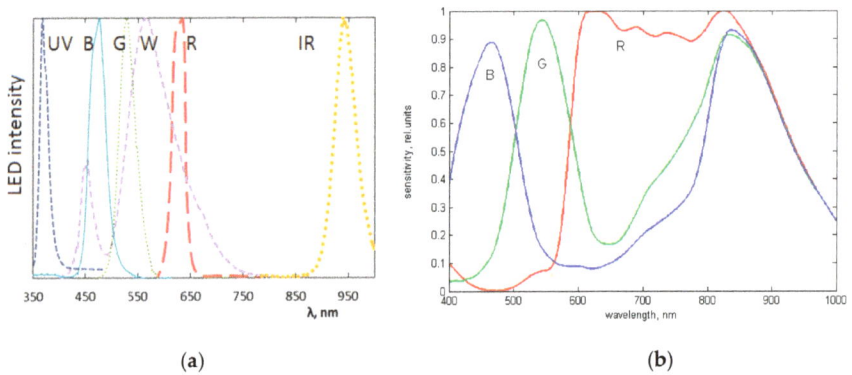

(a) (b)

Figure 14. The measured emission bands of the exploited LEDs (**a**) and spectral sensitivity bands of the CMOS image sensor (**b**) exploited in the *SkImager* prototype [49].

The spectrally-specific skin illumination is performed by a ring of LEDs, surrounding the objective of image sensor—Figure 13b. In total 24 LEDs are operated—six sets of four diodes, emitting at six various wavelength bands (peaks at 365 nm, 450 nm, 540 nm, 660 nm, 940 nm and white—Figure 14a). Each set of equal LEDs is powered separately by the 6-channel LED driver (Figure 13c), in order to provide the same illumination intensity and constant signal output by the visible and NIR emitting diodes. In order to minimize detection of the surface-reflected light, crossed film polarizers cover the LED ring and camera objective (S-Mount M12 × 0.5), respectively. To keep fixed 55 mm distance to the skin, two easily changeable conical tips are used, with the target field diameters 34 mm and 11 mm, respectively. The latter is intended for more curved skin locations, e.g., on nose. Internal surfaces of the tips are black coated and multiple-step shaped, in order to suppress any side-reflected light. The RGB CMOS (Aptina Imaging, Nampa, ID, USA) image sensor with resolution of 2048 × 1536 pixels and maximal framerate 25 frames/s is used. Spectral sensitivity bands of the CMOS sensor (with removed NIR filter) are shown in Figure 14b. More details on the *SkImager* prototype and its test results are provided in [49,50].

2.4.2. The Modular Multimodal Skin Imager

Another prototype for multimodal skin imaging has been designed as a 3D-printed modular device that comprises three main modules (Figure 15):

1. Processing, wireless transmission and power block,
2. Camera and lens block,
3. Illumination block.

The first (processing and communication) module uses embedded computer—Raspberry Pi [51] as the main processing unit. Wireless connections are realized by WiPi USB dongles, and rechargeable battery is used as the power source. Charging is performed by connecting USB cable, similar as for mobile phones. All elements use standard interfaces and can be replaced just by plugging cable to the new device. The second (imaging) module holds an IDS uEye UI-3581LE-C-HQ camera [52] and the Lensagon BVM8020014 lens. Camera uses USB interface and allows upgrading to a new camera without any changes in hardware and software. IDS camera manufacturer was preferred since it has wide range of cameras and all of them share the same physical and software design. By using two lens mounts—"C type" and "S type"—lenses can be interchanged easily, as well.

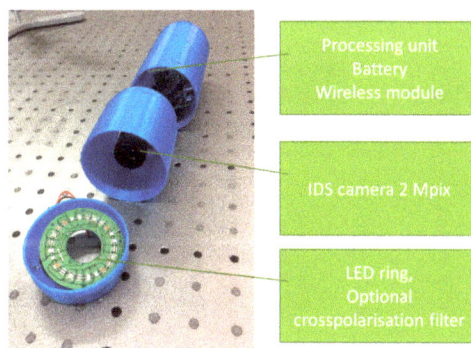

Processing unit
Battery
Wireless module

IDS camera 2 Mpix

LED ring,
Optional
crosspolarisation filter

Figure 15. Photo of the 3D-printed modular multimodal imaging prototype [53].

The third (illumination) module ensures three imaging modes: multispectral imaging of diffuse reflectance (spectral bands with maxima at 435 nm, 535 nm, 660 nm, 740 nm and 940 nm), fluorescence spectral imaging (excitation at 405 nm) and 635 nm laser speckle imaging. Custom printed board was created for managing skin illumination by narrowband LEDs. It uses standard interface for selecting current illumination band, therefore light source change requires less effort than in fully customized existing designs.

By using her/his own smartphone or laptop, the user connects to the device's WiFi network and controls imaging process through the Internet browser. During the first step, the operating system's procedure for connecting to the WiFi network (with a password-controlled access) is performed. On the step two users selects whether he/she requires a new image capture or wishes to view the previous results. During the third step user targets the skin region to be captured by viewing live video stream from the camera. Image is captured by pressing a physical button located on the device. The capturing process can be repeated a number of times. After all skin images are acquired, user can switch to the last—results viewing step. Typical time delay between finishing the image capture procedure and obtaining the results is less than 10 s. More details on this device and its tests are presented in [53].

3. Results

The developed skin imaging prototypes were initially tested in laboratory and then in real clinical environments. All clinical studies were performed with written consent of the involved volunteers under official approval by the local ethics committee. Some results of the clinical measurements, aimed at checking functionality and appropriateness of the prototypes, are briefly presented below.

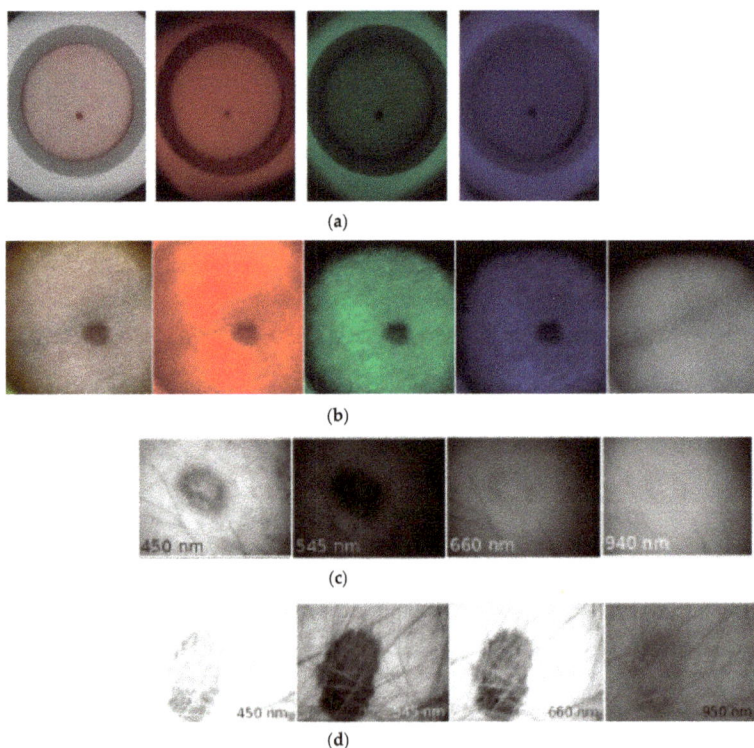

Figure 16. Spectral images of skin malformations taken by different prototypes: (**a**) nevus taken by smartphone—RGB LED prototype at white, red, green and blue illumination [18]; (**b**) nevus taken by SkImager at white, red, green, blue and NIR illumination [49]; (**c**) papilloma taken by modified video-microscope at blue, green, red and NIR illumination [23]; (**d**) melanoma taken by modified video-microscope at blue, green, red and NIR illumination [23].

3.1. Clinical Spectral Images and Chromophore Maps of Skin

Figure 16a illustrates spectral images of a skin nevus taken under white, red, green, and blue illumination of the RGB-LED system by *NEXUS5* smartphone camera, in comparison with spectral images of another nevus, taken under similar illumination by the *SkImager* prototype (Figure 16b). Qualitative agreement of nevi spectral images in the visible range can be observed. *SkImager* and the modified video-microscope provide also NIR spectral images at peak wavelength 940–950 nm which penetrates in skin deeper than the visible light [54]. If the NIR images of skin nevus, papilloma and melanoma are compared (Figure 16b–d), notable differences are seen. Nevus and papilloma images in NIR practically disappear while the melanoma NIR-image still has sufficient contrast, indicating to pathology in deeper skin layers accordingly to the clinical expectations [55].

Nine vascular and pigmented skin lesions were examined by the mobile laser illuminator system [28]. Aim of this study was to check ability of the prototype to provide physiologically feasible skin pigmentation information on already diagnosed skin malformations. After processing the clinical images, skin chromophore maps were constructed and changes of malformation's chromophore content with respect to the adjacent healthy skin evaluated. As initially expected, we observed notable melanin content increase in all cases of both pigmented malformations—nevi and seborrheic keratosis, without essential changes in the hemoglobin content. Increase of oxy-hemoglobin content and decrease of deoxy-hemoglobin (if compared to the surrounding healthy skin) was observed in all examined vascular malformations—hemangiomas, without notable changes in skin melanin content (Figure 17). This result is a good illustration of increased arterial blood supply in skin hemangiomas and confirms functionality of the multi-laser prototype.

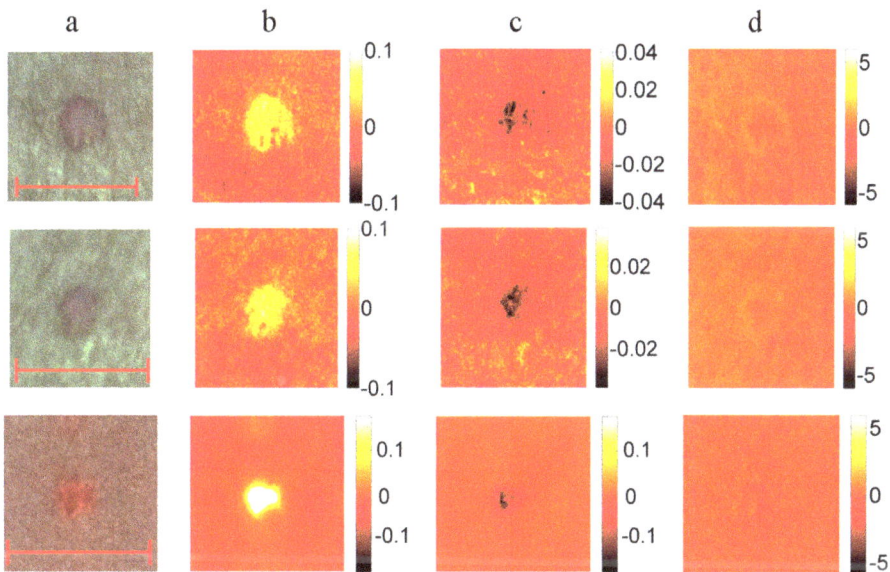

Figure 17. RGB image ((**a**) scale bar 5 mm) and the corresponding maps of chromophore concentration changes for three cases of a vascular hemangioma: (**b**)—oxy-hemoglobin; (**c**)—deoxy-hemoglobin; (**d**)—melanin. Units of the color scale-milimoles [28].

3.2. Fluorescent and Photo-Bleaching Rate Images of Skin Tumors

Overall 50 patients with 150 different skin neoplasms were inspected with the smartphone based fluorescence imager. For more detailed image analysis 13 basal cell carcinomas (BCC) and 1 atypical nevus were selected [39]. In order to visualize the skin AF intensity decrease rates during the photo-bleaching, the following image processing expression was applied:

$$N(C) = (I_{t0}[C] - I_t[C])/I_{t0}[C] \qquad (2)$$

where N(C) represents normalized AF intensity decrease map for each pixel (or pixel group) during the excitation period, $I_{t0}[C]$—AF image at the excitation start moment, $I_t[C]$—AF image after 20 s of continuous excitation and C—color component of the RGB image—red (R), green (G) and blue (B), respectively. The values of RGB components were defined from the image data by a special program developed in MATLAB®.

In all BCC cases (confirmed by cytological examination) the fluorescent images showed lowered AF intensity in malignant tissue as compared with the healthy surrounding skin, which may be attributed to lower concentration of fluorophores and increased blood perfusion caused by the malignant process. A case of solid BCC is illustrated in Figure 18. The G-band AF intensity image (Figure 18b) shows relatively low intensity within the tumor area, with clear margins between tumor and surrounding healthy skin. The tumor area also shows higher AF intensity photobleaching rate (Figure 18c) in comparison with the surrounding healthy skin. Both AF intensity and photobleaching images appear to be useful for non-contact delineation of skin tumor margins.

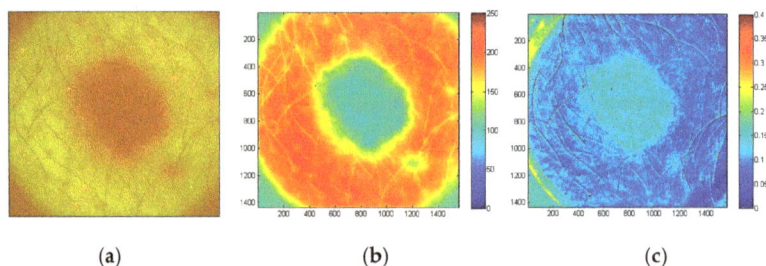

(a)   (b)   (c)

Figure 18. Images of solid BCC: filtered AF color image at the excitation start moment (**a**), the corresponding G-band fluorescence image (**b**) and normalized map of AF photo-bleaching rates (**c**) [39].

The examined atypical nevus (Figure 19) before surgical excision was suspected as melanoma. Histological analysis of the removed tissue sample revealed three different types of tissue cells within the lesion area. Specifically, the upper part of the pathology mostly prevailed by intradermal nevus, the middle part by dysplastic nevus, and the lower part by junctional nevus. Not visible by naked eye, such triple structure of in-vivo skin malformation can be clearly seen in the image of autofluorescence photobleaching rates (Figure 19c). Normalized AF decrease distribution map before surgery/histology showed the fastest intensity decrease in the lower (junctional nevus) and upper side (intradermal nevus), while the middle part (dysplastic nevus) of lesion photo-bleached slower. This example confirms promising potential of the proposed AFPB rate imaging technique for non-contact diagnostics of oncological changes in skin.

3.3. Skin Blood Perfusion Measurements With the PPGI Prototypes

In order to evaluate ability of the double-wavelength PPGI prototype (Figure 10) to discriminate between cutaneous superficial and deep plexus perfusion, hyperemia of superficial plexus was induced by vasodilatory liniment (Transvasin, Seton, UK) [46]. PPGI signal amplitudes at both spectral bands of illumination (peak wavelengths 530 nm and 810 nm) were recorded; Laser Doppler imaging (LDI) signals were captured in parallel by a certified commercial device. Ten healthy volunteers (five males and five females, skin type II) were recruited to participate.

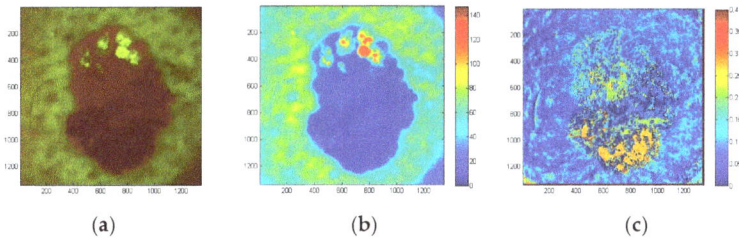

Figure 19. Color filtered AF image of skin atypical nevus at the excitation start moment (**a**), the corresponding G-band fluorescence image (**b**) and normalized AF photo-bleaching rates (**c**) [39].

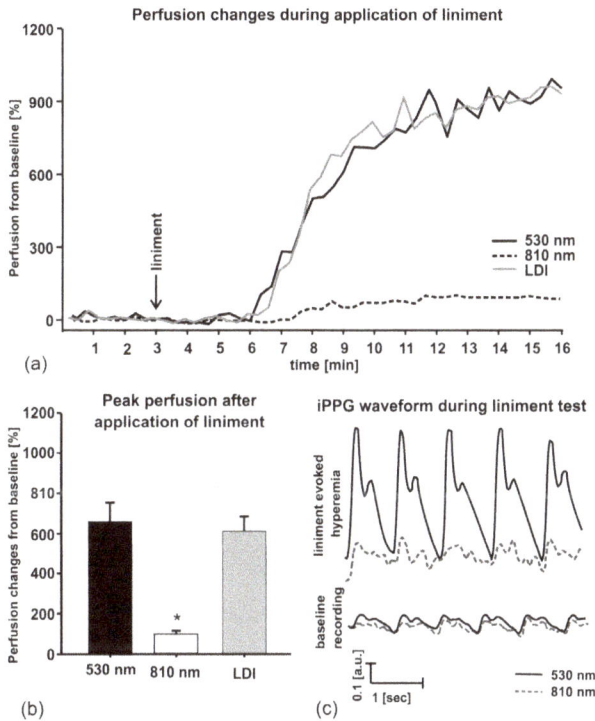

Figure 20. Liniment-induced skin perfusion changes as registered with the double-wavelength PPGI prototype and commercial LDI device (**a**), peak perfusion increase from the baseline (**b**) and the PPGI signal waveforms before and after provocation (**c**) [46].

The subjects were seated on a comfortable reclined chair with the right hand at the dorsal aspect, fixed on the vacuum pillow support (Figure 10b) and kept at heart level, with fingers tightly fitted to avoid movements. The protocol involved 3-min recording of the baseline followed by topical application of liniment and signal recording for 12 min. Within three to four min after application of liniment the reddening of skin appeared, indicating to hyperemia. Green PPGI measurements showed essential (about six times) increase of superficial skin perfusion, well correlated to that measured by the LDI device, while the NIR PPGI signal amplitude (reflecting arterial blood perfusion in deeper dermal layers) only slightly increased—see Figure 20. This result convincingly demonstrates the functional abilities of the developed double-wavelength prototype for non-contact skin microcirculation monitoring.

Local anesthesia affects the sympathetic vascular tone, resulting in vasodilation and raised skin blood perfusion. This increases the amplitude of fast-varying signal detected by the PPGI prototypes—see Figure 21 for illustration. Such physiological response makes possible to detect remotely, if and when anesthesia works just by following the changes in amplitude of the detected PPG signals.

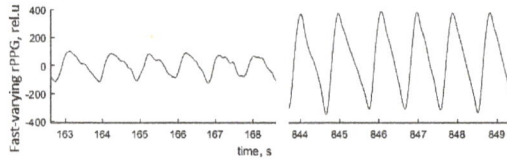

Figure 21. The palm PPGI signal waveforms before (**left**) and after (**right**) administration of local anesthetic [47].

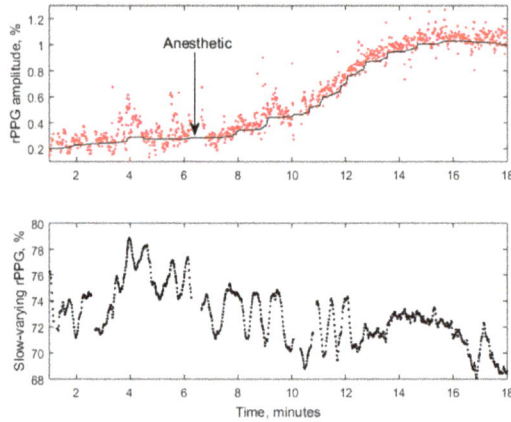

Figure 22. The averaged amplitude of fast-varying PPG signal (**above**) and slow-varying signal (**below**) during the regional anestesia procedure [47].

Figure 22 presents the PPG signal amplitude dynamics in response to regional anesthesia of patient's palm before surgery, as detected by the PPGI prototype attached to the surgical lamp (Figure 12). The graph above shows the beat-to-beat amplitude dynamics while the graph below represents temporal variation of the slow-varying PPGI component. Gradual increase of perfusion with subsequent rise of the PPGI signal amplitude (the upper graph) was observed few min after the administration of local anesthetics. The plateau phase—stable increased skin perfusion induced by the anesthetic—was reached approximately 10 min later and indicated the possible surgery starting time.

Figure 23 shows several screenshots of palm video fused with PPG-amplitude (PPGA) maps during anesthetic action before the surgery. As the local anesthetic affected four different nerves, subsequent microcirculation changes at four different palm skin zones (dermatomes) were observed. The PPGA maps showed increased microcirculation in dermatomes immediately after the local anesthetic was administered (stages 2–6). To conclude, the obtained results confirm clinical efficiency of the developed PPGI prototypes for remote patient anesthesia monitoring before and during surgeries.

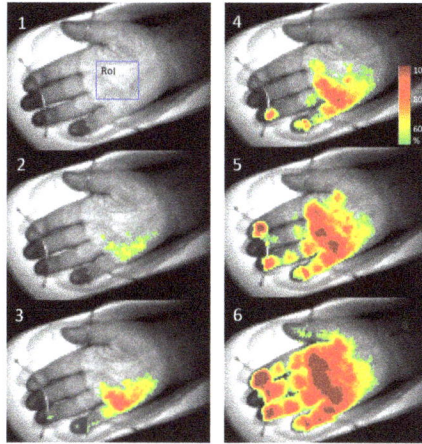

Figure 23. PPGA maps before (1) and after the administration of local anesthetic: 2—1 min, 3—3 min, 4—5 min, 5—6 min, 6—7 min later [47].

4. Discussion

The principles of operation and design features of ten recently developed prototype devices for diagnostic skin imaging have been presented, along with some clinical test results confirming their practical applicability. The laboratory-made prototypes were mainly intended as proof-of-principle devices, able to examine suitability of the developed design concepts and software solutions for further implementation in real clinical environments. Diagnostic sensitivity/specificity, influence of skin color, epidermal thickness and/or optical clearing have not been considered at this stage, as they can be evaluated only after statistically representative clinical trials.

Tests of the multispectral skin imaging prototypes led to conclusions on critical conditions to be met for successful extraction of skin parametric maps (e.g., chromophore distribution maps) from the captured spectral images. The most important ones are uniformity of skin illumination at all used spectral bands, long-term repeatability of all spectral illumination parameters, possibly narrow spectral bandwidths (monochromatic spectral images preferred) and short image acquisition time (single snapshot mode preferred). The developed designs are intended for imaging of relatively flat skin areas; the curved ones (e.g., nose, fingers) still remain an issue due to uneven illumination and varying focal distance. Speckle free multi-laser illumination [33] seems to be a good challenge for multi-spectral skin diagnostic imaging in future. If smartphones or consumer cameras are used for skin image capturing, all automatic settings must be switched off to avoid unexpected artifacts. Besides hardware, also the spectral image processing software has a lot of space for improvements, in order to speed up the image conversion processes and to use more adequate algorithms for calculation of clinically significant parameters.

Fluorescent skin imaging is relatively less complicated non-contact diagnostics technique. It was shown that even a simple and inexpensive smartphone-illuminator system (Figure 9) can provide clinically interesting data for skin tumor identification and margin delineation. Imaging of skin autofluorescence photo-bleaching rates certainly has a good potential for such clinical applications. A technical challenge to be solved is ensuring motionless conditions during the recording of fluorescent images for at least 15 s from any location of the body. The camera-skin motions can be easily avoided if the skin surface is relatively flat (e.g., on the back), while obtaining high quality fluorescent video-files from curved body locations (e.g., face, arms) would require further developments of special holders and skin spacers. Like in the case of multi-spectral imaging, software development for fast and accurate fluorescent image processing is still an issue, as well.

The developed photoplethysmography imaging prototypes and software have revealed new challenges for distant non-contact monitoring of skin blood perfusion changes at different vascular depths and under anesthesia. The latter application seems to be most successful if the camera is attached to the surgical lamp or originally integrated there. Stabilized DC power supply to the lamp is preferred, but the AC supply also does not influence the results much if the video frame rate is selected equal to the light pulsation frequency. Fusion of PPGA images with real body images (Figure 22) seems to be efficient for future on-line monitoring of the anesthesia process details.

Tests of the developed multimodal imaging prototypes have confirmed their proposed functionality. However, from the point of clinical users the number of offered options seems to be too high and more specialized devices based on the tested concepts eventually might be more successful in the medical device market.

Implementation of new design ideas and practical tests of the prototypes will promote better understanding of the challenges and drawbacks of in-vivo skin imaging technologies. Their clear advantages are remote and nearly real-time operation, as well as ability of quantitative pathology documentation. On the other hand, image-based clinical criteria for skin pathology diagnostics either do not exist or are in very early stage of development. Routine healthcare needs "golden standards" for fair assessment of patient's condition and for setting up the recovery strategy, and from this point optical imaging techniques still have to be checked at numerous clinical measurements before becoming a standard of care. Even if some of the above-described skin imaging prototypes would appear clinically acceptable, lots of efforts will be needed in future to establish and validate specific image parameters related to clinically significant threshold levels of particular skin pathologies.

Acknowledgments: Preparation of this review was mainly supported by the Latvian national research program SOPHIS under the grant agreement #10-4/VPP-4/11. The prototypes were developed also in frame of projects funded by the European Regional Development Fund. Author is deeply grateful to all collaborators (co-authors of the below-listed papers and patent applications) for their significant contributions. Fruitful discussions of the results in frame of the EC COST action BM1205 are highly appreciated.

Conflicts of Interest: The authors declare no conflict of interest.

References

1. MoleMate Siascope Handheld Melanoma Screening System. Available online: http://www.wms.co.uk/Dermatology/Dermatoscopes,Lights_and_Magnifiers/MoleMate_Siascope_Handheld_Melanoma_Screening_System (accessed on 9 April 2017).
2. MelaFind. Available online: http://www.melafind.com/melafind/ (accessed on 9 April 2017).
3. Que, S.K.T.; Grant-Kels, J.M.; Rabinovitz, H.S.; Oliveiro, M.; Scope, A. Application of handheld confocal microscopy for skin cancer diagnosis. *Dermatol. Clin.* **2016**, *34*, 469–475. [CrossRef] [PubMed]
4. DermaInspect. Available online: http://www.jenlab.de/DermaInspect.29.0.html?&L=en%3E%22 (accessed on 9 April 2017).
5. Dermlight. Available online: https://dermlite.com/ (accessed on 9 April 2017).
6. Dlite Microscope. Available online: http://skinandhairscope.com/Products/Dlite/Dlite.php (accessed on 9 April 2017).
7. Skinvision. Available online: https://www.skinvision.com/technology-skin-cancer-melanoma-mobile-app (accessed on 12 March 2017).
8. Vidovič, L.; Milanič, M.; Randeberg, L.L.; Majaron, B. Quantitative characterization of traumatic bruises by combined pulsed photothermal radiometry and diffuse reflectance spectroscopy. *Proc. SPIE* **2015**, *9303*, 930307. [CrossRef]
9. Spigulis, J. Biophotonic technologies for noninvasive assessment of skin condition and blood microcirculation. *Latv. J. Phys. Techn. Sci.* **2012**, *49*, 63–80.
10. Multispectral Imaging. Available online: http://www.imaging.org/site/PDFS/Reporter/Articles/REP27_4_CIC20_TOMINAGA_p177.pdf (accessed on 12 March 2017).
11. Jakovels, D.; Spigulis, J.; Rogule, L. RGB mapping of hemoglobin distribution in skin. *Proc. SPIE* **2011**, *8087*, 80872B.

12. Jakovels, D.; Kuzmina, I.; Berzina, A.; Valeine, L.; Spigulis, J. Noncontact monitoring of vascular lesion phototherapy efficiency by RGB multispectral imaging. *J. Biomed. Opt.* **2013**, *18*, 126019. [CrossRef] [PubMed]
13. Jakovels, D.; Spigulis, J. 2-D mapping of skin chromophores in the spectral range 500–700 nm. *J. Biophoton.* **2010**, *3*, 125–129. [CrossRef] [PubMed]
14. Jakovels, D.; Spigulis, J. RGB imaging device for mapping and monitoring of hemoglobin distribution in skin. *Lith. J. Phys.* **2012**, *52*, 50–54. [CrossRef]
15. Philips Vital Signs Camera. Available online: http://www.vitalsignscamera.com/ (accessed on 12 March 2017).
16. The Best Heart Disease iPhone & Android Apps of the Year. Available online: http://www.healthline.com/health-slideshow/top-heart-disease-iphone-android-apps#5 (accessed on 12 March 2017).
17. Spigulis, J.; Lacis, M.; Kuzmina, I.; Lihacovs, A.; Upmalis, V.; Rupenheits, Z. Method and Device for Smartphone Mapping of Tissue Compounds. Lv. Patent WO 2017012675 A1, 26 January 2017.
18. Kuzmina, I.; Lacis, M.; Spigulis, J.; Berzina, A.; Valaine, L. Study of smartphone suitability for mapping of skin chromophores. *J. Biomed. Opt.* **2015**, *20*, 090503. [CrossRef] [PubMed]
19. Dino-Lite for Healthcare. Available online: http://www.dino-lite.com/applications_list.php?index_id=8 (accessed on 12 March 2017).
20. Dino-Lite AM4115-FUT. Available online: http://www.dino-lite.com/products_detail.php?index_m1_id=0&index_m2_id=0&index_id=61 (accessed on 12 March 2017).
21. Rubins, U.; Zaharans, J.; Lihacova, I.; Spigulis, J. Multispectral video-microscope modified for skin diagnostics. *Latv. J. Phys. Techn. Sci.* **2014**, *51*, 65–70. [CrossRef]
22. Diebele, I.; Kuzmina, I.; Lihachev, A.; Spigulis, J.; Kapostinsh, J.; Derjabo, A.; Valaine, L. Clinical evaluation of melanomas and common nevi by spectral imaging. *Biomed. Opt. Express* **2012**, *3*, 467–472. [CrossRef] [PubMed]
23. Bekina, A.; Diebele, I.; Rubins, U.; Zaharans, J.; Derjabo, A.; Spigulis, J. Multispectral assessment of skin malformations by modified video-microscope. *Latv. J. Phys. Techn. Sci.* **2012**, *49*, 4–8.
24. Bekina, A.; Rubins, U.; Lihachova, I.; Zaharans, J.; Spigulis, J. Skin chromophore mapping by means of a modified video-microscope for skin malformation diagnosis. *Proc. SPIE* **2013**, *8856*, 88562G.
25. Spigulis, J.; Elste, L. Method and Device for Imaging of Spectral Reflectance at Several Wavelength Bands. Lv. Patent WO2013135311 A1, 19 September 2013.
26. Spigulis, J.; Jakovels, D.; Rubins, U. Multi-spectral skin imaging by a consumer photo-camera. *Proc. SPIE* **2010**, *7557*, 75570M.
27. Spigulis, J.; Oshina, I. Snapshot RGB mapping of skin melanin and hemoglobin. *J. Biomed. Opt.* **2015**, *20*, 050503. [CrossRef] [PubMed]
28. Spigulis, J.; Oshina, I.; Berzina, A.; Bykov, A. Smartphone snapshot mapping of skin chromophores under triple-wavelength laser illumination. *J. Biomed. Opt.* **2017**, *22*, 091508. [CrossRef] [PubMed]
29. Prahl, S. Tabulated Molar Extinction Coefficient for Hemoglobin in Water. Available online: http://omlc.ogi.edu/spectra/hemoglobin/summary.html (accessed on 30 November 2016).
30. Sarna, T.; Swartz, H.M. The Physical Properties of Melanin. Available online: http://omlc.ogi.edu/spectra/melanin/eumelanin.html (accessed on 30 November 2016).
31. Spigulis, J.; Elste, L. Single-snapshot RGB multispectral imaging at fixed wavelengths: proof of concept. *Proc. SPIE* **2014**, *8937*, 89370L.
32. Spigulis, J.; Oshina, I. Method and Device for Chromophore Mapping under Illumination by Several Spectral Lines. Lv. Patent 15106 B, 20 March 2016.
33. Rubins, U.; Kviesis-Kipge, E.; Spigulis, J. Device for Obtaining Speckle-Free Images at Illumination by Scattered Laser Beams. Lv. Patent P-17-17, 10 May 2017.
34. Oshina, I.; Spigulis, J.; Rubins, U.; Kviesis-Kipge, E.; Lauberts, K. Express RGB mapping of three to five skin chromophores. *OSA Tech. Dig.* **2017**, in press.
35. Lihachev, A.; Lesins, J.; Jakovels, D.; Spigulis, J. Low power cw-laser signatures on human skin. *Quant. Electron.* **2010**, *40*, 1077–1080. [CrossRef]
36. Lihachev, A. Kinetics of Laser-Excited In-Vivo Skin Autofluorescence and Remission. Ph.D. Thesis, University of Latvia, Riga, Latvia, 2010.
37. Lesinsh, J.; Lihachev, A.; Rudys, R.; Bagdonas, S.; Spigulis, J. Skin autofluorescence photobleaching and photo-memory. *Proc. SPIE* **2011**, *8092*, 80920N.

38. Spigulis, J.; Lihachev, A.; Erts, R. Imaging of laser-excited tissue autofluorescence bleaching rates. *Appl. Opt.* **2009**, *48*, D163–D168. [CrossRef] [PubMed]

39. Lihachev, A.; Derjabo, A.; Ferulova, I.; Lange, M.; Lihacova, I.; Spigulis, J. Autofluorescence imaging of Basal Cell Carcinoma by smartphone RGB camera. *J. Biomed. Opt.* **2015**, *20*, 120502. [CrossRef] [PubMed]

40. Allen, J. Photoplethysmography and its application in clinical physiological measurement. *Physiol. Meas.* **2007**, *28*, R1. [CrossRef] [PubMed]

41. Spigulis, J. Optical non-invasive monitoring of skin blood pulsations. *Appl. Opt.* **2005**, *44*, 1850–1857. [CrossRef] [PubMed]

42. Rubins, U.; Upmalis, V.; Rubenis, O.; Jakovels, D.; Spigulis, J. Real-time photoplethysmography imaging system. *Proc. IFMBE* **2011**, *34*, 183–186.

43. Rubins, U.; Spigulis, J.; Miscuks, A. Photoplethysmography imaging algorithm for continuous monitoring of regional anesthesia. In Proceedings of the 2016 ACM/IEEE 14th Symposium on Embedded Systems for Real-Time Multimedia, Pittsburgh, PA, USA, 6–7 October 2016. [CrossRef]

44. Rubins, U.; Spigulis, J.; Miscuks, A. Application of color magnification technique for revealing skin microcircuration changes under regional anaesthetic input. *Proc. SPIE* **2013**, *9032*, 903203.

45. Spigulis, J.; Gailite, L.; Lihachev, A.; Erts, R. Simultaneous recording of skin blood pulsations at different vascular depths by multi-wavelength photoplethysmography. *Appl. Opt.* **2007**, *46*, 1754–1759. [CrossRef] [PubMed]

46. Marcinkevics, Z.; Rubins, U.; Zaharans, J.; Miscuks, A.; Urtane, E.; Ozolina-Moll, L. Imaging photoplethysmography for clinical assessment of cutaneous microcirculation at two different depths. *J. Biomed. Opt.* **2016**, *21*, 35005. [CrossRef] [PubMed]

47. Rubins, U.; Miscuks, A.; Lange, M. Simple and convenient remote photoplethysmography system for monitoring regional anesthesia effectiveness. In Proceedings of the EMBEC-NBC2017, Tampere, Finland, 12–15 June 2017, in press.

48. Spigulis, J.; Garancis, V.; Rubins, U.; Zaharans, E.; Zaharans, J.; Elste, L. A device for multimodal imaging of skin. *Proc. SPIE* **2013**, *8574*, 85740J.

49. Spigulis, J.; Rubins, U.; Kviesis-Kipge, E.; Rubenis, O. SkImager: A concept device for in-vivo skin assessment by multimodal imaging. *Proc. Est. Acad. Sci.* **2014**, *63*, 213–220. [CrossRef]

50. Spigulis, J.; Rubins, U.; Kviesis-Kipge, E. Multimodal Imaging Device for Non-Contact Skin Diagnostics. Lv. Patent 14749 B, 20 November 2013.

51. Embedded Linux on Board Computer Description. Available online: https://www.raspberrypi.org/ (accessed on 12 March 2017).

52. Industrial USB Cameras Description. Available online: https://en.ids-imaging.com/ (accessed on 12 March 2017).

53. Bliznuks, D.; Jakovels, D.; Saknite, I.; Spigulis, J. Mobile platform for online processing of multimodal skin optical images: Using online Matlab server for processing remission, fluorescence and laser speckle images, obtained by using novel handheld device. In Proceedings of the 2015 International Conference on BioPhotonics (BioPhotonics), Florence, Italy, 20–22 May 2015. [CrossRef]

54. Anderson, R.R.; Parrish, J.A. The optics of human skin. *J. Invest. Dermatol.* **1981**, *77*, 13–19. [CrossRef] [PubMed]

55. Rigel, S.D.; Robinson, K.J.; Ross, I.M.; Friedman, R. *Cancer of the Skin: Expert Consult*, 2nd ed.; Elsevier Health Sciences: Amsterdam, The Netherlands, 2011; pp. 99–123.

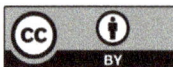

sensors

MDPI

Article

Optical Detection of Ketoprofen by Its Electropolymerization on an Indium Tin Oxide-Coated Optical Fiber Probe

Robert Bogdanowicz [1], Paweł Niedziałkowski [2], Michał Sobaszek [1], Dariusz Burnat [3], Wioleta Białobrzeska [2], Zofia Cebula [2], Petr Sezemsky [4], Marcin Koba [3,5], Vitezslav Stranak [4], Tadeusz Ossowski [2] and Mateusz Śmietana [3,*]

[1]   Faculty of Electronics, Telecommunications and Informatics, Gdansk University of Technology, Narutowicza 11/12, 80-233 Gdansk, Poland; rbogdan@eti.pg.gda.pl (R.B.); micsobas@pg.edu.pl (M.S.)
[2]   Department of Analytical Chemistry, Faculty of Chemistry, University of Gdansk, Wita Stwosza 63, 80-308 Gdansk, Poland; pawel.niedzialkowski@ug.edu.pl (P.N.); wioleta.bialobrzeska@phdstud.ug.edu.pl (W.B.); zofia.jelinska@phdstud.ug.edu.pl (Z.C.); tadeusz.ossowski@ug.edu.pl (T.O.)
[3]   Institute of Microelectronics and Optoelectronics, Warsaw University of Technology, Koszykowa 75, 00-662 Warszawa, Poland; drkbrt@o2.pl (D.B.); marcinkoba@gmail.com (M.K.)
[4]   Institute of Physics and Biophysics, Faculty of Science, University of South Bohemia, Branisovska 1760, 370 05 Ceske Budejovice, Czech Republic; petr.sezemsky@gmail.com (P.S.); stranv00@centrum.cz (V.S.)
[5]   National Institute of Telecommunications, Szachowa 1, 04-894 Warszawa, Poland
*   Correspondence: M.Smietana@elka.pw.edu.pl; Tel.: +48-22-234-6364

Received: 28 February 2018; Accepted: 23 April 2018; Published: 27 April 2018

Abstract: In this work an application of optical fiber sensors for real-time optical monitoring of electrochemical deposition of ketoprofen during its anodic oxidation is discussed. The sensors were fabricated by reactive magnetron sputtering of indium tin oxide (ITO) on a 2.5 cm-long core of polymer-clad silica fibers. ITO tuned in optical properties and thickness allows for achieving a lossy-mode resonance (LMR) phenomenon and it can be simultaneously applied as an electrode in an electrochemical setup. The ITO-LMR electrode allows for optical monitoring of changes occurring at the electrode during electrochemical processing. The studies have shown that the ITO-LMR sensor's spectral response strongly depends on electrochemical modification of its surface by ketoprofen. The effect can be applied for real-time detection of ketoprofen. The obtained sensitivities reached over 1400 nm/M (nm·mg^{-1}·L) and 16,400 a.u./M (a.u.·mg^{-1}·L) for resonance wavelength and transmission shifts, respectively. The proposed method is a valuable alternative for the analysis of ketoprofen within the concentration range of 0.25–250 µg mL^{-1}, and allows for its determination at therapeutic and toxic levels. The proposed novel sensing approach provides a promising strategy for both optical and electrochemical detection of electrochemical modifications of ITO or its surface by various compounds.

Keywords: ketoprofen; anti-inflammatory drug; drug analysis; optical fiber sensor; reactive magnetron sputtering thin film; indium tin oxide (ITO); lossy-mode resonance (LMR); electrochemistry; electropolymerization

---

1. Introduction

Demand for nonprescription drugs, such as 2-(3-benzoylphenyl)-propanoic acid (ketoprofen, KP) is expected to increase in the near future. KP is a nonsteroidal anti-inflammatory drug, widely used for the treatment of various kinds of pains, rheumatoid arthritis and osteoarthritis [1]. KP exhibits analgesic and antipyretic activity, which is mainly caused by the inhibition of prostaglandin synthesis by inhibiting cyclooxygenase [2]. The widespread and growing volume of human and veterinary prescriptions needs to be followed by the development of analytical techniques allowing for detection of KP traces in various biofluids or sludge water.

Several methods have already been reported for quantitative determination of KP, including liquid chromatography-mass spectrometry [3], UV-fluorescence [4], ion chromatography [5], flow injection with chemiluminescence [6], or electrochemical detection [7]. Both chromatographic and non-chromatographic techniques usually require rigorous sample preparation and expensive extraction methods (including solid-phase extraction) when real samples are considered. Mass spectrometry in turn requires analyte signal suppression or enhancement during electrospray ionization, especially for analysis of multi-compound samples. Application of all these methods is time-consuming and requires expensive and highly specialized setups which are only available in well-equipped research laboratories. Among other techniques, fluorescence at porous SnO_2 nanoparticles was applied for KP detection using combined ion chromatography with photodetection. The limit of detection (LOD) in human serum, urine, and canal water samples was 0.1 µg/kg, 0.5 µg/kg, and 0.39 µg/kg, respectively [5]. However, photometric UV and fluorescence-based methods commonly suffer from low sensitivity and selectivity, while the latter require specific chemicals or compounds (e.g., nanoparticles) in the detection procedure.

Electrochemical studies of KP have already been performed using the polarographic method [8,9] or simultaneously cyclic voltammetry and coulometry techniques at the mercury dropping electrode surface [8,10]. Kormosh et al. [11] developed ion-selective electrodes for potentiometric analysis of KP in piroxicam based on Rhodamine 6G in a membrane plasticizer. The measurements of KP using direct current stripping voltammetry as well as spectrophotometric methods were also reported by Emara et al. [9]. With dropping mercury electrode and using different supporting electrolytes at different pH values it was possible to reach a LOD as low as 5.08×10^{-4} ng mL^{-1}. A similar electrode was utilized by Ghoneim and Tawfik [10], and in a Britton-Robinson buffer (pH 2.0) the LOD was 0.10 ng mL^{-1}. Next, a setup containing glassy carbon (GC) electrode with multiwalled carbon nanotubes/ionic liquid/chitosan composite for covalent immobilization of the ibuprofen by specific aptamer was proposed [7].

It can be concluded that the electrochemical methods offer reliability and accuracy, enabling development of simple, rapid, and cost-effective approaches for the detection of electroactive compounds. However, electrodes for KP detection usually need complex pre-treatment in order to reach high repeatability and environmental stability. Furthermore, KP shows poor solubility in water, a tendency to adsorb and block electrodes, and a rapid metabolization to by-products [12]. Thus, conventional electrochemical assay procedures are not well-suited for this specific application.

To overcome the limitations listed above, we propose a novel approach for KP detection, where together with an electrochemical method an indium tin oxide (ITO)-coated optical fiber sensor is used. ITO is known for its high optical transparency and low electrical resistivity. Moreover, thanks to its band-gap, it is a good candidate for an electrochemical electrode, and it can be used for optical measurements as well. Contrary to other transparent electrode materials, such as boron-doped diamond, thin ITO films can be deposited at a relatively low temperature on various substrates and shapes [13]. Plasma-assisted deposition is often used for obtaining high quality ITO films. An ITO overlay was applied as a standard working electrode, where KP was electropolymerized with the cyclic voltammetry technique. Thanks to the adjustment of both ITO's electrochemical and optical properties, lossy-mode resonance (LMR) effect in optical fiber sensor can also be applied for KP detection. LMR is a thin-film-based optical effect, which takes place when a certain relation between electric permittivity of the film, substrate, and external medium is fulfilled, namely the real part of the film's electric permittivity must be positive and higher in magnitude than both the thin film's permittivity imaginary part and the permittivity of the analyte [14]. Any variation in optical properties of the analyte, especially its refractive index (RI), has an influence on resonance conditions and can thus be detected. Since in visible spectral range ITO shows relatively high RI (n_D ~2 RIU) and non-zero extinction coefficient (corresponding to optical absorption), it has already been successfully applied in LMR-based sensing devices [15]. There have been reported applications of other thin films supporting the LMR effect such as diamond-like carbon [16], SiN$_x$ [17], TiO$_2$ [18], and polymers [19], but among these materials only ITO offers low electrical resistivity and can be applied as an electrode material. Until now both the electrical conductivity of ITO and supported by its thin film LMR effect have been applied only with the purpose of inducing a high voltage change in properties of an electro-optic material deposited on ITO surface [20], and for electropolymerization of a chemical compound on the ITO surface [21]. As an alternative to the conventional assay procedures, the developed opto-electrochemical probe can offer a KP detection method free from pre-treatment of the electrode's surface, as well as prolonged analysis time and sophisticated experimental setup.

The application of opto-electrochemical probes is a novel approach. To the best of our knowledge, in this paper we discuss for the first time the application of LMR phenomenon at the ITO-coated optical fiber for electrochemically-induced KP detection. The developed opto-electrochemical probe offers capability for label-free KP detection with no need of the electrode's surface pre-treatment. Additionally, the GC electrode has been modified by KP for reference.

2. Materials and Methods

KP (2-(3-benzoylphenyl) propionic acid) of purity greater than 98% was obtained from Cayman Company (Ann Arbor, MI, USA) and used without any further purification. A KP solution with a concentration of 2 mM was prepared in a 0.1 M phosphate buffer saline (pH = 7.0). Na$_2$SO$_4$ and K$_3$[Fe(CN)$_6$] were purchased from POCh (Gliwice, Poland).

2.1. ITO Optical Probe Fabrication and Testing

The LMR structures were fabricated using approx. 15 cm-long polymer-clad silica fiber samples of 400/840 µm core/cladding diameter, where 2.5 cm of polymer cladding was removed in the fiber central section [22]. Next, the electrically conductive and optically transparent ITO films were deposited by reactive magnetron sputtering of ITO target (In$_2$O$_3$-SnO$_2$—90/10 wt % and purity of 99.99%). The magnetron, whose axis was perpendicular to the substrate, was supplied by a Cito1310 (13.56 MHz, 300 W) RF source (Comet AG, Flamatt, Switzerland). The experiments were carried out at pressure p = 1.0 Pa in a reactive N$_2$/Ar atmosphere, gas flows were 15 and 0.5–1.0 sccm for Ar and N$_2$, respectively. The overlays were deposited on fibers rotated in the chamber during the process. Simultaneously, Si wafers and glass slides were also coated for reference. Both of the end-faces of the fiber sample were mechanically polished before the optical testing.

To determine RI sensitivity of the fabricated ITO-LMR devices, they were investigated in the air and mixtures of water/glycerin with n$_D$ = 1.33–1.45 RIU. The RI of the mixtures was measured using an AR200 automatic digital refractometer (Reichert Inc., Buffalo, NY, USA). The optical transmission of the ITO-LMR structure was interrogated in the range of λ = 350–1050 nm using an HL-2000 white light source (Ocean Optics Inc., Largo, FL, USA) and an Ocean Optics USB4000 spectrometer. The optical transmission (*T*) in the specified spectral range was detected as counts in specified integration time (up to 100 ms). The temperature of the solutions was stabilized at 25 °C to avoid thermal shift of the RI.

2.2. Electrochemical Setup and Electropolymerization of KP

Cyclic voltammetry measurements were performed with a PGSTAT204 potentiostat/galvanostat (Metrohm, Herisau, Switzerland) controlled by Nova 1.1 software, and using the ITO-LMR probe as a working electrode (WE), a platinum wire as counter electrode (CE), and an Ag/AgCl/0.1 M KCl as a reference electrode (REF). The ITO-LMR working electrode was electrochemically processed in 0.1 M phosphate buffer saline containing from 1×10^{-6} to 1×10^{-3} M of KP at scan rate 50 mV·s^{-1} for 6 cycles. The process allowed for anodic electrooxidation of KP in the potential ranging from 0.3 to 2.0 V vs. Ag/AgCl/0.1 M KCl electrode. The reference GC and ITO electrodes were processed under the same conditions as the ITO-LMR electrode, but for the GC electrode the modification took

10 cycles. Next, the electrodes were washed in water and methanol, and dried under a stream of air. The electrode examinations before and after modification with cyclic voltammetry were performed in 5 mM of $K_3[Fe(CN)_6]$ in 0.5 M Na_2SO_4 solution at scan rate of 100 mV·s^{-1}. The setup used in this experiment is schematically shown in Figure 1.

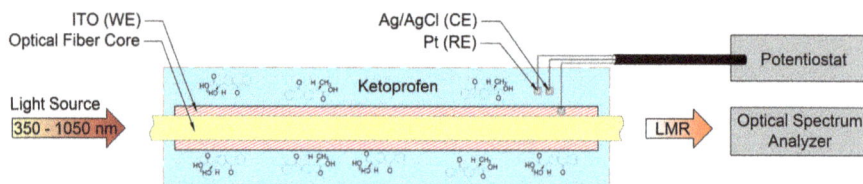

Figure 1. The schematic representation of the experimental setup with ITO-LMR probe used for combined optical and electrochemical KP detection. The electrodes were denoted as working (WE), reference (RE), and counter (CE).

2.3. X-ray Photoelectron Spectroscopy Surface Studies

X-ray Photoelectron Spectroscopy (XPS) studies were carried out using an ESCA300 XPS setup (Scienta Omicron GmbH, Taunusstein, Germany) with a high resolution spectrometer equipped with a monochromatic Kα source. Measurements were done at 10 eV pass energy and 0.05 eV energy step size. A flood gun was used for charge compensation purpose. Finally, the calibration of XPS spectra was performed for carbon peak C1s at 284.6 eV [23,24].

3. Results and Discussion

3.1. The RI Sensitivity of the ITO-LMR Probe

First, the optical probes were studied in an optical setup only. This part of the experiment was done in order to estimate the sensitivity of the device to changes of optical properties at the ITO surface. The probes were installed in a setup allowing one to record the transmission spectra, while the sensor was consecutively immersed in different RI solutions. In Figure 2 a well-defined resonance can be seen that experiences a shift towards higher wavelengths when the external RI increases. It is worth noting that the applied ITO coatings provide relatively narrow resonance. The full width at half maximum (FWHM) obtained for the resonances is approx. 110 nm. When the probe is immersed in the higher RI, the FWHM of the resonance slightly increases. Based on the obtained results, two ways of sensor interrogation can be selected, namely tracking of resonance wavelength (λ_R) or monitoring transmission at discrete wavelength, the most effectively chosen at the resonance slope. In the case of this experiment, the transmission was monitored at λ = 600 nm (T_{600}). Both the λ_R and T_{600} were plotted vs. RI in the inset of Figure 2. The shift is positive for both of the interrogation schema, but for tracking λ_R the dependence is less linear (the sensitivity increases with RI) than for the T_{600}.

The measurements of reference Si samples allowed to estimate the thickness of the coating to 260 nm. According to theoretical studies [25], a low order LMR may be observed for such thickness of ITO. It is known that low order LMRs offer the highest sensitivity to changes in external RI [14], as well as changes in properties of a layer formed on the ITO surface [26].

The standard commercial ITO electrodes undergo thermal annealing to decrease both optical absorption and electrical resistivity, most likely due to the crystallization processes [27]. The LMR-satisfying properties of non-annealed, as fabricated ITO films are attributed to unique advantages of the applied discharge during deposition process. Our previous research clearly showed that optimization of the deposition pressure 0.5 Pa < p < 1.0 Pa induces collisions of the sputtered particles [28,29]. The application of magnetron sputtering is advantageous and allows to tailor the optical and electrical properties of the deposited ITO films with no additional post-deposition annealing as it is often required in case of other deposition methods [30].

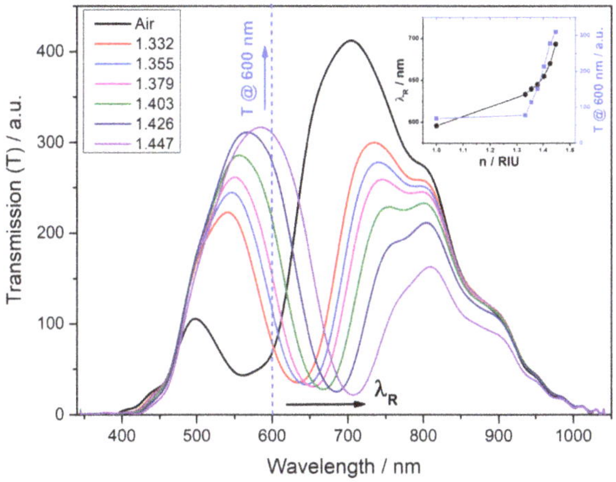

Figure 2. Spectral response of ITO-LMR probe to changes in external RI (n). The changes of resonance wavelength (λ_R) and transmission (T) at $\lambda = 600$ nm are shown in the inset.

3.2. Electrodeposition of KP on GC, ITO and ITO-LMR Electrodes

The electrochemical deposition of KP on GC, ITO and ITO-LMR electrodes was made by anodic oxidation. The redox behavior of KP molecule at the GC and ITO electrode has not been reported yet. However, the anodic oxidation of KP was observed at the boron doped diamond electrode. The current peak measured for this electrode during the electrodeposition processes is associated with the oxidation of carboxyl group in KP [31]. Moreover, the mechanism of the electrochemical reduction of KP have been until now examined only at the mercury electrode and requires transfer of two electrons. This reduction leads to formation of 2-(3-benzhydrolyl)-propionic acid [8] (Scheme 1). The mechanism of reduction of KP—benzophenone-3 has been described elsewhere [32].

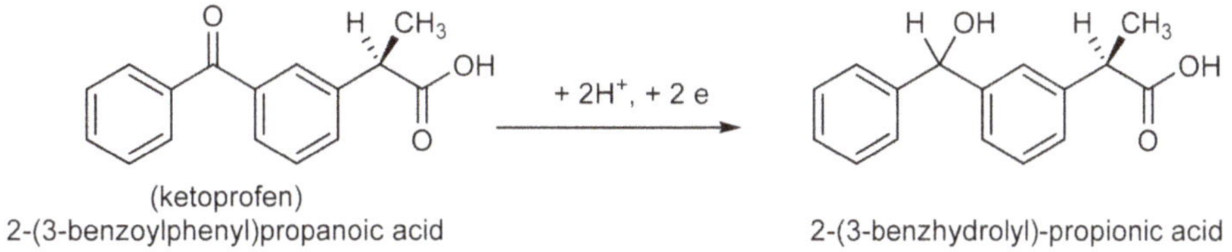

Scheme 1. Chemical structure of KP and mechanism of its electrochemical reduction.

Anodic oxidation by electron transfer leads to deactivation of electrode surface and its modification by adsorption of oxidized polymeric products of the reaction. This effect has been used in this work for modification of different types of electrodes, i.e., GC, ITO, and ITO-LMR. It must be emphasized that only ITO-LMR electrode allows for simultaneous optical and electrochemical monitoring of the modification processes by KP.

The cyclic voltammetry is a very valuable and convenient tool to monitor the electrode surface properties before and after each step of modification [33]. The electrochemical responses of the bare GC, ITO and ITO-LMR electrodes were investigated in a solution of 0.5 M Na_2SO_4 containing 5 mM $[Fe(CN)_6]^{3-/4-}$. The comparison of cyclic voltammograms of modified and bare electrodes is presented in Figure 3. For the bare GC electrode, well-defined reversible redox peaks corresponding to one-electron reversible reaction and the peak to peak separation value of 95 mV were reported [34]. This redox reaction of KP completely blocked the GC electrode after 10 scans. The current peak observed in the first scan (Figure 3a) can be attributed to the oxidation of carboxyl group of the KP [35]. The absence of any current for the GC electrode cycled in presence of KP suggests that KP-based layer was formed on the GC surface (Figure 3b). Polymerized KP film the most likely prevents from the penetration of the electroactive substance towards the electrode surface [36]. This phenomenon has been commonly observed for a series of compounds and different electrode material [37,38].

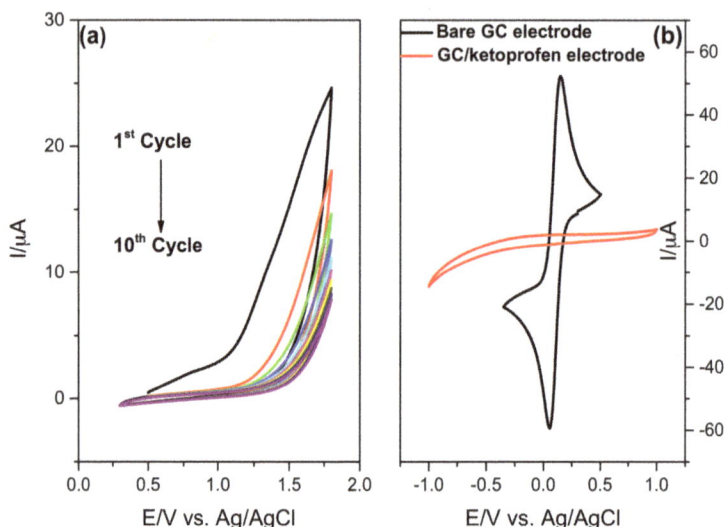

Figure 3. Cyclic voltammetry curves recorded for (**a**) GC electrode in 0.1 M phosphate buffer saline containing 2 mM of KP for 10 cycles, scan rate of 50 mV·s^{-1}; and (**b**) bare GC and GC/KP electrode in 0.5 M Na$_2$SO$_4$ containing of 5 mM [Fe(CN)$_6$]$^{3-/4-}$. The scan rate was set to 100 mV·s^{-1}.

Next, a reference ITO electrode deposited on a glass slide underwent a similar modification procedure. In Figure 4a the cyclic voltammetry curves recorded for ITO electrode in 0.1 M phosphate buffer saline containing 2 mM of KP in 10 cycles are shown. For the bare ITO electrode a redox response with peak to peak potential separation reached 245 mV. Significant differences between the electrochemical response for bare and modified electrodes recorded in 0.5 M Na$_2$SO$_4$ solution containing 5 mM [Fe(CN)$_6$]$^{3-/4-}$ were observed. The decrease in peak current and increase in peak to peak potential separation of up to 511 mV, indicate that the modification of the electrode surface by KP was effective (Figure 4b). This phenomenon also suggests that the surface of the ITO electrode was blocked by KP, which is observed in the disappearance of the anodic and cathodic peak [39].

The ITO-LMR probe was coated with KP during only six anodic oxidation cycles in the potential range from 0.3 to 2.0 V and with a scan rate of 50 mV·s^{-1} (Figure 5a). After this process, the electrode was extensively washed with water and methanol. It is worth noting that for the modification by KP of GC and ITO electrodes, 10 cycles were applied. In the case of ITO-LMR electrode, six cycles were enough to completely cover the electrode. In Figure 5b the cyclic voltammetry response to 0.5 M Na$_2$SO$_4$ containing 5 mM [Fe(CN)$_6$]$^{3-/4-}$ is shown for bare and KP-modified ITO-LMR electrode. Bare and modified ITO-LMR electrodes show redox responses with peak to peak potential separation reaching 419 mV and 628 mV, respectively. Moreover, for the KP-modified ITO-LMR electrode the redox current peaks significantly increased. This effect suggests that the electrode has a more developed active surface area than the one before modification [40]. This was only observed for anodic oxidation of

KP on the ITO-LMR electrode. In the other cases, namely reference ITO and GC electrodes, the current peaks for redox couple decreased significantly as a result of modification by KP.

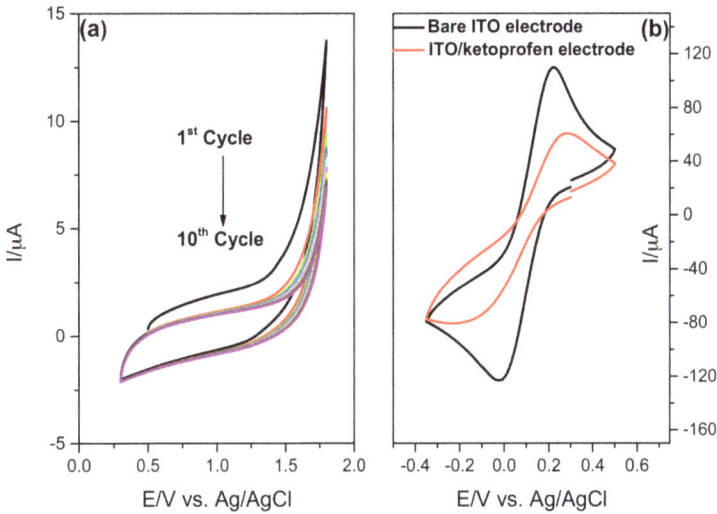

Figure 4. Cyclic voltammetry curves recorded for (**a**) ITO electrode in 0.1 M phosphate buffer saline containing 2 mM of KP (10 cycles, scan rate of 50 mV·s^{-1}) and (**b**) ITO and ITO/KP electrode in 0.5 M Na$_2$SO$_4$ containing 5 mM [Fe(CN)$_6$]$^{3-/4-}$, scan rate 100 mV·s^{-1}.

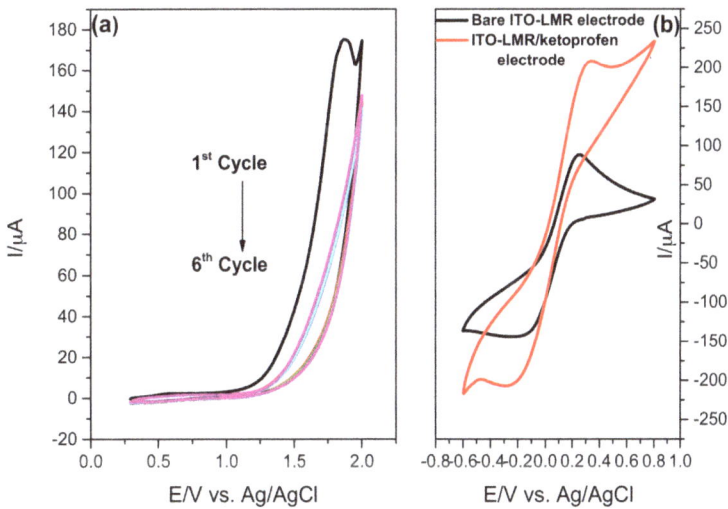

Figure 5. Cyclic voltammetry curves recorded for (**a**) ITO-LMR electrode in 0.1 M phosphate buffer saline containing 2 mM of KP for 6 cycles at scan rate of 50 mV·s^{-1}; and (**b**) bare for and KP-modified ITO-LMR in 0.5 M Na$_2$SO$_4$ containing 5 mM [Fe(CN)$_6$]$^{3-/4-}$, scan rate 100 mV·s^{-1}.

In Table 1 are summarized the electrochemical results obtained for the samples before and after KP modification. The peak splitting difference between bare ITO and ITO-LMR electrodes, i.e., ΔE reaching 245 mV and 419 mV, respectively, can originate from two effects. First, the ITO deposition on cylindrical shape, such as optical fiber, is more challenging than on a flat surface and has an impact on size, crystallinity and morphology of the electrode active surface. Second, the KP modifies the shape of the cyclic voltammetry curves and the peak to peak separations ΔE from 511 to 628 mV for ITO and ITO-LMR electrode, respectively. The diffusion of electrons through the KP is disturbed, revealing slightly reduced electrocatalytic activities, which can be attributed to its structural features and electrochemical properties.

Table 1. Electrochemical parameters of the reactions for $[Fe(CN)_6]^{3-/4-}$ on the surface of bare and KP modified ITO electrodes.

Sample	E_{red} (mV)	E_{ox} (mV)	ΔE (mV)	$E_{1/2}$ (mV)
Bare ITO electrode	−24	221	245	123
KP/ITO electrode	−230	281	511	230
Bare ITO-LMR electrode	−165	254	419	210
KP/ITO-LMR electrode	−285	343	628	314

3.3. XPS Studies of KP-Modified ITO Surface

High-resolution XPS spectra, analyzed within the energy range of C1s and O1s peaks, make it possible to verify successful KP modification of ITO surface at the level of 10^{-3} M. Survey of the XPS spectrum presented in Figure 6 reveals significant contribution from ITO background seen as tin, indium, and oxygen peaks, and smaller contribution from electropolymerized thin KP layer on ITO surface. The high-resolution XPS spectra were also acquired, in the energy range characteristic for C1s and O1s peaks. The high-resolution analysis allows for verification of successful KP modification of ITO surface at the level of 10^{-3} M. Recorded spectra with their deconvolution are shown in the inset of Figure 6 and extracted data are summarized in Table 2.

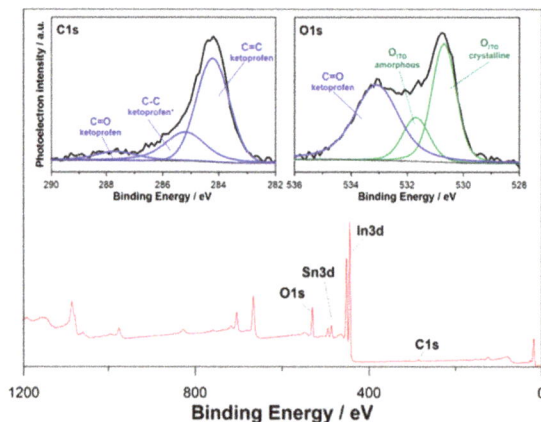

Figure 6. XPS survey spectrum and high-resolution XPS spectra registered for C1s and O1s energy range. Peaks underwent spectral deconvolution are superimposed with colors depending on their origination (blue for KP and green for ITO). The KP concentration was 1×10^{-3} M.

The C1s spectrum was deconvoluted with three peaks, each denoting a different chemical state of carbon. The primary component is located at +284.2 eV and is characteristic for aromatic C=C bonds in KP. The second and third type of interaction can be associated with aliphatic C-C and C=O bonds. Their energy shift versus the primary spectral component is +1.0 for C−C and +3.5 eV for C=O type of bonds and highly correlates with other results found in the literature [41–43]. Furthermore, the XPS analysis carried out within the O1s energy region confirmed the pronounced presence of peak located at 533.1 eV, which is characteristic for carbonyl bonds. Finally, the acquired C=C:C−C:C=O ratio of 6.5:2.8:1 corresponds to the known for KP 6:1:1. A slight excess of C–C contribution can be explained by the presence of adventitious carbon coming from sample storage in atmospheric conditions. The amount of adventitious carbon found at bare ITO electrode did not exceed 5 at.% and was excluded from further analysis.

Table 2. Comparison of chemical composition of bare ITO and ITO/KP electrode.

XPS Photopeak	Chemical State	Binding Energy (eV)	Chemical Composition (at.%)	
			Bare ITO Electrode	ITO/KP Electrode
C1s	C=C	284.2	-	27.8
	C–C *	285.2	-	9.9
	C=O	287.7	-	4.3
O1s	ITO$_{cryst}$	530.7	40.5	13.6
	ITO$_{amorph}$	531.7	12.8	5.5
	C=O	533.1	-	17.3
In	ITO$_{cryst}$	444.1	29.8	9.8
	ITO$_{amorph}$	445.1	11.8	9.2
Sn	ITO$_{cryst}$	486.1	3.7	1.4
	ITO$_{amorph}$	487.0	1.4	1.2

* Indicates the influence of adventitious carbon in total chemical composition of C–C chemical state.

We have also performed detailed XPS analysis of peaks located in In3d5 and Sn3d5 energy range. The results of the analysis were also summarized in Table 2. According to literature survey, ITO analysis are typically based on spectral deconvolution using two sub-peaks—often ascribed to be contribution from crystalline and amorphous ITO. The observed peak shift between crystalline and amorphous phases—1.0 eV for In and 0.9 eV for Sn peaks—was found to stay in agreement with literature survey [44–46].

3.4. ITO-LMR-Based KP Electropolymerization Monitoring

The electrochemically-induced polymerization of KP was monitored optically using ITO-LMR probe. As shown in Figure 7, there were changes in the spectral response during cyclic voltammetry electropolymerization of KP for its two concentrations in the solution, i.e., the lowest and the highest. Obviously, for high KP concentration (1×10^{-3} M) results in electropolymerization of denser film which is followed by more pronounced changes in the optical spectrum (Figure 7B). Nevertheless, as low KP concentration as 1×10^{-6} M can be observed in optical response (Figure 7A). For all the applied concentrations, the most noticeable changes in the spectrum can be observed for the resonance at approx. λ_R ~650 nm, where a shift towards longer wavelengths takes place with the process progress. On top of tracking the resonant wavelength shift, in the discussed case also changes in T can be monitored at specific wavelength. For these resonance conditions, as previously when response to RI has been analyzed, we picked $\lambda = 600$ nm that is in the middle of the resonance slope. Due to the limited resolution of the spectrometer, T monitoring may deliver more accurate data than λ_R.

The saturation of KP polymerization process was noticed for the ITO-LMR probe during the second CV cycle. The scan rate was set to 100 mV·s^{-1} in the range 0–2 V what resulted in 40 s per one cycle. The full range optical transmission was recorded with integration time up to 100 ms for 3500 data set. Thus, the entire optical analysis took 6 minutes. However, the wavelength range could be limited to e.g., 50 nm (approx. 250 data points) resulting in 25 seconds-long analysis. Summarizing, the result of KP determination was achieved with response time below 1 minute with no additional pretreatment, labeling, or incubation required.

Variations of the two parameters, namely λ_R and T versus progress in the electrodeposition process are shown for all the KP concentrations in Figure 8. As in the case of an increase in external RI, both of them increase with progress of the electrodeposition process. The effect can be explained as a mass transfer of KP, i.e., densification of the medium at the ITO surface, resulting in the growth of the KP polymer film. A similar shift has already been reported for aptamer immobilization or swelling of poly-acrylic acid (PAA) and polyallylamine hydrochloride (PAH) polymeric coatings on ITO deposited on a fiber [26,47]. The increase in both parameters depends on the concentration of KP and surely has an impact on the thickness of the electrodeposited film. The effect of KP deposition on the electrode was revealed earlier by XPS studies (Figure 6) and recognized by a shift of peaks characteristic for aromatic C=C and aliphatic C–C and C=O bonds existing in this compound.

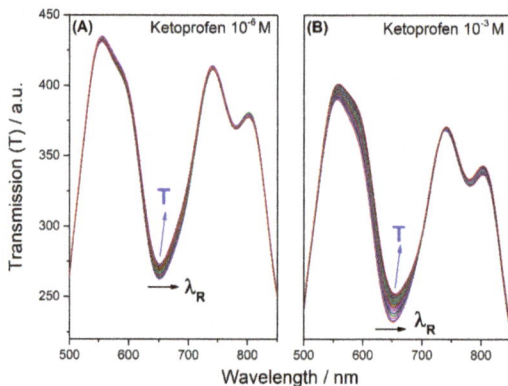

Figure 7. Changes in optical response of the ITO-LMR probe recorded during electropolymerization of KP on ITO surface for two KP concentrations, namely (**A**) 1×10^{-6} M and (**B**) 1×10^{-3} M.

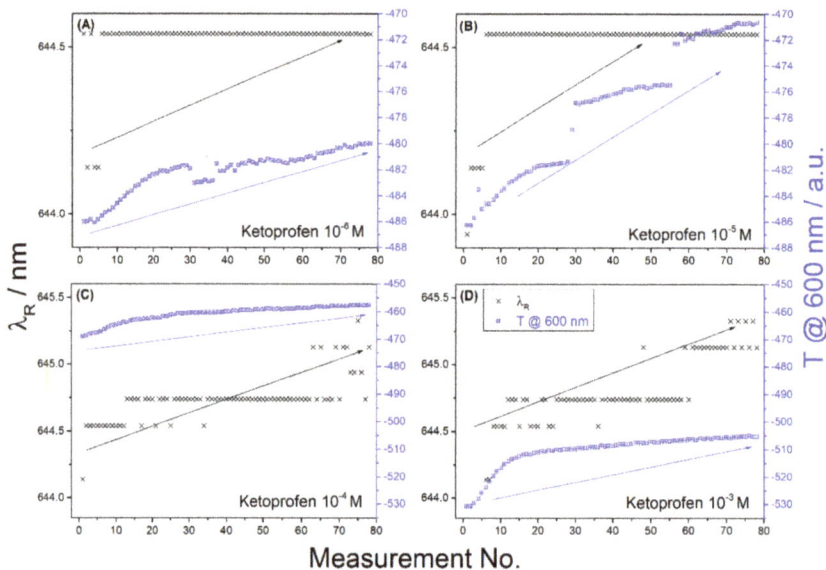

Figure 8. Change in resonance wavelengths (λ_R) {×} and transmission (*T*) at 600 nm {□} with progress of KP electropolymerization process on ITO-LMR probe for KP concentration (**A**) 1×10^{-6} M; (**B**) 1×10^{-5} M; (**C**) 1×10^{-4} M; and (**D**) 1×10^{-3} M.

The relative changes of λ_R and *T* at $\lambda = 600$ nm are summarized in Table 3 using data shown in Figure 8. The final values of the achieved parameters after 80 measurements (approx. 120 s) were plotted versus the KP concentration. It must be noted that both the parameters linearly depend on the concentration with an average correlation coefficient R^2 higher than 0.93. The sensitivities have been considered as ratios of the slopes reaching 1400.86 nm/M (nm·mg^{-1}·L) and 16,422.46 a.u./M (a.u·mg^{-1}·L) for resonance wavelengths (λ_R) and T, respectively. The calculated LOD of KP is 0.536 or 0.575 mM using λ_R and T, respectively. The application of enhanced resolution equipment and standardized solutions at lower concentration would allow us to enhance this value as well as the LOD. The KP detection experiments were performed three times using separately deposited ITO-LMR probes. They were used to determine 1 mM KP solution with an average RSD value 8.5%, which indicates the satisfactory reproducibility and repeatability of the approach.

Table 3. The relative changes of λ_R and T at 600 nm of ITO-LMR probe recorded vs. KP concentration.

KP Concentration	ΔT (a.u.)	$\Delta\lambda$ (nm)
1×10^{-3} M	255.2	1.98
1×10^{-4} M	123.2	0.99
1×10^{-5} M	113.9	0.6
1×10^{-6} M	60.4	0.4

Analytical capability for KP determination with bare ITO-LMR electrode and other previously used nanomaterials is compared in Table 4. It can be concluded that the measurements with the ITO-LMR probe offer competitive sensitivity mainly when higher KP concentrations are considered. At these conditions standard electrochemical sensors are not effective due to adsorption at the electrode surface. The sensing concept can be further developed towards detection of other polymerizing agents. Fabrication of such sensors can be easily scaled-up keeping physical homogeneity and electrochemical performance. Summarizing, the application of the ITO-LMR probe offers competitive response toward KP detection mainly when larger concentrations are considered and standard electrochemical sensors are oversaturated by adsorption. The sensing concept can be further developed for future studies of other polymerizing agents.

Table 4. Comparison of KP linear measurement range and LOD achieved with different methods.

Technique	Details	Linear Range	Limit of Detection	Reference
Adsorptive Stripping Square Wave	Mercury electrode	1×10^{-8}–3×10^{-7} M	0.1 ng mL^{-1}	[10]
LC-APCI-MS	Single Ion Monitoring mode (SIM)	100–500 ng/mL	1.0 ng/mL	[3]
IC-FLD	SnO$_2$ nanoparticles	0.1 μg/kg	0.2–1.5 mg/kg	[5]
Differential Pulse Voltammetry	Aptamer and glassy carbon electrode	70 pM–6 μM	20 pM	[7]
Potentiometry	PVC electrode	0.0001–0.05 mol/L	6.3×10^{-5} mol/L	[11]
Microdialisys	Short polymeric columns (SPE)	25–5000 ng/mL	3 ng/mL	[48]
Flow injection	Flow injection with chemiluminescence	5.0×10^{-8}–3.0×10^{-6} mol/L	2.0×10^{-8} mol/L	[6]
High-Performance Liquid Chromatography	Single-pass intestinal perfusion method	12.5–200 ng/mL	0.05 ng/mL	[49]
Rp-HPLC	PDA detector	872.5 nM	4.85–9.7×10^5	[2]
Differential Pulse Polarography	Dropping-mercury electrode	1×10^{-5}–5×10^{-4} M	9.8×10^{-6} mol/L	[8]
Polarography	Dropping-mercury electrode	10^{-8}–10^{-6}M	2.0×10^{-9} mol/L	[8]
Stripping voltammetry	Mercury electrode	1×10^{-8}–1×10^{-7} M	2.0×10^{-9} mol/L	[9]
ITO-LMR probe	ITO electrode	1×10^{-6}–1×10^{-3} M	0.5×10^{-3} mol/L	This work

4. Conclusions

In this study we have developed an optical fiber sensor based on the LMR effect supported by a thin ITO overlay and used it for real-time optical monitoring of electrochemical deposition of KP. The developed highly conductive ITO overlay was deposited on an optical fiber core and applied as a working electrode in cyclic voltammetry electrochemical setup. We have found that electrodeposition of KP on the ITO surface induces a significant change in the LMR response. The variation in optical transmission for the ITO-LMR sensor gradually follows the progress in the electrochemical deposition process. The sensor can be interrogated by tracing transmission at discrete wavelength as well as resonant wavelength shifts. Optical setup enables LMR monitoring of the KP concentration down to 1×10^{-6} M. Thus, the proposed method is a valuable alternative for the analysis of KP within the concentration range of 0.25–250 µg mL^{-1}, allowing its determination at therapeutic and toxic levels. The sensing concept can be applied for detection of various other pharmaceuticals, as well as organics or biocompounds that are capable for electropolymerization at ITO surface. It is worth noting that this effect was obtained at bare ITO electrodes fabricated by magnetron sputtering. This deposition method is known for scalability and thus is widely applied as an industrial technology for a wide range of applications. The obtained devices are cheap in large-scale production, disposable, and can be applied in low-power, portable point-of-care devices or microchips. Moreover, the probes can be interrogated with simplified and limited in wavelength range systems based on LED source and Si photodiode with a bandpass filter.

Author Contributions: R.B., P.N., M.S., V.S., T.O. and M.Ś. conceived and designed the experiments; D.B., W.B., Z.C. and P.S. performed the experiments; R.B., P.N. and M.Ś. analyzed the data; M.K. developed measurement setup elements and data acquisition and analysis tools; R.B., P.N. and M.Ś. wrote the paper.

Funding: This research was funded by NATO grant number SPS G5147, National Science Centre (NCN), Poland grant numbers 2014/14/E/ST7/00104 and 2016/21/B/ST7/01430, and Faculty of Electronics, Telecommunications and Informatics of the Gdansk University of Technology (DS funds).

Conflicts of Interest: The authors declare no conflict of interest.

References

1. Sakeena, M.H.F.; Yam, M.F.; Elrashid, S.M.; Munavvar, A.S.; Aznim, M.N. Anti-inflammatory and Analgesic Effects of Ketoprofen in Palm Oil Esters Nanoemulsion. *J. Oleo Sci.* **2010**, *59*, 667–671. [CrossRef] [PubMed]
2. Asanuma, M.; Asanuma, S.N.; Gómez-Vargas, M.; Yamamoto, M.; Ogawa, N. Ketoprofen, a non-steroidal anti-inflammatory drug prevents the late-onset reduction of muscarinic receptors in gerbil hippocampus after transient forebrain ischemia. *Neurosci. Lett.* **1997**, *225*, 109–112. [CrossRef]
3. Abdel-Hamid, M.E.; Novotny, L.; Hamza, H. Determination of diclofenac sodium, flufenamic acid, indomethacin and ketoprofen by LC-APCI-MS. *J. Pharm. Biomed. Anal.* **2001**, *24*, 587–594. [CrossRef]
4. Patrolecco, L.; Ademollo, N.; Grenni, P.; Tolomei, A.; Barra Caracciolo, A.; Capri, S. Simultaneous determination of human pharmaceuticals in water samples by solid phase extraction and HPLC with UV-fluorescence detection. *Microchem. J.* **2013**, *107*, 165–171. [CrossRef]
5. Muhammad, N.; Li, W.; Subhani, Q.; Wang, F.; Zhao, Y.-G.; Zhu, Y. Dual application of synthesized SnO$_2$ nanoparticles in ion chromatography for sensitive fluorescence determination of ketoprofen in human serum, urine, and canal water samples. *New J. Chem.* **2017**, *41*, 9321–9329. [CrossRef]
6. Zhuang, Y.; Song, H. Sensitive determination of ketoprofen using flow injection with chemiluminescence detection. *J. Pharm. Biomed. Anal.* **2007**, *44*, 824–828. [CrossRef] [PubMed]
7. Roushani, M.; Shahdost-fard, F. Covalent attachment of aptamer onto nanocomposite as a high performance electrochemical sensing platform: Fabrication of an ultra-sensitive ibuprofen electrochemical aptasensor. *Mater. Sci. Eng. C* **2016**, *68*, 128–135. [CrossRef] [PubMed]
8. Amankwa, L.; Chatten, L.G. Electrochemical reduction of ketoprofen and its determination in pharmaceutical dosage forms by differential-pulse polarography. *Analyst* **1984**, *109*, 57–60. [CrossRef] [PubMed]
9. Emara, K.M.; Ali, A.M.; Abo-El Maali, N. The polarographic behaviour of ketoprofen and assay of its capsules using spectrophotometric and voltammetric methods. *Talanta* **1994**, *41*, 639–645. [CrossRef]
10. Ghoneim, M.M.; Tawfik, A. Voltammetric studies and assay of the anti-inflammatory drug ketoprofen in pharmaceutical formulation and human plasma at a mercury electrode. *Can. J. Chem.* **2003**, *81*, 889–896. [CrossRef]
11. Kormosh, Z.; Hunka, I.; Bazel, Y.; Matviychuk, O. Potentiometric determination of ketoprofen and piroxicam at a new PVC electrode based on ion associates of Rhodamine 6G. *Mater. Sci. Eng. C* **2010**, *30*, 997–1002. [CrossRef]

12. Cheng, Y.; Xu, T.; Fu, R. Polyamidoamine dendrimers used as solubility enhancers of ketoprofen. *Eur. J. Med. Chem.* **2005**, *40*, 1390–1393. [CrossRef]

13. Paine, D.C.; Whitson, T.; Janiac, D.; Beresford, R.; Yang, C.O.; Lewis, B. A study of low temperature crystallization of amorphous thin film indium–tin–oxide. *J. Appl. Phys.* **1999**, *85*, 8445–8450. [CrossRef]

14. Villar, I.D.; Hernaez, M.; Zamarreño, C.R.; Sánchez, P.; Fernández-Valdivielso, C.; Arregui, F.J.; Matias, I.R. Design rules for lossy mode resonance based sensors. *Appl. Opt.* **2012**, *51*, 4298–4307. [CrossRef] [PubMed]

15. Zamarreño, C.R.; Hernaez, M.; Del Villar, I.; Matias, I.R.; Arregui, F.J. Tunable humidity sensor based on ITO-coated optical fiber. *Sens. Actuators B Chem.* **2010**, *146*, 414–417. [CrossRef]

16. Śmietana, M.; Dudek, M.; Koba, M.; Michalak, B. Influence of diamond-like carbon overlay properties on refractive index sensitivity of nano-coated optical fibres. *Phys. Status Solidi A* **2013**, *210*, 2100–2105. [CrossRef]

17. Michalak, B.; Koba, M.; Śmietana, M. Silicon Nitride Overlays Deposited on Optical Fibers with RF PECVD Method for Sensing Applications: Overlay Uniformity Aspects. *Acta Phys. Pol. A* **2015**, *127*, 1587–1591. [CrossRef]

18. Burnat, D.; Koba, M.; Wachnicki, Ł.; Gierałtowska, S.; Godlewski, M.; Śmietana, M. Refractive index sensitivity of optical fiber lossy-mode resonance sensors based on atomic layer deposited TiO$_x$ thin overlay. In Proceedings of the 6th European Workshop on Optical Fibre Sensors, Limerick, Ireland, 31 May–3 June 2016.

19. Zamarreño, C.R.; Hernáez, M.; Del Villar, I.; Matías, I.R.; Arregui, F.J. Optical fiber pH sensor based on lossy-mode resonances by means of thin polymeric coatings. *Sens. Actuators B Chem.* **2011**, *155*, 290–297. [CrossRef]

20. Ascorbe, J.; Corres, J.M.; Arregui, F.J.; Matías, I.R. Optical Fiber Current Transducer Using Lossy Mode Resonances for High Voltage Networks. *J. Light. Technol.* **2015**, *33*, 2504–2510. [CrossRef]

21. Sobaszek, M.; Dominik, M.; Burnat, D.; Bogdanowicz, R.; Stranak, V.; Sezemsky, P.; Śmietana, M. Optical monitoring of thin film electro-polymerization on surface of ITO-coated lossy-mode resonance sensor. In Proceedings of the 25th International Conference on Optical Fiber Sensors, Jeju, Korea, 24–28 April 2017.

22. Smietana, M.; Szmidt, J.; Dudek, M.; Niedzielski, P. Optical properties of diamond-like cladding for optical fibres. *Diam. Relat. Mater.* **2004**, *13*, 954–957. [CrossRef]

23. Miller, D.J.; Biesinger, M.C.; McIntyre, N.S. Interactions of CO2 and CO at fractional atmosphere pressures with iron and iron oxide surfaces: One possible mechanism for surface contamination? *Surf. Interface Anal.* **2002**, *33*, 299–305. [CrossRef]

24. Wysocka, J.; Krakowiak, S.; Ryl, J. Evaluation of citric acid corrosion inhibition efficiency and passivation kinetics for aluminium alloys in alkaline media by means of dynamic impedance monitoring. *Electrochim. Acta* **2017**, *258*, 1463–1475. [CrossRef]

25. Villar, I.D.; Zamarreño, C.R.; Sanchez, P.; Hernaez, M.; Valdivielso, C.F.; Arregui, F.J.; Matias, I.R. Generation of lossy mode resonances by deposition of high-refractive-index coatings on uncladded multimode optical fibers. *J. Opt.* **2010**, *12*, 095503. [CrossRef]

26. Zubiate, P.; Zamarreño, C.R.; Sánchez, P.; Matias, I.R.; Arregui, F.J. High sensitive and selective C-reactive protein detection by means of lossy mode resonance based optical fiber devices. *Biosens. Bioelectron.* **2017**, *93*, 176–181. [CrossRef] [PubMed]

27. Dominik, M.; Siuzdak, K.; Niedziałkowski, P.; Stranak, V.; Sezemsky, P.; Sobaszek, M.; Bogdanowicz, R.; Ossowski, T.; Śmietana, M. Annealing of indium tin oxide (ITO) coated optical fibers for optical and electrochemical sensing purposes. In Proceedings of the 2016 Electron Technology Conference, Wisla, Poland, 11–14 September 2016.

28. Śmietana, M.; Sobaszek, M.; Michalak, B.; Niedziałkowski, P.; Białobrzeska, W.; Koba, M.; Sezemsky, P.; Stranak, V.; Karczewski, J.; Ossowski, T.; et al. Optical Monitoring of Electrochemical Processes with ITO-Based Lossy-Mode Resonance Optical Fiber Sensor Applied as an Electrode. *J. Light. Technol.* **2018**, *36*, 954–960. [CrossRef]

29. Stranak, V.; Bogdanowicz, R.; Sezemsky, P.; Wulff, H.; Kruth, A.; Smietana, M.; Kratochvil, J.; Cada, M.; Hubicka, Z. Towards high quality ITO coatings: The impact of nitrogen admixture in HiPIMS discharges. *Surf. Coat. Technol.* **2018**, *335*, 126–133. [CrossRef]

30. Del Villar, I.; Zamarreño, C.R.; Hernaez, M.; Sanchez, P.; Arregui, F.J.; Matias, I.R. Generation of Surface Plasmon Resonance and Lossy Mode Resonance by thermal treatment of ITO thin-films. *Opt. Laser Technol.* **2015**, *69*, 1–7. [CrossRef]

31. Feng, L.; Oturan, N.; Hullebusch, E.D.; van Esposito, G.; Oturan, M.A. Degradation of anti-inflammatory drug ketoprofen by electro-oxidation: Comparison of electro-Fenton and anodic oxidation processes. *Environ. Sci. Pollut. Res.* **2014**, *21*, 8406–8416. [CrossRef] [PubMed]

32. Vidal, L.; Chisvert, A.; Canals, A.; Psillakis, E.; Lapkin, A.; Acosta, F.; Edler, K.J.; Holdaway, J.A.; Marken, F. Chemically surface-modified carbon nanoparticle carrier for phenolic pollutants: Extraction and electrochemical determination of benzophenone-3 and triclosan. *Anal. Chim. Acta* **2008**, *616*, 28–35. [CrossRef] [PubMed]

33. Wu, B.; Zhao, N.; Hou, S.; Zhang, C. Electrochemical Synthesis of Polypyrrole, Reduced Graphene Oxide, and Gold Nanoparticles Composite and Its Application to Hydrogen Peroxide Biosensor. *Nanomaterials* **2016**, *6*. [CrossRef] [PubMed]

34. Sun, Y.; Ren, Q.; Liu, X.; Zhao, S.; Qin, Y. A simple route to fabricate controllable and stable multilayered all-MWNTs films and their applications for the detection of NADH at low potentials. *Biosens. Bioelectron.* **2013**, *39*, 289–295. [CrossRef] [PubMed]

35. Muruganathan, M.; Latha, S.S.; Bhaskar Raju, G.; Yoshihara, S. Anodic oxidation of ketoprofen—An anti-inflammatory drug using boron doped diamond and platinum electrodes. *J. Hazard. Mater.* **2010**, *180*, 753–758. [CrossRef] [PubMed]

36. Yang, H.; Zhu, Y.; Chen, D.; Li, C.; Chen, S.; Ge, Z. Electrochemical biosensing platforms using poly-cyclodextrin and carbon nanotube composite. *Biosens. Bioelectron.* **2010**, *26*, 295–298. [CrossRef] [PubMed]

37. Kannan, P.; Chen, H.; Lee, V.T.-W.; Kim, D.-H. Highly sensitive amperometric detection of bilirubin using enzyme and gold nanoparticles on sol–gel film modified electrode. *Talanta* **2011**, *86*, 400–407. [CrossRef] [PubMed]

38. Oztekin, Y.; Tok, M.; Bilici, E.; Mikoliunaite, L.; Yazicigil, Z.; Ramanaviciene, A.; Ramanavicius, A. Copper nanoparticle modified carbon electrode for determination of dopamine. *Electrochim. Acta* **2012**, *76*, 201–207. [CrossRef]

39. Radi, A.-E.; Muñoz-Berbel, X.; Lates, V.; Marty, J.-L. Label-free impedimetric immunosensor for sensitive detection of ochratoxin A. *Biosens. Bioelectron.* **2009**, *24*, 1888–1892. [CrossRef] [PubMed]

40. Rahman, M.M.; Jeon, I.C. Studies of electrochemical behavior of SWNT-film electrodes. *J. Braz. Chem. Soc.* **2007**, *18*, 1150–1157. [CrossRef]

41. Nikitin, L.N.; Vasil'kov, A.Y.; Banchero, M.; Manna, L.; Naumkin, A.V.; Podshibikhin, V.L.; Abramchuk, S.S.; Buzin, M.I.; Korlyukov, A.A.; Khokhlov, A.R. Composite materials for medical purposes based on polyvinylpyrrolidone modified with ketoprofen and silver nanoparticles. *Russ. J. Phys. Chem. A* **2011**, *85*, 1190–1195. [CrossRef]

42. Bosselmann, S.; Owens, D.E.; Kennedy, R.L.; Herpin, M.J.; Williams, R.O. Plasma deposited stability enhancement coating for amorphous ketoprofen. *Eur. J. Pharm. Biopharm.* **2011**, *78*, 67–74. [CrossRef] [PubMed]

43. Zhuo, N.; Lan, Y.; Yang, W.; Yang, Z.; Li, X.; Zhou, X.; Liu, Y.; Shen, J.; Zhang, X. Adsorption of three selected pharmaceuticals and personal care products (PPCPs) onto MIL-101(Cr)/natural polymer composite beads. *Sep. Purif. Technol.* **2017**, *177*, 272–280. [CrossRef]

44. Thøgersen, A.; Rein, M.; Monakhov, E.; Mayandi, J.; Diplas, S. Elemental distribution and oxygen deficiency of magnetron sputtered indium tin oxide films. *J. Appl. Phys.* **2011**, *109*, 113532. [CrossRef]

45. Brumbach, M.; Veneman, P.A.; Marrikar, F.S.; Schulmeyer, T.; Simmonds, A.; Xia, W.; Lee, P.; Armstrong, N.R. Surface Composition and Electrical and Electrochemical Properties of Freshly Deposited and Acid-Etched Indium Tin Oxide Electrodes. *Langmuir* **2007**, *23*, 11089–11099. [CrossRef] [PubMed]

46. Li, Y.; Zhao, G.; Zhi, X.; Zhu, T. Microfabrication and imaging XPS analysis of ITO thin films. *Surf. Interface Anal.* **2007**, *39*, 756–760. [CrossRef]

47. Sanchez, P.; Zamarreño, C.R.; Hernaez, M.; Villar, I.D.; Fernandez-Valdivielso, C.; Matias, I.R.; Arregui, F.J. Lossy mode resonances toward the fabrication of optical fiber humidity sensors. *Meas. Sci. Technol.* **2012**, *23*, 014002. [CrossRef]

48. Pickl, K.E.; Magnes, C.; Bodenlenz, M.; Pieber, T.R.; Sinner, F.M. Rapid online-SPE-MS/MS method for ketoprofen determination in dermal interstitial fluid samples from rats obtained by microdialysis or open-flow microperfusion. *J. Chromatogr. B* **2007**, *850*, 432–439. [CrossRef] [PubMed]

49. Zakeri-Milani, P.; Barzegar-Jalali, M.; Tajerzadeh, H.; Azarmi, Y.; Valizadeh, H. Simultaneous determination of naproxen, ketoprofen and phenol red in samples from rat intestinal permeability studies: HPLC method development and validation. *J. Pharm. Biomed. Anal.* **2005**, *39*, 624–630. [CrossRef] [PubMed]

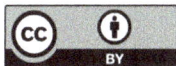

sensors

MDPI

Article

Low-Coherence Interferometric Fiber-Optic Sensors with Potential Applications as Biosensors

Marzena Hirsch [1,†], **Daria Majchrowicz** [1,†], **Paweł Wierzba** [1], **Matthieu Weber** [2], **Mikhael Bechelany** [2] **and Małgorzata Jędrzejewska-Szczerska** [1,*]

1   Department of Metrology and Optoelectronics, Faculty of Electronics, Telecommunications and Informatics, Gdańsk University of Technology, Narutowicza Street 11/12, 80-233 Gdańsk, Poland; hirsch.marzena@gmail.com (M.H.); majchrowiczdaria@gmail.com (D.M.); pwierzba@eti.pg.gda.pl (P.W.)
2   Institut Européen des Membranes, UMR-5635, Université de Montpellier, École Nationale Supérieure de Chimie de Montpellier, Centre national de la recherche scientifique, Place Eugène Bataillon, Montpellier 34095, France; matthieu.weber@umontpellier.fr (M.W.); mikhael.bechelany@univ-montp2.fr (M.B.)
*   Correspondance: mjedrzej@eti.pg.gda.pl; Tel.: +48-58-347-1361
†   These authors contributed equally to this work.

Academic Editor: Vittorio M. N. Passaro
Received: 22 December 2016; Accepted: 24 January 2017; Published: 28 January 2017

Abstract: Fiber-optic Fabry-Pérot interferometers (FPI) can be applied as optical sensors, and excellent measurement sensitivity can be obtained by fine-tuning the interferometer design. In this work, we evaluate the ability of selected dielectric thin films to optimize the reflectivity of the Fabry-Pérot cavity. The spectral reflectance and transmittance of dielectric films made of titanium dioxide (TiO_2) and aluminum oxide (Al_2O_3) with thicknesses from 30 to 220 nm have been evaluated numerically and compared. TiO_2 films were found to be the most promising candidates for the tuning of FPI reflectivity. In order to verify and illustrate the results of modelling, TiO_2 films with the thickness of 80 nm have been deposited on the tip of a single-mode optical fiber by atomic layer deposition (ALD). The thickness, the structure, and the chemical properties of the films have been determined. The ability of the selected TiO_2 films to modify the reflectivity of the Fabry-Pérot cavity, to provide protection of the fibers from aggressive environments, and to create multi-cavity interferometric sensors in FPI has then been studied. The presented sensor exhibits an ability to measure refractive index in the range close to that of silica glass fiber, where sensors without reflective films do not work, as was demonstrated by the measurement of the refractive index of benzene. This opens up the prospects of applying the investigated sensor in biosensing, which we confirmed by measuring the refractive index of hemoglobin and glucose.

Keywords: Fabry-Pérot interferometers; atomic layer deposition; titanium dioxide thin film; fiber-optic sensor; interference

1. Introduction

Optoelectronic instruments based on spectroscopic techniques (e.g., absorption [1,2], Raman [3,4], optical tomography [5,6]) are currently applied in medicine, especially for diagnosis and imaging. However, these measurement methods are expensive, as they often require high-end measurement equipment, expensive consumables (e.g., reagents, dedicated trays, or substrates) and complex methods of sample preparation. Moreover, highly skilled laboratory staff is needed in order to ensure the quality of the measurements performed, which considerably restricts the use of optoelectronic methods in medical diagnosis.

Therefore, there is a real need to develop relatively inexpensive measuring devices that can be used by hospital staff, preferably at the point-of-care (e.g., bedside).

The use of fiber-optic sensors as low-cost measuring devices in biology and medicine represent an attractive alternative. This type of sensor has been the subject of intense research, as it offers several advantages over conventional sensors, such as very high resolution, high accuracy, and small dimensions [7,8]. In fact, fiber-optic sensors possess several advantages in comparison to electronic sensors. Their design often makes use of dielectric materials, which makes them insensitive to electric and magnetic fields generated by other medical devices. Furthermore, they are resistant to most chemical reagents and ionizing radiations. Fiber-optic sensors can be tailored to measure various species and quantities, and they are inexpensive to produce. Finally, the small dimensions of such sensors (below hundreds of micrometers) reduce their impact on the investigated area, allowing for extremely precise measurements [9,10].

Low-coherence interferometry is an excellent detection technique, as it enables the fiber-optic sensors to be insensitive to changes in the intensity of optical signal in the transmission system (because all the information about the measured values is included in the frequency component of the measuring signal spectrum [11,12]). Fiber-optic Fabry-Pérot interferometers (FPI) can be used as efficient optical sensors, and excellent measurement sensitivity can be obtained by the fine-tuning of the interferometer design [13–15].

In the recent years, the advancement of nanotechnology has opened new routes to manufacture thin-films, nanostructures, and nanocomposites materials. Innovative techniques which exploit these routes allow for the elaboration of precise (nano)structures to be achieved, stimulating interest in the properties of these materials and their potential applications.

Atomic layer deposition (ALD) is a vapor phase deposition technique enabling the synthesis of ultrathin films of inorganic materials, with a subnanometer thickness control [16]. ALD can be used to coat 3D substrates with a conformal and uniform film of a high-quality material, a unique capability amongst thin film deposition techniques. Consequently, ALD-grown materials can be applied in various applications such as microelectronics [17], photovoltaics [18], or optical sensing [19]. ALD is based on self-limiting reactions taking place at the surface of the substrate in a cycle-wise fashion. A typical ALD cycle consists of alternate pulses of a precursor and co-reactant gasses in the reactor chamber, separated by purge steps. The properties of the synthetized nanostructures can be tuned by adjusting the process conditions—e.g. the chemistry of the precursor(s) and the co-reactants, the temperature, the number of cycles, or the nature of the substrate [20–23].

Novel interferometer layouts can be considered (as depicted in Figure 1), where a thin film is grown on the end-face of a standard single-mode (SM) fiber. This film deposition creates two distinctive layouts. In the first layout, the deposited film itself is the sensing cavity of the Fabry-Pérot interferometer (Figure 1a). In the second layout, the deposited film acts as a partially transparent mirror improving the reflection at the boundary between the extrinsic cavity and the optical fiber (Figure 1b). Another view of this second layout is the fact that an extrinsic cavity is delimited by two single-mode fibers with the deposited films (Figure 1c).

In this work, we investigated the possible applications of ALD-grown films on SM fibers in low-coherence fiber-optic Fabry-Pérot sensing interferometers. We evaluate the ability of different thin films—namely titanium dioxide (TiO_2) and aluminum oxide (Al_2O_3)—with different thicknesses to tune the reflectivity of the Fabry-Pérot cavity, and we illustrate this modelling work with an experimental fiber using a TiO_2 film.

We first introduce the theory behind the concepts of FPI. Our theoretical modelling work is focused on the first interferometer layout (as shown in Figure 1a), since its properties bring a valuable insight to the expected performance of the other layout, especially the one depicted in Figure 1b. Next, as the best modelling results were obtained with TiO_2 films, we experimentally investigated the ability of an ALD-grown TiO_2 thin film to tune the reflectivity of the FPI cavity, by measuring the influence of TiO_2 thin films on the intensity of reflected interfering beams. Following that, we performed measurements of the refractive index of water, benzene, hemoglobin, and glucose. The main objective of this part of the study was assessment of suitability of the sensor for applications in biosensing. Short-term stability of the TiO$_2$ layers was checked and the refractive index values were compared with reference values to ascertain the correct operation of the sensor.

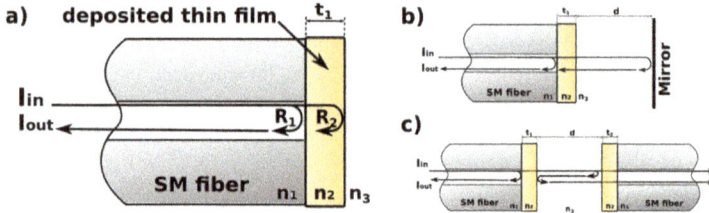

Figure 1. Different designs of fiber-optic Fabry-Pérot interferometers: (**a**) Interferometer with thin film sensing cavity; (**b**) and (**c**) Interferometers with extrinsic sensing cavity operating in reflective and transmission modes, respectively. n_1—refractive index of the fiber; n_2—refractive index of the film; n_3—refractive index of the medium in the cavity; t_1, t_2—thickness of the thin films; d—length of the cavity.

The investigated materials Al$_2$O$_3$ and TiO$_2$ belong to the metal oxides group. These materials are both transparent, and they recently became the subject of growing interest for electronic and optoelectronic sensors. In fact, the sensing properties of oxide thin films are exploited as gas, humidity, and temperature sensors, as well as biosensors [24–26].

2. Theory

The Fabry-Pérot interferometers (FPIs) presented in Figure 1b,c can be considered as multi-cavity interferometers. The propagation of optical radiation in such interferometers is often described using the Gaussian beam formalism. However, FPIs with cavities formed by films manufactured by ALD can be analyzed using a simplified model. As the thickness of the deposited films is limited and as the refractive index difference between the film and the media is relatively small, the Gaussian beam propagating in such films does not expand appreciably. Consequently, in the model, the films manufactured by ALD can be replaced by planar reflective surfaces, whose reflection and transmission coefficients can be calculated using the plane wave approach [27]. This results in a tractable single-cavity model in which the information about the cavities formed by the deposited films is preserved in the values of corresponding reflection and transmission coefficients.

The reflectivity R_1 at the boundary of the optical fiber and the deposited film, and the reflectivity R_2 at the boundary between the film and the surrounding medium, can be calculated using the Fresnel equations:

$$R_1 = \left(\frac{n_2 - n_1}{n_1 + n_2}\right)^2, \tag{1}$$

$$R_2 = \left(\frac{n_3 - n_2}{n_2 + n_3}\right)^2 \tag{2}$$

Using (1) and (2), the reflectivity $\Re$ of the deposited film can be expressed as:

$$\Re = \frac{R_1 + R_2 - 2\sqrt{R_1 R_2}\cos\delta}{1 + R_1 R_2 - 2\sqrt{R_1 R_2}\cos\delta} \tag{3}$$

The phase difference introduced in the interferometer is expressed by Equation (4):

$$\delta = \frac{4\pi}{\lambda}tn_2 \tag{4}$$

where λ—wavelength; t—thickness of the deposited film; $n_{1,2,3}$—refractive indices of the optical fiber core, the deposited film, and the surrounding media (as shown in Figure 1).

Establishing a precise value of the refractive index for the thin films is challenging, as it depends on the thickness and the growth conditions. Furthermore, some materials exhibit birefringence in the bulk form, whereas the thin films behave as isotropic materials [28–30].

Considering Al$_2$O$_3$ material, the values of the refractive index reported in the literature exhibit a substantial dependence on the deposition method and growth conditions [18–20]. In our model, the refractive index of Al$_2$O$_3$ was based on our group experimental data and calculated from Equation (5) [23,31]:

$$n^2_{Al_2O_3} = 1 + \frac{1.4313493\lambda^2}{\lambda^2 - (0.0726631)^2} + \frac{0.65054713\lambda^2}{\lambda^2 - (0.1193242)^2} + \frac{5.3414021\lambda^2}{\lambda^2 - (18.028251)^2}. \qquad (5)$$

Next, the Refractive index of TiO$_2$ was calculated, using Equation (6) below [32]:

$$n^2_{TiO_2} = 5.193 + \frac{0.2441}{\lambda^2 - 0.0803}. \qquad (6)$$

The wavelengths λ are expressed in µm in Equations (5) and (6).

3. Modelling

The spectral characteristics of the TiO$_2$ and Al$_2$O$_3$ thin films have been calculated using the equations presented in Section 2 for various thicknesses (30, 80, 120, 170, and 220 nm). The refractive index of the medium in the cavity n$_3$ was set to 1.00. The reflectance and transmission have been studied for wavelengths in the range from 500 nm to 1700 nm. The results obtained for TiO$_2$ and Al$_2$O$_3$ films are presented in Figures 2 and 3, respectively.

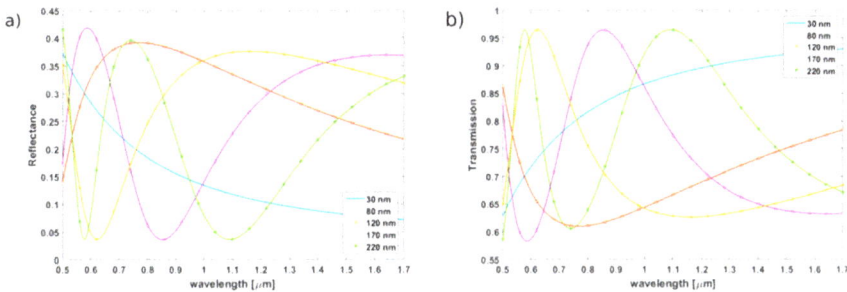

Figure 2. (**a**) Calculated reflectance and (**b**) calculated transmission for TiO$_2$ films of thicknesses ranging from 30 to 220 nm.

For the thinnest films of both oxides (30 nm), it can be seen that the spectral reflectance slowly decreases when increasing the wavelength. However, for thicker films, the optical behavior is different, as wide but distinct fringes can be noticed (for both oxides). Considering the same film thickness, the fringes of the reflectance appear faster for materials presenting higher refractive indexes (in our calculations, the assumed values of n are 2.46 for TiO$_2$ and 1.75 for Al$_2$O$_3$ (at 1300 nm)). The fringes present in the spectra obtained for thicker films are due to the interferences taking place in the film. This effect can be exploited for the design of an interferometer where the thin film itself acts as the sensing medium. However, the measurement techniques most commonly used to process signals from FPI require that the spectrum of the source should cover at least half of the fringe [27]. This condition is difficult to fulfil for the investigation of thin films, as it would require a broadband source with a spectral width over 150 nm, which is difficult to implement. The wavelength range considered is also not very convenient for standard telecommunication optical fibers. Therefore, extracting the data from a FPI sensor using such a thin film as an active medium would require adapting the standard technologies currently used for spectral analysis. However, when considering the sensitivity of TiO$_2$ thin films to humidity, temperature, and specific chemical compounds, this material could find applications in such Fabry-Pérot sensors.

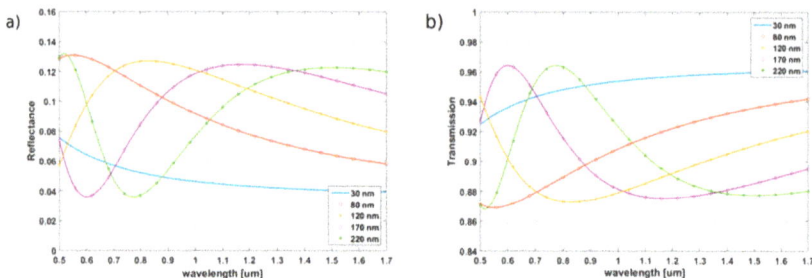

Figure 3. (**a**) Calculated reflectance and (**b**) calculated transmission for Al$_2$O$_3$ films of thicknesses ranging from 30 to 220 nm.

The maximum reflectance obtained is higher for TiO$_2$ (up to 0.417) then for Al$_2$O$_3$ (R_{max} = 0.131). However, even if the reflectance value predicted for Al$_2$O$_3$ thin films is lower than the one of TiO$_2$, it still provides significantly higher level of reflection than a simple boundary between an optical fiber and air cavity (R = 0.036), especially for films thicker than 100 nm.

When considering standard single-mode optical fibers such as SMF-28, wavelengths between 1200 and 1600 nm are typically used. In this range, the maximum reflectance is achieved for films presenting thicknesses between 120 and 220 nm (Table 1).

Table 1. Comparison of calculated values of reflectance and optimal film thickness *t* chosen for the highest reflection at selected wavelengths.

λ (nm)	R_{TiO_2}	$R_{Al_2O_3}$
900	0.3769, *t* = 80 nm	0.1258, *t* = 120 nm
1300	0.3679, *t* = 120 nm	0.1226, *t* = 170 nm
1550	0.3663, *t* = 220 nm	0.1225, *t* = 220 nm

The numerical values presented in the Table 1 were determined for the highest reflectance at selected wavelengths (the ones that are most commonly used when working with optical fibers). However, even if a much thinner film is used, the reflectance of the interferometer's mirror will significantly increase compared to the one of a clean-cut fiber.

Considering the time-consuming nature of the ALD process, where the thickness of the layer depends on the number of performed cycles, using a thinner film allows us to considerably minimize the time required for the fabrication of the sensor. Taking this point into consideration for the experimental evaluation of the performance of ALD layer in optical fiber FPI, a thin TiO$_2$ film of 80 nm thickness has been prepared on the tip of an optical fiber.

4. Materials

4.1. ALD of TiO$_2$

All depositions have been carried out in a custom-built ALD reactor described elsewhere [33]. Titanium isopropoxide ((iPrO)$_4$Ti) precursor was purchased from Sigma Aldrich and used as received. The co-reactant was millipore water. The substrates used were p-type (100) silicon wafers

(MEMC Korea Company, Cheonan, South Korea) and SMF-28 optical fibers (Thorlabs, Newton, MA, USA). To remove the organic contaminants, the substrates were pre-cleaned in acetone and ethanol, and de-ionized water for 5 min in an ultrasonic bath before the depositions.

ALD of TiO_2 was achieved using sequential exposures of $(iPrO)_4Ti$ and H_2O at 120 °C separated by purge steps of argon with a flow rate of 100 sccm. The process consisted of 5 s pulse $((iPrO)_4Ti)$, 30 s exposure, and 40 s purge with dry argon and a 3 s pulse (H_2O), 30 s exposure and 60 s purge. 4000 ALD cycles were carried out in order to achieve the deposition of TiO_2 of ≈80 nm.

Interestingly, it has been shown in previous studies that the amorphous, anatase, and rutile phases of TiO_2 can be obtained by tuning the ALD process parameters, and that the films with different crystallinity phases presented different optical properties [34]. Furthermore, the refractive index of the film has been determined by spectroscopic ellipsometry and a value of 2.0 has been obtained (at lambda = 633 nm). This value is in agreement with the ones found in the literature for TiO_2 films prepared with similar ALD processes (n increases typically from 2.0 to 2.5 with the increasing deposition temperature).

4.2. Characterization of the Films

Chemical and structural characterizations have been performed using Scanning Electron Microscopy (SEM, Hitachi S-4800, Tokyo, Japan), X-ray diffraction (PANAlytical Xpert-PRO diffractometer equipped with an X'celerator detector using Ni-filtered Cu-radiation, Almelo, The Netherlands), and Raman (Raman OMARS 89 (DILOR), Kyoto, Japan). To determine the TiO_2 film thickness after the ALD deposition, ex-situ spectroscopic ellipsometry (SE) measurements were carried out using a Semilab GES5E visible ellipsometer (1.2–5.0 eV) at an angle of incidence of 70.1°. For all the films, the empirical Cauchy dispersion formula has been adopted to model the optical properties and the thicknesses.

4.3. Properties of the TiO_2 Film

Figure 4a shows the SEM image of a ALD-grown TiO_2 film deposited on Si substrate after 4000 ALD cycles. The conformal coating of the Si substrate by the ALD TiO_2 film can be clearly seen.

Spectroscopic ellipsometry (SE) measurements were carried out to evaluate the TiO_2 film thickness as well, and for this specific sample, a thickness of 82 ± 2 nm has been obtained.

The crystallinity study that we carried out showed that the ALD films prepared were amorphous. In fact, grazing-incidence XRD measurements have been realized and the absence of peaks in the spectra obtained suggested that the as-deposited TiO_2 film at 120 °C was amorphous. The formation the amorphous TiO_2 phase was further confirmed by Raman spectroscopy (Figure 4b), since the Raman spectra of the TiO_2 films deposited did not show any peaks either.

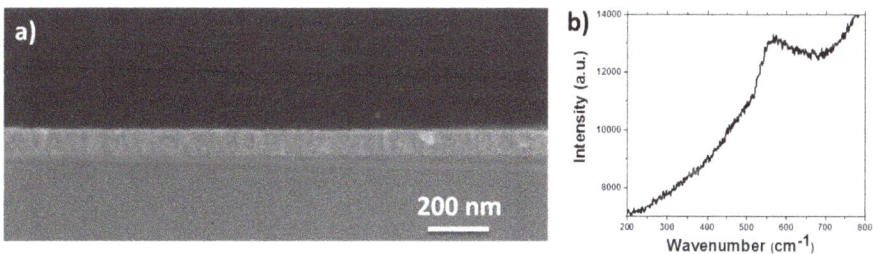

Figure 4. (**a**) SEM cross section image of TiO_2 films deposited by ALD on Si substrates and (**b**) Raman spectrum of TiO_2 films deposited by ALD.

This result is in agreement with previous studies that showed that TiO_2 films deposited by ALD below 200 °C are amorphous, and that annealing at temperatures above 300 °C are typically required to obtain the crystallization of the films. Crystalline TiO_2 typically exhibits the anatase phase, but the rutile phase can also be achieved by ALD, using ozone or plasmas as coreactants [33,35,36]. The relative density of the ALD TiO$_2$ has been reported elsewhere to be 3.6 g/cm^3 [37].

5. Measurements

After the deposition of an 80 nm TiO$_2$ film on SMF-28 optical fibers (Thorlabs, Newton, MA, USA) has been carried out, the performance of the this ALD film in a Fabry-Pérot interferometer has been tested. For this purpose, a low-coherence interferometric sensor has been used (the design of this experimental sensor is depicted in Figure 5). The sensor consists of a Fabry-Pérot interferometer working in reflective mode, an optical spectrum analyzer (Ando AQ6319, Tokyo, Japan), broadband NIR-radiation sources (S1300-G-I-20: λ = 1290 nm, $\Delta\lambda_{FWHM}$ = 50 nm and S-1550-G-I-20: λ = 1550 nm, $\Delta\lambda_{FWHM}$ = 45 nm Superlum), and a single-mode 2 × 2 coupler with 50: 50 power splitting ratio. The standard telecommunication single-mode optical fiber (SMF-28, Thorlabs) coated by ALD is used to connect all components of the setup.

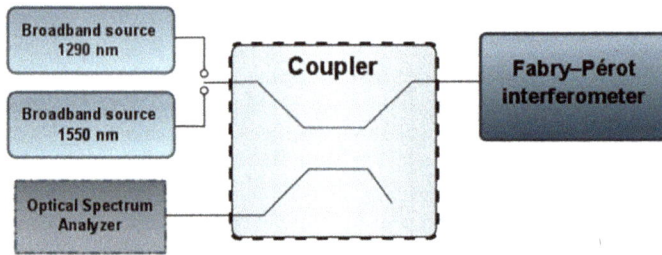

Figure 5. Design of the experimental sensor.

In our study, two Fabry-Pérot interferometers working in reflective mode and having a tunable cavity length were used. The first one had an 80 nm TiO$_2$ thin film deposited on the fiber end face, as shown in Figure 1b. The second FPI had no film deposited and was used as the reference. The measurement was performed in two steps. First, the cavity of the FPI was set to a known length. Then, the spectrum of the light reflected from the FPI was recorded. The measurements were performed for cavity lengths ranging from 50 μm to 500 μm, yielding a series of spectra for each interferometer.

6. Results

In this study, the influence of TiO$_2$ thin films on the quality of the spectrum reflected from the Fabry-Pérot interferometers was investigated. As the optimization function, the visibility V of the measured signal was used. V was defined as:

$$V = \frac{I_{max} - I_{min}}{I_{max} + I_{min}} \tag{7}$$

where I_{max} is the maximum intensity of the optical signal, I_{min} the minimum intensity of the optical signal.

This choice of the optimization function is dictated by the fact that FPI used in low-coherence sensors with spectral detection should be manufactured in such a way that the peaks on the spectral characteristics recorded by the detection setup have the maximum amplitude, i.e., maximum visibility V defined by (7) (in an ideal case V should be equal to 1.0). This contributes to the maximum accuracy of data processing algorithms in these sensors. When V decreases, the accuracy of these algorithms may degrade, although not significantly, as long as V is above 0.7–0.8. Values of V corresponding to optimal cavity length l_{opt} and to 50% and 200% of l_{opt} are shown in Table 2, for each interferometer and each wavelength.

It is important to note that the optimal length l_{opt} of the cavity of the Fabry-Pérot interferometer with TiO$_2$ thin film is around 100 μm and for the Fabry-Pérot interferometer with no film is around 200 μm. The corresponding visibility values are at least 0.95 for both light sources.

Table 2. Visibility of the measured signal in the Fabry-Pérot interferometer.

Fabry-Pérot Interferometer Made by	Length of the Fabry-Pérot Cavity	Central Wavelength of Light Source 1290 nm	Central Wavelength of Light Source 1550 nm
Optical fiber	100 μm	0.75	0.70
	200 μm	0.96	0.95
	400 μm	0.77	0.87
Optical fiber with TiO$_2$ thin film	50 μm	0.89	0.84
	100 μm	0.99	0.98
	200 μm	0.8	0.88

It can be seen that the visibility does not fall steeply. In particular, the visibility for 0.5 l_{opt} and 2.0 l_{opt} does not decrease below 0.7 for any investigated Fabry-Pérot interferometer. This indicates that the cavity length of such an interferometer can be varied in a relatively broad range, up to 4:1, without significant degradation of the performance of the sensor. The measured spectra obtained with the cavity length equal to 100 μm and 200 *u*m are presented in Figures 6 and 7.

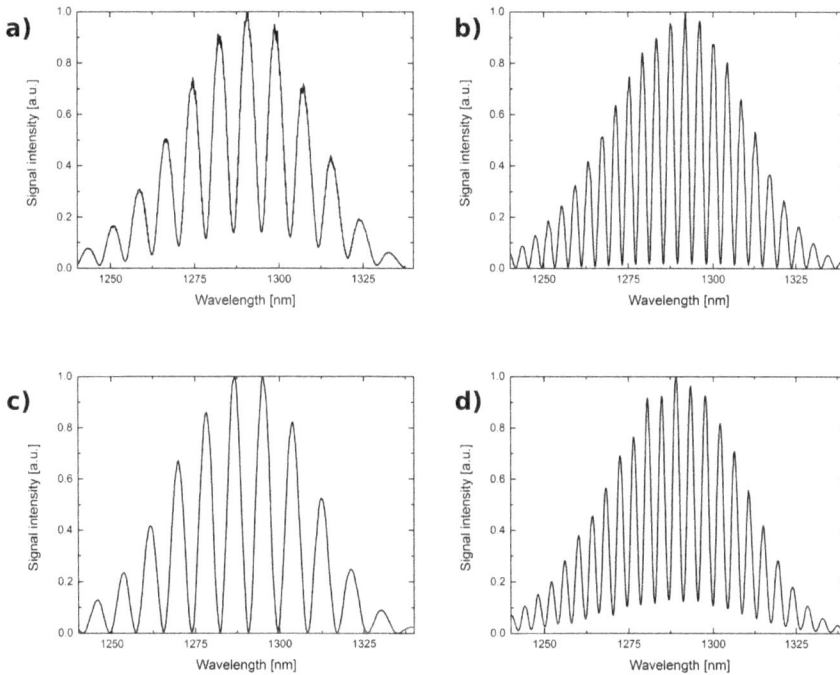

Figure 6. The measurement signal for the 1290 nm source. The Fabry-Pérot interferometer made by: optical fiber and cavity length: (**a**) 100 μm; (**b**) 200 μm; optical fiber with TiO$_2$ thin film and cavity length: (**c**) 100 μm; (**d**) 200 μm.

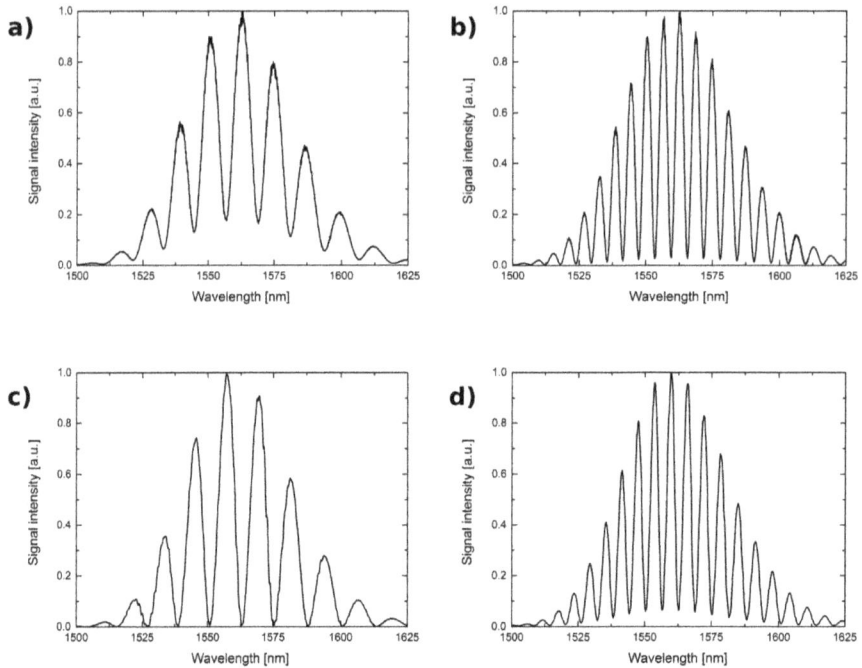

Figure 7. The measurement signal for the 1550 nm source. The Fabry-Pérot interferometer made by: optical fiber and cavity length: (**a**) 100 μm; (**b**) 200 μm; optical fiber with TiO$_2$ thin film and cavity length: (**c**) 100 μm; (**d**) 200 μm.

In order to confirm that proposed ALD-enhanced FPI can be used for measurements of the materials with refractive index close to that of silica glass, sensor response was examined for measurements of benzene (refractive index equal 1.4769 at 1550 nm, while for the core of SMF-28 optical fiber it is 1.468). The calculated value of refractive index obtained from recorded spectra and the reference data are shown to be in good agreement, with difference below 0.029. Following, the measurements were performed for pure water. The value of refractive index measured by our sensor was within 0.032 of the reference value.

To further explore the potential of presented construction in the biosensing applications, the fabricated sensor head was tested with sample of glucose and hemoglobin solution, obtaining refractive index values of 1.3940 and 1.2958, respectively. All of the measurements were performed with the 1550 nm source, the obtained spectra are presented in Figure 8.

The visibility V of the measured signals has decreased in all cases, which was expected as the cavity length was optimized for mediums with a refractive index of 1.0. However, this reduced visibility should not degrade the accuracy of the refractive index calculations.

For each sample, the measurements were performed during a 7-h period. The spectra recorded for each liquid remained stable during this time period. This initial stability test indicated that there was no degradation in the sensing properties of the TiO$_2$ film.

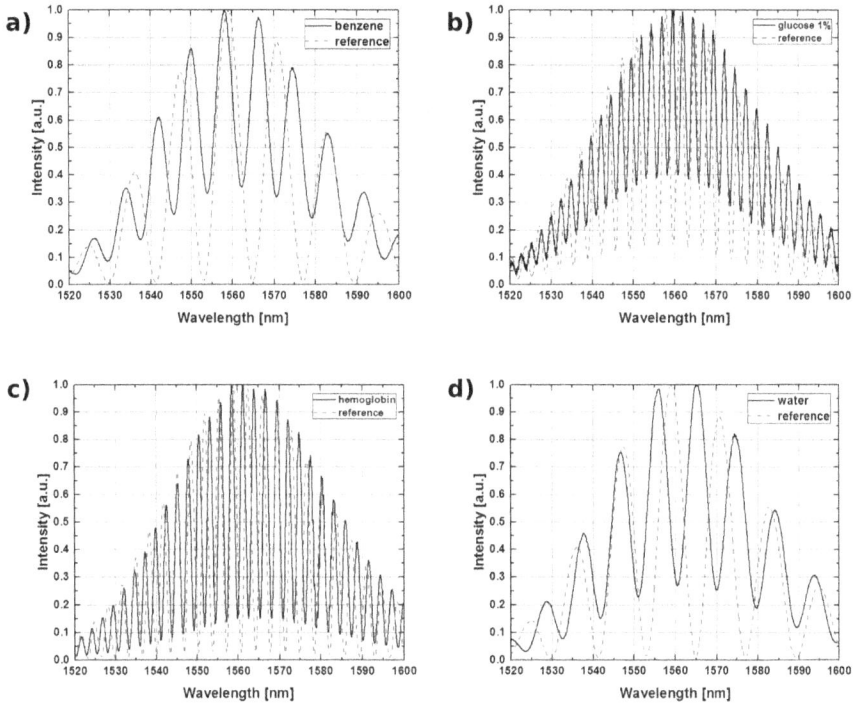

Figure 8. Measurements of Fabry-Pérot interferometer carried out with an optical fiber coated with TiO$_2$ layer when the cavity is filled with: (**a**) benzene; (**b**) glucose (1% solution); (**c**) hemoglobin (13.4 g/dL); and (**d**) water.

7. Conclusions

In the present study, the application of oxide ultrathin films in low coherence fiber-optic Fabry-Pérot sensing interferometers was investigated. The thin films on the tip of SM fibers were aimed to tune the reflectivity of the FPI cavity. The reflectance and transmission spectra were modelled for TiO$_2$ and Al$_2$O$_3$ films of various thicknesses. The obtained results indicate that it is possible to use thin TiO$_2$ film of a thickness around 200–300 nm as active medium in a Fabry-Pérot interferometer. However, the measurements require either an extremely broadband source or a specific adapted signal processing technique. TiO$_2$ and Al$_2$O$_3$ thin films of 100–200 nm deposited on the tip of the optical fiber can also be used as semi-reflective surfaces in order to improve the performance of extrinsic Fabry-Pérot interferometers.

Experiments with a Fabry-Pérot interferometer working in reflective mode were performed in order to illustrate and to verify the modelling presented. The cavity of the interferometer was delimited by an 80 nm TiO$_2$ film deposited by ALD on the fiber end face and by a silver mirror. The cavity length of the interferometer corresponding to the maximum fringe visibility was 100 μm. The reference interferometer (without the TiO$_2$ film) presented an optimal length of 200 μm. Moreover, the level of the signal reflected from the coated interferometer was two times higher than the one from the reference interferometer.

The measurement of refractive index of benzene, which is close to that of silica glass fiber, did not result in any appreciable signal deterioration and yielded a result within 0.029 from the reference value. This confirms the ability of the presented sensor to operate in the refractive index range close to that of silica glass, where sensors without reflective films do not work. Based on the measurement results of refractive index of air and water it can be concluded that the measurement range of our sensor extends from 1.0 to at least 1.5, which gives the sensor good application prospects in biosensing. These prospects were further enhanced by measuring the refractive index of hemoglobin and glucose, during which no degradation in the sensing properties of the TiO_2 film was observed.

Acknowledgments: This study was partially supported by the DS Programs of the Faculty of Electronics, Telecommunications and Informatics of the Gdańsk University of Technology.

Author Contributions: M.H. and M.J.-S. conceived and designed the experiments; D.M. and M.H. performed the experiments; P.W. and M.J.-S. analyzed the data; M.B. and M.W. contributed TiO_2 layers; M.J.-S., D.M., M.H., P.W., M.B. and M.W. wrote the paper.

Conflicts of Interest: The authors declare no conflict of interest.

References

1. Tuchin, V.V. *Handbook of Optical Biomedical Diagnostics*; SPIE Press: Bellingham, WA, USA, 2002.
2. Jakovels, D.; Kuzmina, I.; Berzina, A.; Valeine, L.; Spigulis, J. Noncontact monitoring of vascular lesion phototherapy efficiency by RGB multispectral imaging. *J. Biomed. Opt.* **2013**, *18*, 126019. [CrossRef] [PubMed]
3. Pandey, R.; Paidi, S.K.; Kang, J.W.; Spegazzini, N.; Dasari, R.R.; Valdez, T.A.; Barman, I. Discerning the differential molecular pathology of proliferative middle ear lesions using Raman spectroscopy. *Sci. Rep.* **2015**, *5*, 13305. [CrossRef] [PubMed]
4. Pandey, R.; Dingari, N.C.; Spegazzini, N.; Dasari, R.R.; Horowitz, G.L.; Barman, I. Emerging trends in optical sensing of glycemic markers for diabetes monitoring. *TrAC Trends Anal. Chem.* **2015**, *64*, 100–108. [CrossRef] [PubMed]
5. Głowacki, M.J.; Gnyba, M.; Strąkowska, P.; Gardas, M.; Kraszewski, M.; Trojanowski, M.; Strąkowski, M.R. OCT and Raman spectroscopic investigation of sol-gel derived hydroxyapatite enhaced with silver nanoparticles. *Metrol. Meas. Syst.* **2017**, in press.
6. Brezinski, M.E. *Optical Coherence Tomography*, 1st ed.; Academic Press: Cambridge, MA, USA, 2006.
7. Rao, Y.-J. Recent progress in fiber-optic extrinsic Fabry–Perot interferometric sensors. *Opt. Fiber Technol.* **2006**, *12*, 227–237. [CrossRef]
8. Kirkendall, C.K.; Dandridge, A. Overview of high performance fibre-optic sensing. *J. Phys. Appl. Phys.* **2004**, *37*, R197–R216. [CrossRef]
9. Grattan, K.T.; Meggitt, B.T. *Optical Fiber Sensor Technology*; Kluwer Academic Publisher: Boston, MA, USA, 2000.
10. Islam, M.R.; Ali, M.M.; Lai, M.-H.; Lim, K.-S.; Ahmad, H. Chronology of Fabry-Perot interferometer fiber-optic sensors and their applications: A review. *Sensors* **2014**, *14*, 7451–7488. [CrossRef] [PubMed]
11. Wierzba, P.; Jedrzejewska-Szczerska, M. Optimization of a Fabry-Perot Sensing Interferometer Design for an Optical Fiber Sensor of Hematocrit Level. *Acta Phys. Pol. A* **2013**, *124*, 586–588. [CrossRef]
12. Jędrzejewska-Szczerska, M. Response of a New Low-Coherence Fabry-Perot Sensor to Hematocrit Levels in Human Blood. *Sensors* **2014**, *14*, 6965–6976. [CrossRef] [PubMed]
13. Milewska, D.; Karpienko, K.; Jędrzejewska-Szczerska, M. Application of thin diamond films in low-coherence fiber-optic Fabry Pérot displacement sensor. *Diam. Relat. Mater.* **2016**, *64*, 169–176. [CrossRef]
14. Majchrowicz, D.; Hirsch, M.; Wierzba, P.; Bechelany, M.; Viter, R.; Jędrzejewska-Szczerska, M. Application of Thin ZnO ALD Layers in Fiber-Optic Fabry-Pérot Sensing Interferometers. *Sensors* **2016**, *16*, 416. [CrossRef] [PubMed]
15. Majchrowicz, D.; Hirsch, M. Fiber optic low-coherence Fabry-Pérot interferometer with ZnO layers in transmission and reflective mode: Comparative study. *Proc. SPIE* **2016**, *9917*, 99171C.
16. Leskelä, M.; Ritala, M. Atomic Layer Deposition Chemistry: Recent Developments and Future Challenges. *Angew. Chem. Int. Ed.* **2003**, *42*, 5548–5554. [CrossRef] [PubMed]
17. Auth, C.; Allen, C.; Blattner, A.; Bergstrom, D.; Brazier, M.; Bost, M.; Buehler, M.; Chikarmane, V.; Ghani, T.; Glassman, T.; et al. A 22nm high performance and low-power CMOS technology featuring fully-depleted tri-gate transistors, self-aligned contacts and high density MIM capacitors. In Proceedings of the 2012 Symposium on VLSI Technology (VLSIT), Honolulu, HI, USA, 12–14 June 2012; pp. 131–132.

18. Dingemans, G.; Kessels, W.M.M. Status and prospects of Al2O3-based surface passivation schemes for silicon solar cells. *J. Vac. Sci. Technol. A* **2012**, *30*, 40802. [CrossRef]

19. Jędrzejewska-Szczerska, M.; Wierzba, P.; Chaaya, A.A.; Bechelany, M.; Miele, P.; Viter, R.; Mazikowski, A.; Karpienko, K.; Wróbel, M. ALD thin ZnO layer as an active medium in a fiber-optic Fabry–Perot interferometer. *Sens. Actuators A Phys.* **2015**, *221*, 88–94. [CrossRef]

20. George, S.M. Atomic Layer Deposition: An Overview. *Chem. Rev.* **2010**, *110*, 111–131. [CrossRef] [PubMed]

21. Weber, M.J.; Verheijen, M.A.; Bol, A.A.; Kessels, W.M.M. Sub-nanometer dimensions control of core/shell nanoparticles prepared by atomic layer deposition. *Nanotechnology* **2015**, *26*, 94002. [CrossRef] [PubMed]

22. Weber, M.J.; Mackus, A.J.M.; Verheijen, M.A.; van der Marel, C.; Kessels, W.M.M. Supported Core/Shell Bimetallic Nanoparticles Synthesis by Atomic Layer Deposition. *Chem. Mater.* **2012**, *24*, 2973–2977. [CrossRef]

23. Chaaya, A.A.; Viter, R.; Baleviciute, I.; Bechelany, M.; Ramanavicius, A.; Gertnere, Z.; Erts, D.; Smyntyna, V.; Miele, P. Tuning Optical Properties of Al$_2$O$_3$/ZnO Nanolaminates Synthesized by Atomic Layer Deposition. *J. Phys. Chem. C* **2014**, *118*, 3811–3819. [CrossRef]

24. Snure, M.; Paduano, Q.; Hamilton, M.; Shoaf, J.; Mann, J.M. Optical characterization of nanocrystalline boron nitride thin films grown by atomic layer deposition. *Thin Solid Films* **2014**, *571*, 51–55. [CrossRef]

25. Boudiombo, J.; Boudrioua, A.; Loulergue, J.C.; Malhouitre, S.; Machet, J. Optical waveguiding properties and refractive index analysis of boron nitride (BN) thin films prepared by reactive ion plating. *Opt. Mater.* **1998**, *10*, 143–153. [CrossRef]

26. López, J.; Martínez, J.; Abundiz, N.; Domínguez, D.; Murillo, E.; Castillón, F.F.; Machorro, R.; Farías, M.H.; Tiznado, H. Thickness effect on the optical and morphological properties in Al$_2$O$_3$/ZnO nanolaminate thin films prepared by atomic layer deposition. *Superlattices Microstruct.* **2016**, *90*, 265–273. [CrossRef]

27. Wierzba, P.; Jędrzejewska-Szczerska, M. Spectral reflectance modeling of ZnO layers made with Atomic Layer Deposition for application in optical fiber Fabry-Perot interferometric sensors. *Proc. SPIE* **2015**, *9448*, 944819.

28. Wang, Z.-Y.; Zhang, R.-J.; Lu, H.-L.; Chen, X.; Sun, Y.; Zhang, Y.; Wei, Y.-F.; Xu, J.-P.; Wang, S.-Y.; Zheng, Y.-X.; et al. The impact of thickness and thermal annealing on refractive index for aluminum oxide thin films deposited by atomic layer deposition. *Nanoscale Res. Lett.* **2015**, *10*, 46. [CrossRef] [PubMed]

29. Kumar, P.; Wiedmann, M.K.; Winter, C.H.; Avrutsky, I. Optical properties of Al$_2$O$_3$ thin films grown by atomic layer deposition. *Appl. Opt.* **2009**, *48*, 5407–5412. [CrossRef] [PubMed]

30. Kasikov, A.; Aarik, J.; Mändar, H.; Moppel, M.; Pärs, M.; Uustare, T. Refractive index gradients in TiO$_2$ thin films grown by atomic layer deposition. *J. Phys. Appl. Phys.* **2006**, *39*, 54–60. [CrossRef]

31. Refractive Index of Al$_2$O$_3$ (Aluminium Oxide, Sapphire)—Kischkat. Available online: http://refractiveindex.info/?shelf=main&book=Al2O3&page=Kischkat (accessed on 23 September 2016).

32. Refractive Index of TiO$_2$ (Titanium Dioxide)—Devore-o. Available online: http://refractiveindex.info/?shelf=main&book=TiO2&page=Devore-o (accessed on 23 September 2016).

33. Schlicht, S.; Assaud, L.; Hansen, M.; Licklederer, M.; Bechelany, M.; Perner, M.; Bachmann, J. An electrochemically functional layer of hydrogenase extract on an electrode of large and tunable specific surface area. *J. Mater. Chem. A* **2016**, *4*, 6487–6494. [CrossRef]

34. Profijt, H.B.; van de Sanden, M.C.M.; Kessels, W.M.M. Substrate Biasing during Plasma-Assisted ALD for Crystalline Phase-Control of TiO$_2$ Thin Films. *Electrochem. Solid-State Lett.* **2011**, *15*, G1–G3. [CrossRef]

35. Xie, Q.; Jiang, Y.-L.; Detavernier, C.; Deduytsche, D.; Van Meirhaeghe, R.L.; Ru, G.-P.; Li, B.-Z.; Qu, X.-P. Atomic layer deposition of TiO$_2$ from tetrakis-dimethyl-amido titanium or Ti isopropoxide precursors and H$_2$O. *J. Appl. Phys.* **2007**, *102*, 83521. [CrossRef]

36. Kim, S.K.; Kim, W.-D.; Kim, K.-M.; Hwang, C.S.; Jeong, J. High dielectric constant TiO$_2$ thin films on a Ru electrode grown at 250 °C by atomic-layer deposition. *Appl. Phys. Lett.* **2004**, *85*, 4112–4114. [CrossRef]

37. Triani, G.; Evans, P.J.; Mitchell, D.R.G.; Attard, D.J.; Finnie, K.S.; James, M.; Hanley, T.; Latella, B.; Prince, K.E.; Bartlett, J. Atomic layer deposition of TiO$_2$/Al$_2$O$_3$ films for optical applications. *Proc. SPIE* **2005**, *5870*, 587009.

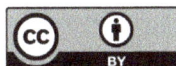

sensors

MDPI

Article

Feasibility of Optical Coherence Tomography (OCT) for Intra-Operative Detection of Blood Flow during Gastric Tube Reconstruction

Sanne M. Jansen [1,2,*,†], Mitra Almasian [1,†], Leah S. Wilk [1], Daniel M. de Bruin [1], Mark I. van Berge Henegouwen [3], Simon D. Strackee [2], Paul R. Bloemen [1], Sybren L. Meijer [4], Suzanne S. Gisbertz [3] and Ton G. van Leeuwen [1]

[1] Department of Biomedical Engineering & Physics, Academic Medical Center, University of Amsterdam, 1105 AZ Amsterdam, The Netherlands; m.almasian@amc.uva.nl (M.A.); l.s.wilk@amc.uva.nl (L.S.W.); d.m.debruin@amc.uva.nl (D.M.d.B.); p.r.bloemen@amc.uva.nl (P.R.B.); t.g.vanleeuwen@amc.uva.nl (T.G.v.L.)
[2] Department of Plastic, Reconstructive & Hand Surgery, Academic Medical Center, University of Amsterdam, 1105 AZ Amsterdam, The Netherlands; s.d.strackee@amc.uva.nl
[3] Department of Surgery, Academic Medical Center, University of Amsterdam, 1105 AZ Amsterdam, The Netherlands; m.i.vanbergehenegouwen@amc.uva.nl (M.I.v.B.H.); s.s.gisbertz@amc.uva.nl (S.S.G.)
[4] Department of Pathology, Academic Medical Center, University of Amsterdam, 1105 AZ Amsterdam, The Netherlands; s.l.meijer@amc.uva.nl
* Correspondence: s.m.jansen@amc.uva.nl; Tel.: +31-20-566-5207
† These authors contributed equally to this work.

Received: 15 March 2018; Accepted: 21 April 2018; Published: 25 April 2018

Abstract: In this study; an OCT-based intra-operative imaging method for blood flow detection during esophagectomy with gastric tube reconstruction is investigated. Change in perfusion of the gastric tube tissue can lead to ischemia; with a high morbidity and mortality as a result. Anastomotic leakage (incidence 5–20%) is one of the most severe complications after esophagectomy with gastric tube reconstruction. Optical imaging techniques provide for minimal-invasive and real-time visualization tools that can be used in intraoperative settings. By implementing an optical technique for blood flow detection during surgery; perfusion can be imaged and quantified and; if needed; perfusion can be improved by either a surgical intervention or the administration of medication. The feasibility of imaging gastric microcirculation in vivo using optical coherence tomography (OCT) during surgery of patients with esophageal cancer by visualizing blood flow based on the speckle contrast from M-mode OCT images is studied. The percentage of pixels exhibiting a speckle contrast value indicative of flow was quantified to serve as an objective parameter to assess blood flow at 4 locations on the reconstructed gastric tube. Here; it was shown that OCT can be used for direct blood flow imaging during surgery and may therefore aid in improving surgical outcomes for patients.

Keywords: flow; monitoring; OCT; optical imaging; surgery; esophagectomy; gastric tube; perfusion; speckle

---

1. Introduction

The viability of cells and tissue mainly depends on blood flow as it transports oxygen and nutrients to the cells. Without oxygen and nutrients, ischemia occurs and tissue becomes necrotic [1]. An esophageal resection with ensuing gastric tube reconstruction is the cornerstone of treatment in patients with esophageal cancer. To be able to pull up the gastric tube, ligation of the left gastric artery, the left gastro-epiploic artery, the short gastric vessels and some branches of the right gastric artery is needed. As a result, perfusion of the tube's gastric tissue after reconstruction relies on the right gastroepiploic artery and some branches of the right gastric artery [2] leaving the future neo-esophageal anastomotic site depending only on collateral blood flow.

Anastomotic leakage (incidence 5–20%) and stricture (10–22%) are major complications following esophagectomy, and mortality is as high as 4% [2]. Perfusion deficiency of the gastric tube is seen as the major risk factor to develop these complications, which, in turn, correlate with high morbidity, IC-unit stay, high costs in healthcare and decreased quality of life [3]. Monitoring perfusion would allow surgeons to make different choices in their surgical design [4] and, if needed, involve anesthesiology interventions to optimize perfusion by the use of fluid or medication [5]. Consequently, intra-operative perfusion monitoring could potentially aid in achieving better patient outcomes after surgery and in decreasing complications and mortality.

Optical techniques are well-suited for intra-operative monitoring due to their minimal-invasive and real-time visualization capabilities [6]. Optical Coherence Tomography (OCT) allows high-resolution, non-invasive, real-time imaging of tissue [7]. It detects backscattered near-infrared light from tissue to obtain depth-resolved, in vivo images. As a result, this technique potentially allows visualization of vasculature in different tissue layers until a depth of approximately 2.5 mm [8]. Moreover, the underlying arteries will not influence the measured perfusion in the overlaying microvascular network, in contrast to other optical imaging techniques like fluorescence imaging, laser speckle contrast imaging or laser Doppler flowmetry [9–11]. Finally, a handheld OCT probe is easy to use in the operation room.

A large number of studies have investigated and established the link between OCT speckle and the flow of the imaged medium, ranging from qualitative detection of flow to quantitative analysis of the flow parameter in very controlled measurement settings [8,12–14]. By analyzing the speckle variance [15] or speckle decorrelation [12] of OCT data, flow can be discriminated from static tissue in order to visualize blood vessels and microcirculation. In previous studies we have shown that OCT speckle decorrelation can be used to obtain a quantitative blood flow parameter [8,14]. However, because of the needed fixation during imaging, these systems are not readily applicable in the operating room. Therefore, for the visualization of flow during surgery, in this study we use speckle contrast in the OCT M-mode scans to distinguish flow from static tissue.

The aim of this study is to research the feasibility of a commercially available OCT system to detect blood vessels in gastric tissue, in patients with esophageal cancer in a clinical setting during esophageal cancer surgery with gastric tube reconstruction. 3D OCT scans are obtained to image tissue layers in the reconstructed gastric tube and compared to histopathological slides, yielding information about tissue structure and blood vessel locations. In this paper, speckle contrast, the ratio of speckle variance over the mean, is calculated from OCT M-mode scans to distinguish areas with flow from static tissue. The percentage of pixels indicative of flow is used as an objective parameter to compare blood flow at different locations, ranging from normal perfusion, near the remaining right gastroepiploic artery and/or branches of the right gastric artery, to decreased perfusion, near the future anastomotic side.

2. Materials and Methods

This prospective, observational, in vivo pilot study of 26 patients with esophageal cancer who underwent an esophageal resection with gastric tube reconstruction was approved by the medical ethics committee (NL52377.018.15) of the Academic Medical Center of Amsterdam, and submitted at the clinicaltrials.gov database (NCT02902549) [16]. Patients were included in this study between October 2015 and June 2016 in the Academic Medical Center (Amsterdam, The Netherlands). Written informed consent was obtained at least one week before surgery. Surgery was performed by two experienced upper-gastrointestinal surgeons (MIvBH, SSG).

Usually, patients undergo a minimally invasive Ivor Lewis procedure (2-stage procedure with intra-thoracic anastomosis), however, in case of a mid- or proximal esophageal carcinoma, a minimally invasive McKeown procedure (3-stage procedure with cervical anastomosis) was performed. Mobilization and vascularization of the gastric conduit was the same in both procedures.

The procedures have been described in detail before [5]. In brief, during the abdominal phase a lymphadenectomy and mobilization of the stomach was performed, ligating the left gastric artery, some branches of the right gastric artery at the level of the angulus, the left gastro-epiploic artery and the short gastric vessels (Figure 1). During the thoracic phase a lymphadenectomy was performed, the esophagus was mobilized and after extraction of the specimen and gastric pull-up an intrathoracic or a cervical anastomosis was created. In all patients, a 3–4 cm wide gastric tube was reconstructed using a powered ECHOLON FLEX Stapler (Ethicon, Johnson & Johnson Health Care Systems, Piscataway, NJ, USA). Branches of the right gastric artery supply the remains of the lesser curvature. The right gastro-epiploic artery supplies the greater curvature until the watershed area with the left gastro-epiploic artery.

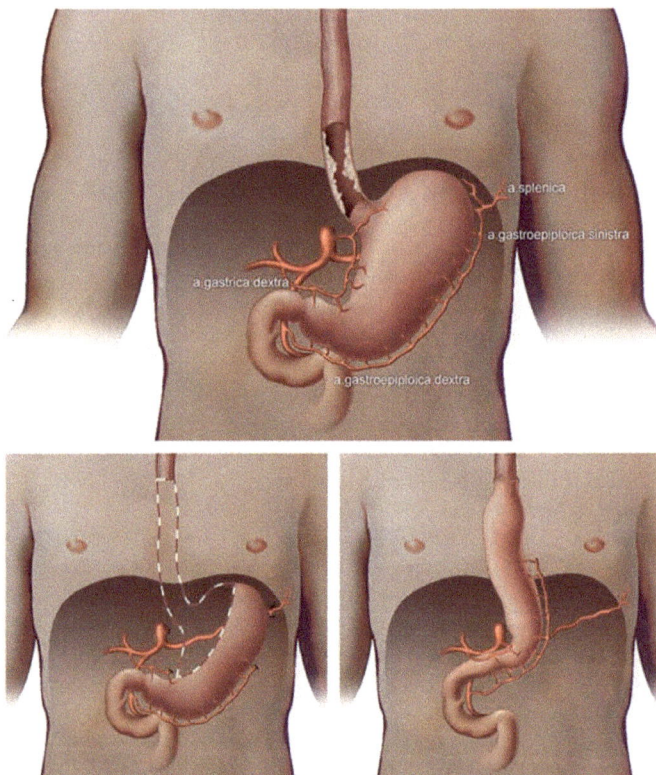

Figure 1. Esophageal cancer with gastric vascularization, esophagectomy and gastric tube reconstruction with only one artery left (gastroepiploic artery).

OCT data were recorded using a commercial 50 kHz IVS 2000 swept source OCT system (THORLABS, Newton, NJ, USA) operating at a center wavelength of ~1300 nm. The full width half maximum axial and lateral resolutions were measured to be ~14 µm and ~25 µm, respectively. Volumetric images (x, y, z) of 10 mm by 10 mm by 2.5 mm, containing 1024 by 1024 by 400 pixels, and M-mode scans (x, y, z) of 0 mm by 10 mm by 2.5 mm, containing 1024, 1024, 400 pixels were collected. The depth axis was corrected for the refractive index of tissue (n_{ref} = 1.4) (Figure 2).

A sterile sheet was placed around the probe for the intra-operative measurements on gastric tissue. Measurements were taken with a hand-held OCT probe directly after preparation of the gastric tube, at four perfusion areas: 3 cm proximal of the level of the watershed between the right and left gastro-epiploic arteries (location 1), at the level of the watershed between the right and left gastro-epiploic arteries (location 2), 3 cm distal to the watershed between the right and left gastro-epiploic arteries (location 3) and at the level of the gastric fundus (location 4), physiologically from normal perfusion to decreased perfusion. Time to obtain data was recorded in the CRF.

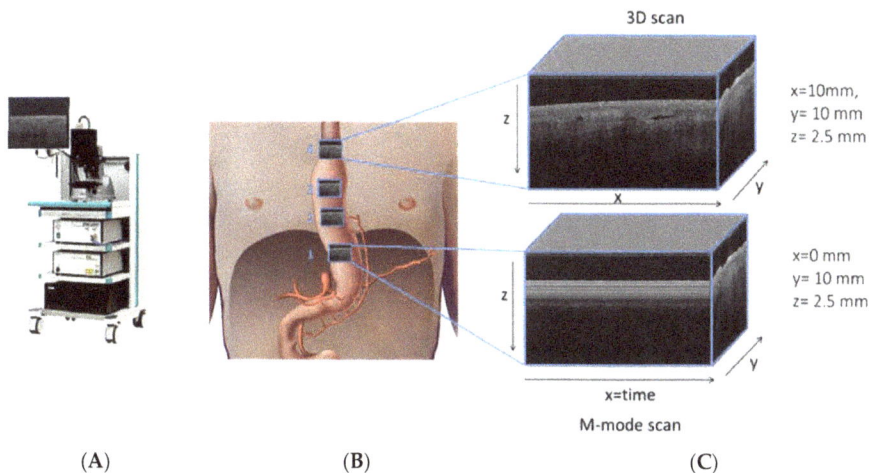

Figure 2. Santec OCT system (panel **A**), schematic figure (panel **B**) of gastric tube with ROI of 10 × 10 mm of OCT grayscale images at four perfusion areas, with shadowing of vessels in cross sectional OCT image (panel **C**).

Tissue from the fundus of the gastric tube was obtained for histology ($n = 5$) in 5 patients during surgery, with the aim to correlate these findings to the OCT scans. After routine processing of the tissue HE-stained, slides were digitized and evaluated by a pathologist (SLM) to define tissue layers and localize different structures, such as blood and lymph vessels. Different tissue layers (serosa, subserosa and muscularis propria) and blood and lymph vessels were annotated and compared to OCT scans.

All data analysis was performed using custom-made scripts written in MATLAB (Mathworks, Natick, MA, USA). Using the M-mode scans, the speckle contrast (C) as a function of time was quantified in order to differentiate regions of flow from regions of static tissue. To this end, the following processing steps were applied to the data (Figure 3). First, a dB mask (−2 dB) was applied to exclude noise from the OCT data, where after a region of interest (ROI) in the Y-Z image is chosen to exclude corrupted parts of the scan, if needed. Second, the pixel-specific speckle contrast is calculated along the time axis for all pixels selected. The speckle contrast is the ratio of the amplitude variance over the mean amplitude [17]. The amplitude of regions with flow on OCT M-mode scans are expected to be Rayleigh distributed and hence have a speckle contrast value of 0.52 [18]. Here, we have used a speckle contrast gate between 0.42 and 0.62 to detect areas with flow. Next, a median filter with a kernel of 7 by 3 pixels is applied to the speckle contrast images. The pixels remaining after filtering are labeled as flow. The boundaries of the speckle contrast gate and the size of the median filter kernel are optimized by comparing the resulting speckle contrast images with the original X-Z M-mode scans by eye in five randomly chosen scans. Finally, an overlay is created using a Y-Z plot of the gated and filtered speckle contrast and the Y-Z grayscale OCT image. The percentage of pixels labelled as flow relative to the total number of pixels is calculated as an objective parameter to indicate the amount of vessels in the analyzed area.

The ability of the proposed method to distinguish pixels with flow from static tissue based on a speckle contrast gate between 0.42 and 0.62 was validated on a tissue mimicking flow phantom [8]. To simulate human perfusion heparinized human whole blood was flown with a velocity of 5 mm/s through a channel with a 100 µm diameter embedded in scattering silicon. The details on the manufacturing of the flow phantom are described elsewhere [8]. Single M-mode OCT scans (400×400 pixels) were collected at a static and flow region of the phantom and the speckle contrast was calculated as a function of depth.

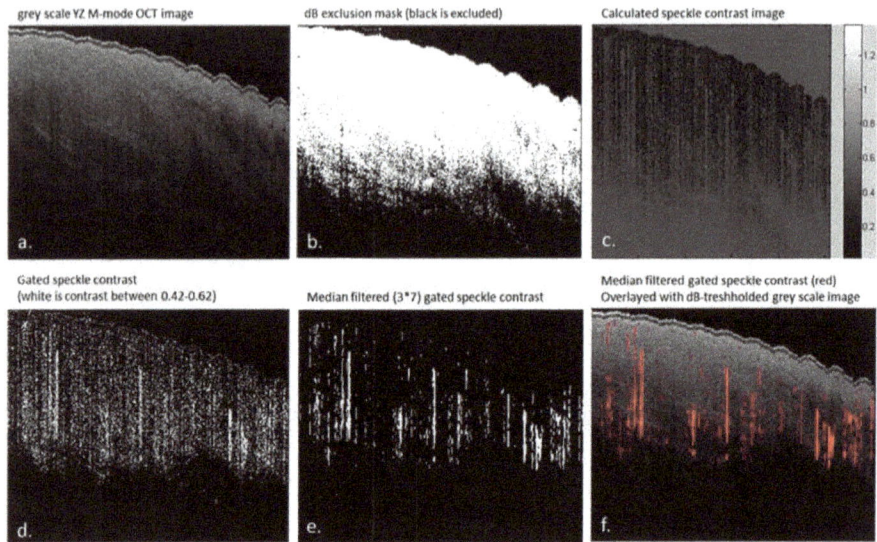

Figure 3. Data analysis steps of OCT M-mode scans, all images are shown from the y-z plane. (**a**) grayscale y-z M-mode scan; (**b**) applied dB mask to exclude noise from the data, the white areas on this image are included as data (**c**) over the time scale calculated speckle contrast values (of regions of included data after the dB threshold (**d**) speckle contrast within the 0.42–0.62 gate plotted in white (**e**) speckle contrast after applying a median filter with a 7×3 pixel kernel (**f**) gated and filtered speckle contrast (red) overlaid with the grayscale OCT image.

3. Results

3.1. Patients and Feasibility of Intra-Operative OCT Imaging

In total, 26 patients signed informed consent. Four patients were excluded based on delay in operation time (measurements interrupted the operation by ±20 min), which made imaging impossible considering patient safety. Therefore 22 patients were included for data acquisition (Figure 4). In all 22 patients, 3D OCT images were acquired at four locations of the gastric tube, from the base to the fundus, the future anastomotic site ($n = 88$). Furthermore, M-mode scans were acquired at the same four locations of the gastric tube, from physiologically expected normal to decreased perfusion ($n = 88$). Speckle contrast analysis was not possible for all acquired M-mode scans due to poor quality of the scans (e.g., specular reflections, out of focus, and crossing zero-delay). In most cases the quality of the scans was hampered by specular reflections from the sterile sheet on top of the tissue. In total 48 M-mode scans were excluded. In four patients ($n = 12$) OCT data acquisition and speckle contrast analysis yielding areas indicative of flow (%) was successful at all four locations.

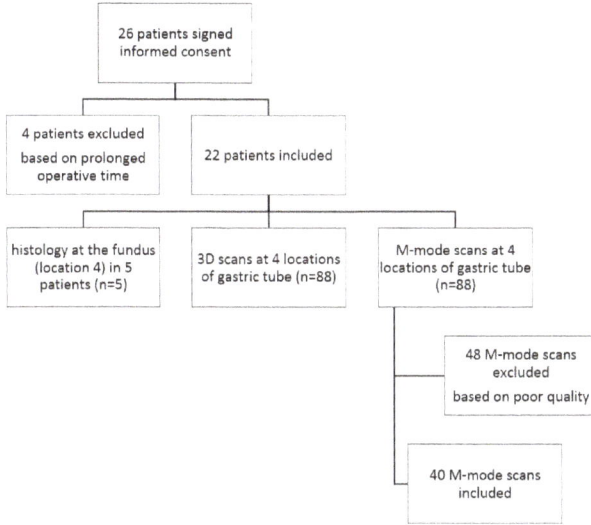

Figure 4. Flow diagram: patient and data inclusion.

3.2. 3D OCT Scans

3D images were obtained at four locations of the gastric tube (Figure 5). On the 3D scans, different tissue layers could be distinguished. By comparison with histopathology slides, these layers could be identified. Importantly, the localization of the blood vessels of the reconstructed gastric tube was similar in OCT images compared to histopathology (Figure 6). Furthermore, because lymph fluid is a low-scattering medium, lymph vessels could be identified in the OCT images as well.

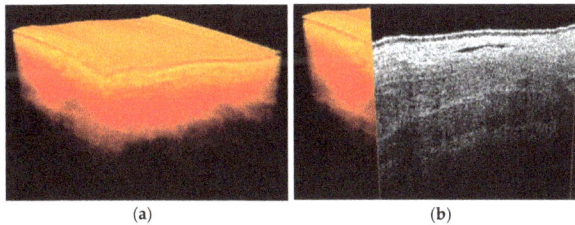

(a) (b)

Figure 5. 3D OCT scan of the gastric tube, (**a**) volumetric representation (**b**) with cross section visualized.

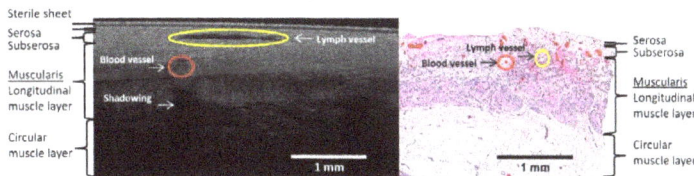

Figure 6. OCT B-scan of location 4, the fundus (at the left panel), and HE stained histology slide (the right panel) obtained at the end of the gastric tube. Blood and lymph vessels are indicated in red and yellow, respectively. The corresponding tissue layers, serosa, subserosa (purple/dark pink) and muscularis propria (light pink) are depicted in both panels. The scale bar depicts a length of 1 mm.

3.3. Speckle Contrast Analysis of M-Mode OCT Scans

Areas indicative of flow could be distinguished from static tissue by calculating the speckle contrast in the M-mode images. As depicted in Figure 7A, the contrast calculated for a single M-mode scan for static tissue was mostly below 0.4, unless the SNR was too low as observed at larger depths. When flow was present in the channel at 0.2 mm below the surface, the speckle contrast was between 0.42 and 0.62 (Figure 7B). Please note that an increase in the speckle contrast was observed below the flow channel as well. Similar effects were observed in the single M-mode scans of the reconstructed gastric tube, as depicted in Figure 7C for the less perfused part of the tissue and in Figure 7D in which a blood vessel was present at a depth of 0.2 mm below the tissue surface.

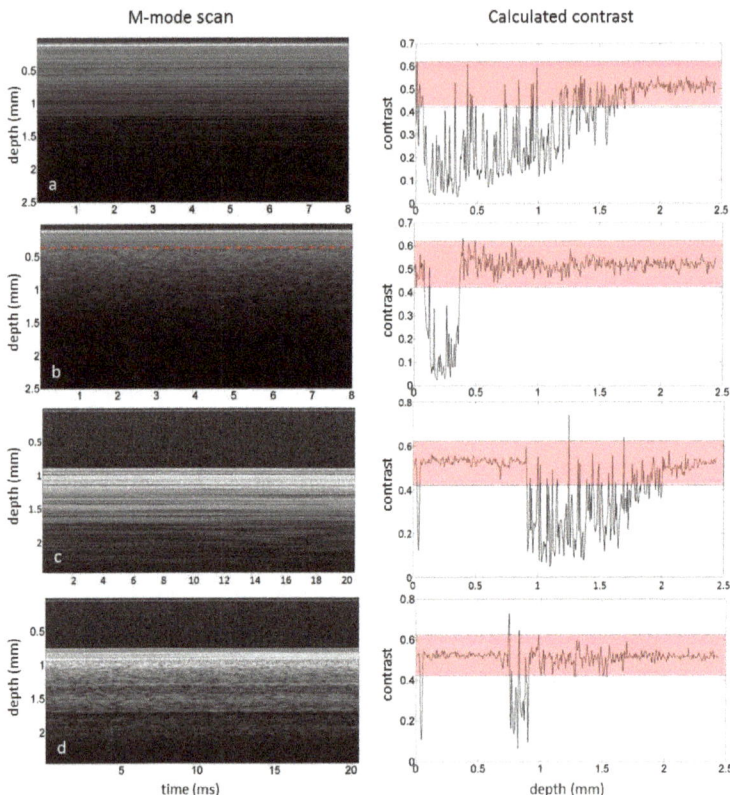

Figure 7. Single M-mode OCT scans (**left**) and the corresponding calculated contrast (**right**) of a. a static region of the flow phantom, b. a region with flow in the flow phantom in which the red line depicts the approximated location of the top of the flow channel, c. a static region of tissue and d. a region with flow in tissue by a blood vessel at approximately 0.2 mm below the tissue surface. The red bar depicts the speckle contrast threshold used in this manuscript.

Calculation of speckle contrast percentage (%) as a parameter for tissue areas with flow was possible in 13 (n = 40) of the 22 included patients (59%) and in all four locations in 4 (n = 12) of the 22 patients (14%) (for data inclusion and exclusion criteria, see first results section and Figure 4). We observed a decrease in speckle contrast percentage (%) from location 1 to location 4 in 6 of the 13 patients (46%) and an increase in 3 of the 13 patients (23%). The speckle contrast percentage data at location 1 or 4 was missing for 3 out of 13 patients.

The results, percentage pixels indicating flow relative to the total number of pixels, per patient and location are summarized in Table 1 and Figure 8. In 10 patients, data analysis was possible for location 4. In 80% of these patients, percentage of flow pixels was lower compared to location 1, 2 or 3.

Table 1. Percentage of pixels indicative of flow per patient per location obtained from the OCT M-mode scans. In red the flow in location 4 of the gastric tube.

Patient	pt2	pt3	pt4	pt5	pt6	pt9	pt12	pt14	pt16	pt17	pt18	pt19	pt20	pt21	pt22
location 1	5	8	18	22	x	24	x	16	x	13	20	8	12	11	15
location 2	x	x	x	x	x	28	2	17	8	10	6	9	4	8	8
location 3	14	8	x	x	x	23	5	14	x	24	x	2	x	x	3
location 4	11	1	14	17	18	16	x	13	x	21	x	0	1	x	x

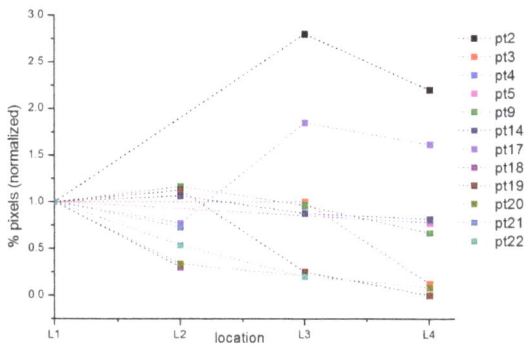

Figure 8. Normalized percentage of pixels per patient per location obtained from the OCT M-mode scans. The values are normalized relative to location 1, hence only the plots for patients with a value for location 1 are shown.

For patients 9, 14, 17 and 19 the speckle contrast analysis was possible on all four locations on the gastric tube. Figure 9 depicts the OCT M-mode scans of all four locations for patients 9, 14 17 and 19. A decrease of areas with speckle contrast indicative of flow (red) is visible towards the fundus in patients 9, 14 and 19. The expected shadowing due to multiple scattering [8] caused by the high scattering coefficient in blood is clearly observed in the images [18].

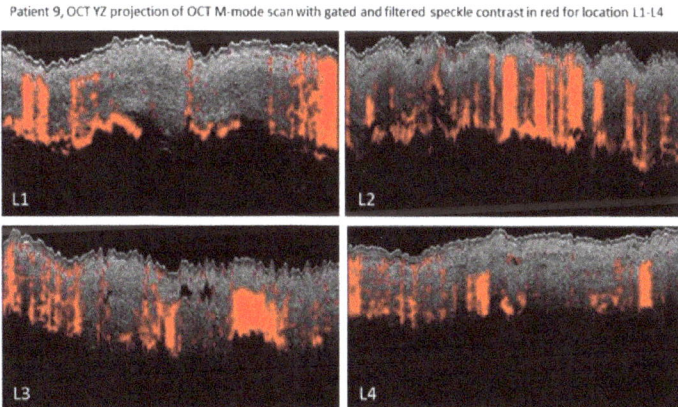

Patient 9, OCT YZ projection of OCT M-mode scan with gated and filtered speckle contrast in red for location L1-L4

Figure 9. *Cont.*

Patient 14, OCT YZ projection of OCT M-mode scan with gated and filtered speckle contrast in red for location L1-L4

Patient 17, OCT YZ projection of OCT M-mode scan with gated and filtered speckle contrast in red for location L1-L4

Patient 19, OCT YZ projection of OCT M-mode scan with gated and filtered speckle contrast in red for location L1-L4

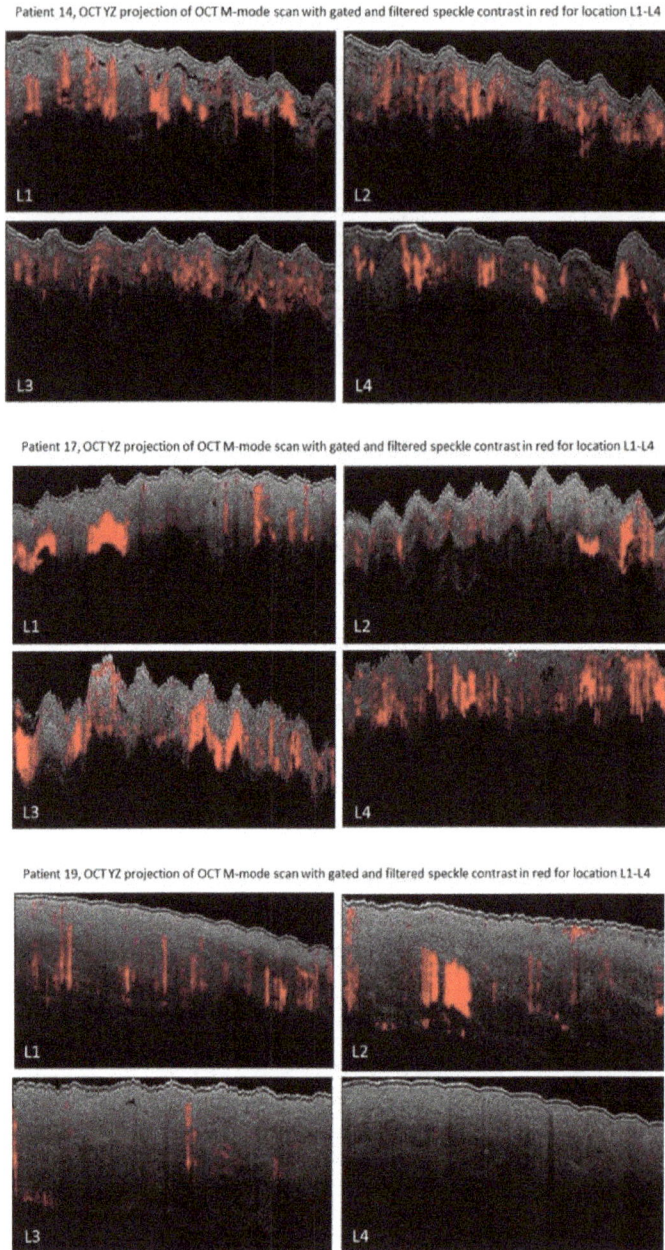

Figure 9. OCT speckle contrast indicative of flow overlaid with OCT grayscale (YZ) images from M-mode scans from location 1 (L1, 3 cm below the watershed), location 2 (L2, watershed), location 3 (L3, 3 cm above the watershed), location 4 (L4, fundus). In patient 9 high speckle contrast indicative of flow is seen in location 2 on the watershed area. In patient 14 and 19 a decreased speckle contrast indicative of flow is observed towards location 4. In patient 17 an increase in speckle contrast indicative of flow from location 1 to 4 is observed.

3.4. Histology Results

Histology of the fundus tissue was available for patients 14, 17 and 19. Figure 10 depicts the OCT M-mode scan of location 4 with speckle contrast in red and the histopathology slide also of location 4 with blood vessels in red and serosa, subserosa (purple/darkpink) and muscularis propria (light pink) tissue layers.

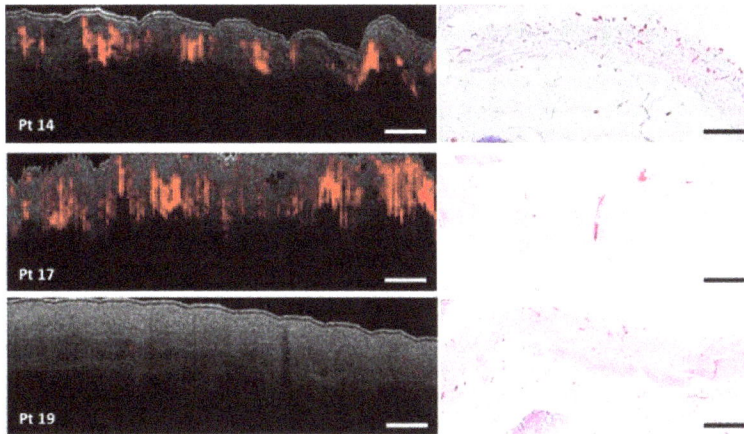

Figure 10. OCT scan of location 4 (fundus), the scale bar depicts a length of 1 mm, and histology slides HE-stained, of patient 14, 17 and 19 with blood vessels in red and tissue layers: serosa, subserosa (purple/dark pink), muscularis propria (light pink).

Although the OCT scan and the histology slide are not one to one correlated, the amount and location of the blood vessels tend to agree per patient. Histology of patient 14 demonstrates many blood vessels localized in the superficial subserosa, which is evidently visible in the OCT scan. Histology of patient 19, in contrary, shows no blood vessels, except for capillaries, which is demonstrated in the OCT scan as well.

4. Discussion

This study is the first that demonstrates OCT imaging of gastric tissue and detection of flow in vivo in patients with esophageal cancer during surgery. We show that intra-operative OCT imaging of gastric tissue and microcirculation is feasible. Moreover, regions of flow could be distinguished from static tissue by calculating speckle contrast in the M-mode scans. The percentage of pixels distinguished as flow was quantified as an objective parameter. This parameter can potentially be used to differentiate normal from decreased perfusion areas.

By comparing OCT data with HE-stained histopathology slides, it was possible to define tissue layers (serosal, subserosal, muscularis propria) and blood vessels. A network of blood vessels was observed in the subserosa. Similar blood vessels, in turn, were depicted in the OCT data exhibiting speckle contrast values between 0.42 and 0.62. Together, these findings substantiate our hypothesis that OCT speckle contrast in M-mode scans can be used to indicate regions of blood flow, while the tissue under study is moving due to the heart beat and respiration.

Lymph vessels were visible as well in the OCT images, assuming that the lymph fluid is a low-scattering medium [19]. Detection and segmentation of the lymphatic vessel, which is outside our scope in the presented work, could potentially add to the analysis of the reconstructed gastric tube OCT data. The clinical value of visualization of lymphatic vessels in the reconstructed gastric tube has yet to be studied.

A limitation of this study is the small number of patients with successful data analysis at all locations. Quality of the images was suboptimal as stabilization of the OCT probe was very difficult. Due to the intra-operative setting, a sterile operational field and hence a sterile drape over the OCT probe was required. This sterile drape introduced specular reflections, which hampered the automated image analysis. This problem could be solved by introducing a sterile probe. Mechanical stability is a general requirement for successful OCT data acquisition and particularly for the quantification of speckle-related parameters. Motion artefacts induced by the surgeon's hand as well as the patient's heartbeat and breathing diminished the quality of the OCT scans by introducing non-flow related speckle decorrelation. Next to visual information, we attempted to visualize blood vessel in the 3D OCT by calculating the speckle decorrelation in adjacent B-scans using the algorithm proposed by Gong et al. [12]. Unfortunately, due to external motion artefacts we were not able to visualize flow in these scans as the speckle in most parts of the scan (also the static tissue) was decorrelated. Previous literature showed better results of microvascular OCT imaging using fixation of the probe [20], which in this study was impossible due to the in vivo, intra-operative setting of this study. Moreover, heartbeat and breathing of the patient will be a problem in imaging intestinal organs, compared to extremities, since the organs are highly perfused and therefore connected to arteries with a large diameter. For future studies, we recommend a probe stabilizer with negative pressure, as is used in SDF imaging, to decrease motion artefacts [21]. Furthermore, optimization of the scanning protocol could increase feasibility of OCT imaging: by using a smaller scanning range, heartbeat and breathing will have less influence on the motions artefacts. Equally, a faster OCT system would decrease the influence of motion in the image and increase speckle stability.

OCT provides depth resolved images with a microscale resolution potentially allowing for visualization of the microvasculature. The visualization of blood vessels located directly underneath other blood vessels is hampered by the shadowing effect caused by multiply scattered photons in the vessels affecting both the OCT intensity and the speckle decorrelation. Red blood cells are highly forward scattering at common OCT wavelengths, which increases the probability of multiple scattering and therefore shadowing. This effect is clearly visible in Figure 7b, in which flow induces the speckle contrast of lower static parts to increase to values similarly to those of flowing blood.

The advantage of OCT over other optical modalities is the depth resolution provided in real-time. Previous research shows the potential benefit of different optical techniques in intra-operative perfusion imaging such as fluorescence imaging [4,22–26], thermography [27], laser speckle contrast imaging [28] and sidestream darkfield microscopy [8,29,30]. Fluorescence imaging creates a wide field overview of the vasculature of the tissue, enabling the surgeon to indicate the perfusion status of an organ or tissue by the intensity measurements of a fluorophore (e.g., indocyanine green, ICG). However, overlaying vessels cannot be distinguished. Therefore, microvascular tissue with impaired perfusion could look highly perfused because of the high flow in an underlying artery. Moreover, for the illumination of vessels with fluorescence imaging, a fluorophore is needed which makes this technique invasive. Thermography and laser speckle contrast imaging are both widely tested in vivo in patients. They both create an overview of the tissue perfusion in a color-coded scale, easily interpreted by clinicians. The disadvantage of thermography for intraoperative perfusion monitoring is the used parameter: temperature, is a parameter exhibiting a slow response to a change in tissue perfusion. Laser speckle contrast imaging, on the other hand, uses perfusion units to estimate the perfusion status, which is an arbitrary unit and therefore not easily interpreted as an absolute value to differentiate good from decreased perfusion. Sidestream darkfield microscopy provides tissue imaging, like OCT, on a millimeter scale. It is able to visualize single erythrocytes flowing through capillaries. However, it can only focus at one imaging depth up to 500 micrometer and surgeons need to focus the camera by hand, which is a challenge considering the motion artefacts discussed previously.

OCT could optimize surgery by improving the understanding of perfusion and intra-operative visualization of the microcirculation. Integration of the software is needed to create real-time evaluation of perfusion in tissue. The proposed speckle analysis algorithm is fast, automated and can be used unsupervised, and can be integrated in the image acquisition software to enable real-time visualization of blood flow during surgery. With this parameter, real-time intra-operative OCT data analysis will be possible. Future studies should focus on the speckle contrast percentage indicative of flow and patient outcome to study a possible correlation and define a threshold value to help the surgeon to decide whether to adjust the surgical plan or not. In the future, OCT-based quantitative perfusion imaging and -evaluation could potentially improve surgical outcome and decrease post-operative complications due to impaired perfusion.

5. Conclusions

This study shows the feasibility of intra-operative OCT-based imaging of gastric tissue and detection of flow in blood vessels in patients with esophageal cancer. Flow was detected by calculating off-line the speckle contrast in M-mode OCT images, from which the percentage of pixels indicative of flow was obtained. This objective parameter was obtained while the bulk tissue was moving and therefor it may be a useful for intra-operative perfusion evaluation. Potentially, surgeons could use a threshold value for quantitative assessment of the perfusion state of tissue and with that improve patient outcome.

Author Contributions: S.M.J., D.M.d.B., T.G.v.L., M.I.v.B.H., S.D.S. and S.S.G. conceived and designed the experiments; S.M.J., M.I.v.B.B., S.S.G. and P.R.B. performed the experiments; S.M.J. and M.A. analyzed the data; L.S.W. and S.L.M. contributed reagents/materials/analysis tools; S.M.J and M.A. wrote the paper with revisions of D.M.d.B., T.G.v.L., M.I.v.B.B., S.D.S., S.L.M. and S.S.G.

Acknowledgments: The authors would like to thank ZonMw for their financial support and Institute Quantivision for their support in trial conception, and I. Kos for her contribution in technical drawings.

Conflicts of Interest: The authors declare no conflict of interest.

References

1. Futier, E.; Robin, E.; Jabaudon, M.; Guerin, R.; Petit, A.; Bazin, J.-E.; Constantin, J.-M.; Vallet, B. Central venous O_2 saturation and venous-to-arterial CO_2 difference as complementary tools for goal-directed therapy during high-risk surgery. *Crit. Care* **2010**, *14*, R193. [CrossRef] [PubMed]
2. Biere, S.S.; van Berge Henegouwen, M.I.; Maas, K.W.; Bonavina, L.; Rosman, C.; Garcia, J.R.; Gisbertz, S.S.; Klinkenbijl, J.H.; Hollmann, M.W.; de Lange, E.S.; et al. Minimally invasive versus open oesophagectomy for patients with oesophageal cancer: A multicentre, open-label, randomised controlled trial. *Lancet* **2012**, *379*, 1887–1892. [CrossRef]
3. Miyazaki, T.; Kuwano, H.; Kato, H.; Yoshikawa, M.; Ojima, H.; Tsukada, K. Predictive value of blood flow in the gastric tube in anastomotic insufficiency after thoracic esophagectomy. *World J. Surg.* **2002**, *26*, 1319–1323. [CrossRef] [PubMed]
4. Zehetner, J.; DeMeester, S.R.; Alicuben, E.T.; Oh, D.S.; Lipham, J.C.; Hagen, J.A.; DeMeester, T.R. Intraoperative Assessment of Perfusion of the Gastric Graft and Correlation With Anastomotic Leaks After Esophagectomy. *Ann. Surg.* **2015**, *262*, 74–78. [CrossRef] [PubMed]
5. Veelo, D.P.; Gisbertz, S.S.; Hannivoort, R.A.; Van Dieren, S.; Geerts, B.F.; Henegouwen, M.I.V.B.; Hollmann, M.W. The effect of on-demand vs deep neuromuscular relaxation on rating of surgical and anaesthesiologic conditions in patients undergoing thoracolaparoscopic esophagectomy (DEPTH trial): Study protocol for a randomized controlled trial. *Trials* **2015**, *331*. [CrossRef] [PubMed]
6. Jansen, S.M.; de Bruin, D.M.; van Berge Henegouwen, M.I.; Strackee, S.D.; Veelo, D.P.; Van Leeuwen, T.G.; Gisbertz, S.S. Optical Techniques for Perfusion Monitoring of the Gastric Tube after Esophagectomy: A review of technologies & thresholds. *Dis. Esophagus* **2018**, in press.
7. Huang, D.; Huang, D.; Swanson, E.A.; Lin, C.P.; Schuman, J.S.; Stinson, W.G.; Chang, W.; Hee, M.R.; Flotire, T.; Gregory, K.; et al. Optical Coherence Tomography. *Science* **1991**, *254*, 1178–1181. [CrossRef] [PubMed]
8. Jansen, S.M.; de Bruin, D.M.; Faber, D.J.; Dobbe, I.J.G.G.; Heeg, E.; Milstein, D.M.J.; Strackee, S.D.; van Leeuwen, T.G. Applicability of quantitative optical imaging techniques for intraoperative perfusion diagnostics: A comparison of laser speckle contrast imaging, sidestream dark-field microscopy, and optical coherence tomography. *J. Biomed. Opt.* **2017**, *22*, 1–9. [CrossRef] [PubMed]

9.   Alander, J.T.; Kaartinen, I.; Laakso, A.; Pätilä, T.; Spillmann, T.; Tuchin, V.V.; Venermo, M.; Välisuo, P. A Review of indocyanine green fluorescent imaging in surgery. *Int. J. Biomed. Imaging* **2012**, *2012*. [CrossRef] [PubMed]

10. Senarathna, J.; Member, S.; Rege, A.; Li, N.; Thakor, N.V. Laser Speckle Contrast Imaging: Theory, Instrumentation and Applications. *IEEE Rev. Biomed. Eng.* **2013**, *6*, 99–110. [CrossRef] [PubMed]

11. Rajan, V.; Varghese, B.; Van Leeuwen, T.G.; Steenbergen, W. Review of methodological developments in laser Doppler flowmetry. *Lasers Med. Sci.* **2009**, *24*, 269–283. [CrossRef] [PubMed]

12. Gong, P.; Es'haghian, S.; Harms, K.A.; Murray, A.; Rea, S.; Kennedy, B.F.; Wood, F.M.; Sampson, D.D.; Mclaughlin, R.A. Optical coherence tomography for longitudinal monitoring of vasculature in scars treated with laser fractionation. *J. Biophotonics* **2016**, *9*, 626–636. [CrossRef] [PubMed]

13. Mariampillai, A.; Leung, M.K.K.; Jarvi, M.; Standish, B.A.; Lee, K.; Wilson, B.C.; Vitkin, A.; Yang, V.X.D. Optimized speckle variance OCT imaging of microvasculature. *Opt. Lett.* **2010**, *35*, 1257–1259. [CrossRef] [PubMed]

14. Weiss, N.; Van Leeuwen, T.G.; Kalkman, J. Localized measurement of longitudinal and transverse flow velocities in colloidal suspensions using optical coherence tomography. *Phys. Rev. E Stat. Nonlinear Soft Matter Phys.* **2013**, *88*, 1–7. [CrossRef] [PubMed]

15. Liu, X.; Zhang, K.; Huang, Y.; Kang, J.U. Spectroscopic-speckle variance OCT for microvasculature detection and analysis. *Biomed. Opt. Express* **2011**, *2*, 2995–3009. [CrossRef] [PubMed]

16. Jansen, S.M.; de Bruin, D.M.; van Berge Henegouwen, M.I.; Strackee, S.D.; Veelo, D.P.; van Leeuwen, T.G.; Gisbertz, S.S. Can we predict necrosis intra-operatively? Real-time optical quantitative perfusion imaging in surgery: Study protocol for a prospective, observational, in vivo pilot study. *Pilot Feasibil. Stud.* **2017**, *3*, 65. [CrossRef] [PubMed]

17. Almasian, M.; van Leeuwen, T.G.; Faber, D.J. OCT Amplitude and Speckle Statistics of Discrete Random Media. *Sci. Rep.* **2017**, *7*, 14873. [CrossRef] [PubMed]

18. Mahmud, M.S.; Cadotte, D.W.; Vuong, B.; Sun, C.; Luk, T.W.H.; Mariampillai, A.; Yang, V.X.D. Review of speckle and phase variance optical coherence tomography to visualize microvascular networks. *J. Biomed. Opt.* **2013**, *18*, 50901. [CrossRef] [PubMed]

19. Gong, P.; Es'haghian, S.; Harms, K.-A.; Murray, A.; Rea, S.; Wood, F.M.; Sampson, D.D.; McLaughlin, R.A. In vivo label-free lymphangiography of cutaneous lymphatic vessels in human burn scars using optical coherence tomography. *Biomed. Opt. Express* **2016**, *7*, 4886. [CrossRef] [PubMed]

20. Liew, Y.M.; McLaughlin, R.A.; Gong, P.; Wood, F.M.; Sampson, D.D. In vivo assessment of human burn scars through automated quantification of vascularity using optical coherence tomography. *J. Biomed. Opt.* **2013**, *18*, 61213. [CrossRef] [PubMed]

21. Balestra, G.M.; Bezemer, R.; Boerma, E.C.; Yong, Z.-Y.; Sjauw, K.D.; Engstrom, A.E.; Koopmans, M.; Ince, C. Improvement of sidestream dark field imaging with an image acquisition stabilizer. *BMC Med. Imaging* **2010**, *10*, 15. [CrossRef] [PubMed]

22. Rino, Y.; Yukawa, N.; Sato, T.; Yamamoto, N.; Tamagawa, H.; Hasegawa, S.; Oshima, T.; Yoshikawa, T.; Masuda, M.; Imada, T. Visualization of blood supply route to the reconstructed stomach by indocyanine green fluorescence imaging during esophagectomy. *BMC Med. Imaging* **2014**, *14*, 14–18. [CrossRef] [PubMed]

23. Shimada, Y.; Okumura, T.; Nagata, T.; Sawada, S.; Matsui, K.; Hori, R.; Yoshioka, I.; Yoshida, T.; Osada, R.; Tsukada, K. Usefulness of blood supply visualization by indocyanine green fluorescence for reconstruction during esophagectomy. *Esophagus* **2011**, *8*, 259–266. [CrossRef] [PubMed]

24. Kubota, K.; Yoshida, M.; Kuroda, J.; Okada, A.; Ohta, K.; Kitajima, M. Application of the HyperEye Medical System for esophageal cancer surgery: A preliminary report. *Surg. Today* **2013**, *43*, 215–220. [CrossRef] [PubMed]

25. Kumagai, Y.; Ishiguro, T.; Sobajima, J.; Fukuchi, M.; Ishibashi, K.; Baba, H.; Mochiki, E.; Kawano, T.; Ishida, H. Indocyanine green fluorescence method for reconstructed gastric tube during esophagectomy. *Dis. Esophagus* **2014**, *27*, 106A. [CrossRef]

26. Yukaya, T.; Saeki, H.; Kasagi, Y.; Nakashima, Y.; Ando, K.; Imamura, Y.; Ohgaki, K.; Oki, E.; Morita, M.; Maehara, Y. Indocyanine Green Fluorescence Angiography for Quantitative Evaluation of Gastric Tube Perfusion in Patients Undergoing Esophagectomy. *J. Am. Coll. Surg.* **2015**, *221*, e37–e42. [CrossRef] [PubMed]

Sensors **2018**, *18*, 1331

27. Pauling, J.D.; Shipley, J.A.; Raper, S.; Watson, M.L.; Ward, S.G.; Harris, N.D.; McHugh, N.J. Comparison of infrared thermography and laser speckle contrast imaging for the dynamic assessment of digital microvascular function. *Microvasc. Res.* **2012**, *83*, 162–167. [CrossRef] [PubMed]

28. Milstein, D.M.J.; Ince, C.; Gisbertz, S.S.; Boateng, K.B.; Geerts, B.F.; Hollmann, M.W.; Van Berge Henegouwen, M.I.; Veelo, D.P. Laser speckle contrast imaging identifies ischemic areas on gastric tube reconstructions following esophagectomy. *Medicine* **2016**, *95*. [CrossRef] [PubMed]

29. De Backer, D.; Hollenberg, S.; Boerma, C.; Goedhart, P.; Büchele, G.; Ospina-Tascon, G.; Dobbe, I.; Ince, C. How to evaluate the microcirculation: Report of a round table conference. *Crit. Care* **2007**, *11*, R101. [CrossRef] [PubMed]

30. De Bruin, A.F.J.; Kornmann, V.N.N.; van der Sloot, K.; van Vugt, J.L.; Gosselink, M.P.; Smits, A.; Van Ramshorst, B.; Boerma, E.C.; Noordzij, P.G.; Boerma, D.; et al. Sidestream dark field imaging of the serosal microcirculation during gastrointestinal surgery. *Color. Dis.* **2016**, *18*, O103–O110. [CrossRef] [PubMed]

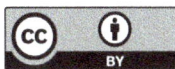

Article

Neuron Stimulation Device Integrated with Silicon Nanowire-Based Photodetection Circuit on a Flexible Substrate

Suk Won Jung [1,2], Jong Yoon Shin [1], Kilwha Pi [1], Yong Sook Goo [3] and Dong-il "Dan" Cho [1,*]

[1] ISRC/ASRI, Department of Electrical and Computer Engineering, Seoul National University, 1 Gwanak-ro, Gwanak-gu, Seoul 08826, Korea; jungsw@keti.re.kr (S.W.J.); jshin33@snu.ac.kr (J.Y.S.); khpi1@snu.ac.kr (K.P.)

[2] Human Care System Research Center, Convergence System R&D Division, Korea Electronics Technology Institute, 25 Saenari-ro, Bundang-gu, Seongnam-si, Gyeonggi-do 13509, Korea

[3] Department of Physiology, College of Medicine, Chungbuk National University, 1 Chungdae-ro, Seowon-gu, Cheongju, Chungbuk 28644, Korea; ysgoo@chungbuk.ac.kr

* Correspondence: dicho@snu.ac.kr; Tel.: +82-2-880-6488

Academic Editors: Dragan Indjin, Željka Cvejić and Małgorzata Jędrzejewska-Szczerska
Received: 7 September 2016; Accepted: 25 November 2016; Published: 1 December 2016

Abstract: This paper proposes a neural stimulation device integrated with a silicon nanowire (SiNW)-based photodetection circuit for the activation of neurons with light. The proposed device is comprised of a voltage divider and a current driver in which SiNWs are used as photodetector and field-effect transistors; it has the functions of detecting light, generating a stimulation signal in proportion to the light intensity, and transmitting the signal to a micro electrode. To show the applicability of the proposed neural stimulation device as a high-resolution retinal prosthesis system, a high-density neural stimulation device with a unit cell size of 110×110 μm and a resolution of 32×32 was fabricated on a flexible film with a thickness of approximately 50 μm. Its effectiveness as a retinal stimulation device was then evaluated using a unit cell in an in vitro animal experiment involving the retinal tissue of retinal Degeneration 1 (*rd1*) mice. Experiments wherein stimulation pulses were applied to the retinal tissues successfully demonstrate that the number of spikes in neural response signals increases in proportion to light intensity.

Keywords: neuron stimulation; silicon nanowire; photodetector; micro electrode; retinal prosthesis

1. Introduction

Impaired connectivity or functional disorders in the neural system hinder the activation of cells or the proper transmission of information. Neural stimulation methods have been extensively investigated as potential cures for a wide range of neurological disorders, such as mental disorders, dementia, motor disabilities, and visual impairment owing to retinal degeneration [1–4]. In such investigations, electrical stimulation using extracellular electrodes is extensively used as the method for activating neurons [5–7]. In conjunction with the use of extracellular electrodes, methods for the activation of neurons using light are also being studied. In these methods, light-sensitive devices are used for generating electrical stimulation signals [8–10]. For instance, in a retinal prosthetic system, image data are acquired from external cameras connected to intraocular micro electrodes through wires [11–14] or from internal photodetectors integrated with intraocular micro electrodes [15–18]. The modulated electrical signals are then transmitted to a micro electrode array (MEA) mounted into retinal cells.

In retinal prostheses, a high-resolution system is required to provide high-quality image perception ability to a visually handicapped patient. A key to successfully developing high-resolution systems is that the stimulation signals generated from image information are individually transmitted to a large number of stimulating electrodes [19]. In the case of retinal prosthesis systems that use external cameras, such an electrical interface becomes very complicated and difficult to implement because a camera and MEA are physically distinct and separate from each other. In fact, many commercialized retinal prostheses that use an external camera, such as the Argus II system [14] from Second Sight Medical Products Inc. (Sylmar, CA, USA) or EpiRet3 [13] of EpiRet GmbH, have a low resolution; these systems have only 60 and 25 stimulating electrodes integrated into the implant device, respectively. On the other hand, in the case of retinal prostheses with embedded photodetectors for image perception within their retinal implant devices instead of using externally worn cameras, the photodetector, the signal processing circuit, and stimulating electrodes are collocated at each cell of retinal implant devices. Much research on this topic is also underway. The US Optobionics Corporation manufactured a subretinal implant device called an 'artificial silicon retina' (ASR) [18] and conducted clinical experiments. The ASR device comprises 5000 cells, where micro photodiodes and stimulating electrodes are integrated on a silicon substrate of approximately 25 μm in thickness. The German Retina Implant AG developed a subretinal implant device using a silicon chip, in which 1500 cells with TiN electrodes are integrated with photodiodes and amplifying circuits fabricated by a CMOS process [15]. It was also reported that, by using the above subretinal implants, patients could recognize things or letters. Furthermore, it has been found from the existing research cases that photodetectors embedded in a device can easily solve the problem of signal line connection to high-density stimulating electrodes, and thus this method is advantageous for the implementation of a high-resolution retinal prosthesis system for a high-level image perception function. Despite the recent results of various studies on the development of a high-resolution retinal prosthesis system, there still remain problems that should be solved to implement a safer and more reliable retinal prosthesis system, such as low flexibility in a retinal stimulator device, the possibility of cell necrosis due to the overheating of a retinal stimulator chip [20], and low biocompatibility of the device material [21].

As a method for light-based activation of neurons that can be applied to high-resolution retinal prosthesis systems by solving the above-described problems, this paper proposes a novel neural stimulation method as well as a flexible neural stimulation device integrated with a silicon nanowire (SiNW)-based photodetection circuit. The SiNW-based photodetection circuit comprises a voltage divider and a current driver that uses a SiNW PD [22], SiNW FETs [19], and micro electrodes. The SiNW FET and the SiNW PD are connected in series via the voltage divider, making a large resistance variation in the SiNW PD desirable because the output voltage changes when the resistance varies when light detection occurs. In the fabricated SiNW PD, the resistance is approximately 5.6 GΩ in a dark environment and approximately 2.9 MΩ at 4040 lux, corresponding to a resistance ratio of approximately 1930, which is sufficiently large and useful over a high dynamic range. Thus, the output voltage of the voltage divider at the supply voltage is 5 V and the illuminance range is 0–10,000 lux, corresponding to a very large swing range of 0.1 V (dark)–4.8 V (10,000 lux). In the current driver, where the SiNW FET and micro electrodes are connected in series, the SiNW FET is driven by the output voltage of the voltage divider and the maximum on-current at the 5 V supply voltage was found to be approximately 480 μA with an on–off ratio of 5×10^4. Thus, the current driver has a sufficient on-current level and on–off characteristics to stimulate neurons via micro electrodes. Based on this preliminary analysis, the proposed process—stimulation signal modulation proportional to light intensity using a neuron stimulation device with a voltage divider and the current driver—could then be validated.

To demonstrate the applicability of the proposed neural stimulation method in high-resolution retinal prosthesis systems, a high-density neural stimulation device with a unit cell size of 110×110 μm and a resolution of 32×32 was fabricated on a flexible film approximately 50 μm thick. Its effectiveness as a light-based retinal stimulation device was evaluated by testing the unit cell in an in vitro animal experiment using the retinal tissue of *rd1* mice. Application of retinal stimulation pulses to the retinal tissue demonstrated that the number of spikes in neural response signals increase in proportion to light intensity.

2. Experimental

2.1. Device Design and Configuration

This paper proposes a neural stimulation device and a method to evoke neural signals through the use of light. Figure 1a shows a block diagram of the unit cell of the proposed neural stimulation device and the process of neural stimulation resulting from the modulation of a stimulation signal according to the intensity of light irradiated onto the neural stimulation device. Figure 1b shows the configuration of the unit cell. The neural stimulation device comprises a SiNW PD, SiNW FETs, and micro electrodes (a stimulation electrode and a ground electrode). The resistance of the SiNW PD decreases as the light illumination intensity increases and the device can be classified as a sort of variable resistor. Thus, the neural stimulation device in Figure 1b can be expressed as the equivalent circuit in Figure 1c, which can functionally be divided into two parts: the voltage divider circuit on the left, and the current driver circuit on the right.

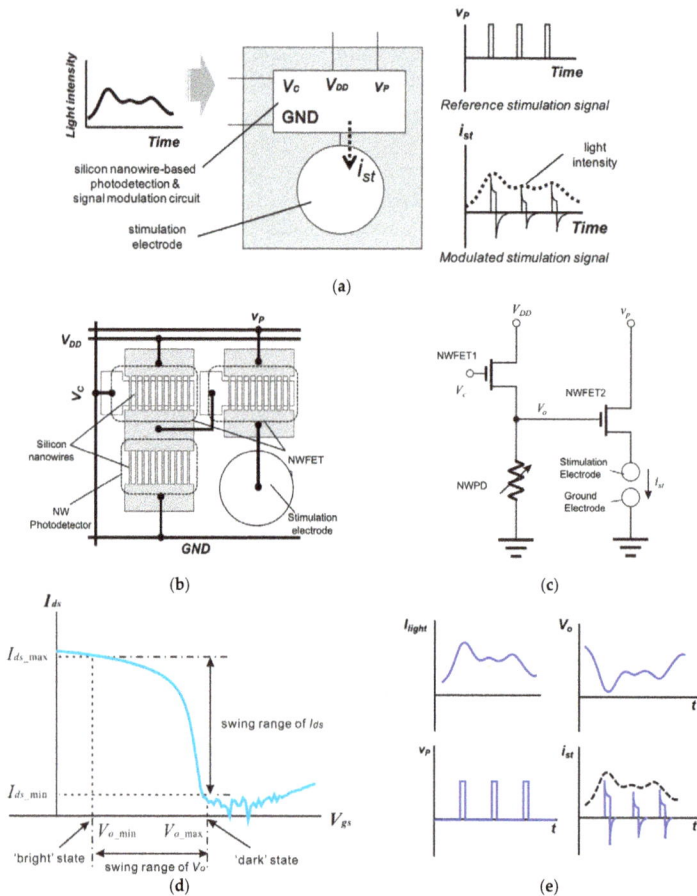

Figure 1. *Cont.*

(f)

Epiretinal implant   Subretinal implant

(g)

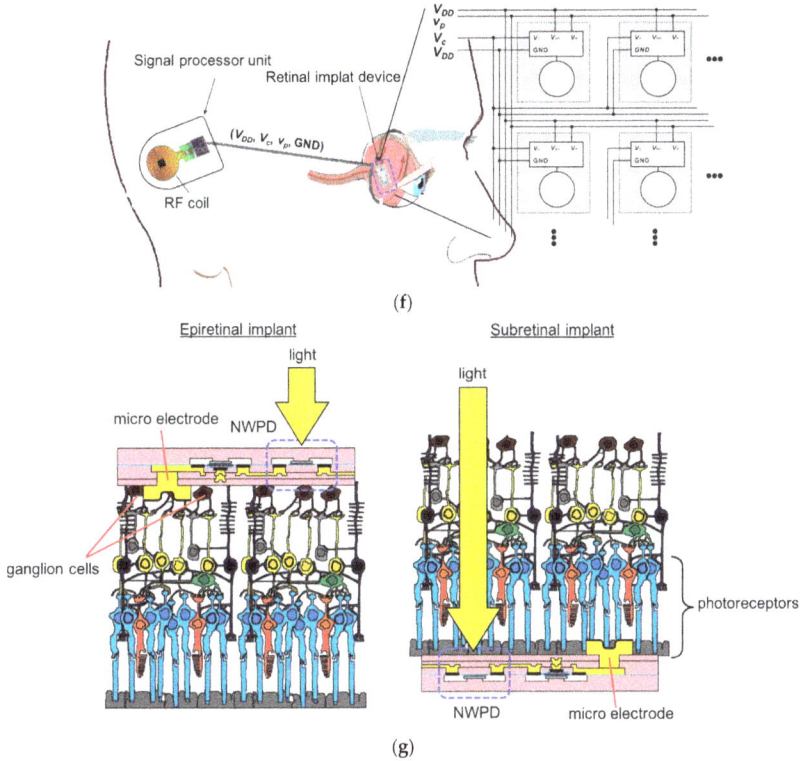

Figure 1. (**a**) Configuration and a block diagram of unit cell of the proposed neuron stimulation device and a modulation procedure of stimulation signal by light detection; (**b**) Configuration of device composed of SiNW FETs, a SiNW PD, and micro electrodes; (**c**) Equivalent circuit of the device; (**d**) V_{gs}-I_{ds} curve of the SiNW FET2 (NWFET2) and the relation between the V_o's swing range and the current swing range of the NWFET2; (**e**) Waveforms of the signals I_{light}, V_o, v_p and i_{st}; (**f**) Configuration of proposed device for a high resolution retinal prosthetic system and internal electrical connection diagram of the retinal prosthetic device; (**g**) Epiretinal and subretinal implantation of the proposed neural stimulation device in an eye ball.

In the voltage divider circuit on the left, the resistance of SiNW FET1 (NWFET1) is controlled by the control voltage (V_c), and the resistance of SiNW PD (NWPD) varies with light illumination intensity. Therefore, the output voltage (V_o) of the voltage divider can be expressed by the following equation:

$$V_o = \frac{R_{NWPD}}{R_{NWFET1} + R_{NWPD}} \cdot V_{DD}, \tag{1}$$

where V_{DD} is the supply voltage, R_{NWFET1} is the resistance of NWFET1, and R_{NWPD} is the resistance of NWPD. In the 'dark' condition with no light illumination, V_o becomes maximum because R_{NWPD} becomes maximum. As the intensity of light irradiated onto NWPD increases, both R_{NWPD} and V_o gradually decrease. If the intensity of light irradiated onto the neural stimulation device varies over time, V_o will have a waveform with a shape inverse to the waveform of light intensity, as shown in Figure 1e.

In the current driver circuit on the right side of the equivalent circuit, NWFET2 is driven by V_o. If NWFET2 has the gate-source voltage to drain-source current (V_{gs}-I_{ds}) characteristics shown in Figure 1d, I_{ds} becomes minimum ($I_{ds} = I_{ds\_min}$) when V_o is maximum ($V_o = V_{o\_max}$, at the dark state), and I_{ds} becomes maximum ($I_{ds} = I_{ds\_max}$) when V_o is minimum ($V_o = V_{o\_min}$, when light intensity is the greatest). Figure 1e illustrates one example of the waveform of v_p. The reference stimulation signal of a unipolar pulse signal with fixed amplitude and frequency is applied to the drain of NWFET2. If NWFET2 is driven by V_o with the wave waveform shown in Figure 1e, the pattern of the stimulation signal that is transmitted to the micro electrodes and neurons has the shape i_{st}, as shown in Figure 1e. It is seen that each pulse of the reference stimulation signal is modulated to have an amplitude proportional to light intensity; in this way, the proposed neural stimulation detects light intensity and can perform stimulation signal modulation in proportion to light intensity.

The proposed neural stimulation device can most effectively be used in retinal prosthetic systems. To do so, it is necessary to fabricate a retinal implant unit integrated with high-density cells. Figure 1f shows a method for high-density integration of the proposed neural stimulation device for application to a high-resolution retinal prosthetic system. The block diagram shows the arrangement of the device's cells in a 2D matrix pattern and the method for the connection of signal lines for each cell. As each unit cell can modulate stimulation signals through the independent detection of light intensity, it is only necessary to connect the four signal lines V_{DD}, v_p, V_c, and a ground (GND) electrode. The retinal implant unit integrated with these high-density neural stimulation cells is connected to a separately fabricated signal processor. The retinal implant unit is easily implantable into the eyeball as it is fabricated in a flexible form that can be bent to fit the curvature of the eye; the signal processor unit, on the other hand, is implanted remotely. An RF coil for communication with external devices and a wireless electric power supply and a signal processing chip for controlling the implant device are embedded into the processor unit. An electrostatic discharge (ESD) protection circuit is required for a practical implementation and it can be integrated in the signal processing chip. The proposed retinal implant unit can be applied to both epiretinal and subretinal implant methods as shown in Figure 1g. In epiretinal implants, the micro electrodes are in contact with ganglion cells and the light is incident on the opposite side where the micro electrodes are formed and reaches the NWPDs. In subretinal implants, the micro electrodes are in contact with photoreceptors and the light is incident on the same side where the micro electrodes are formed and reaches the NWPDs.

2.2. Fabrication and Results

Figure 2 shows the process for fabricating the proposed neural stimulation device into a flexible form and the process for fabrication of the current driver component, in which the silicon nanowire FET and micro electrodes are connected in series. In the first step, silicon nanowires are formed using the top-down method (Figure 2a–e) [23]. Subsequently, polysilicon gates and source and drain electrodes are fabricated (Figure 2f–j). The electric signal lines (V_{DD}, v_p, V_c and GND) are then formed via a multi-layer metallization process (Figure 2k,l). A 5 µm-thick polyimide layer is patterned and Au micro electrodes are then formed via an Au electroplating process (Figure 2m). For biocompatibility, a Pt-black layer can be formed on the surface of the Au electrodes by a successive Pt electroplating process after the Au electroplating process [24]. Theoretically, TiN micro electrodes can be fabricated by TiN sputtering and RIE (Reactive Ion Etching) processes instead of electroplating. In this paper, Pt-black micro electrodes are fabricated and are used for the following in vitro experiments. After the micro electrodes are fabricated, the device wafer is bonded with a dummy wafer using a bonding wax, BGL-7160 (AI Technology Inc., Princeton, NJ, USA), and the device wafer is thinned to approximately 30 µm via a chemical-mechanical planarization (CMP) process (Figure 2n,o). Photoresist (PR) patterning is performed and the silicon is etched by using a deep reactive ion etch (DRIE) process (Figure 2p). The bonding wax is melted by heating the substrate to 160 °C, and the fabrication of the flexible neural stimulation device is completed by separating the neural stimulation device from the dummy substrate (Figure 2q–s).

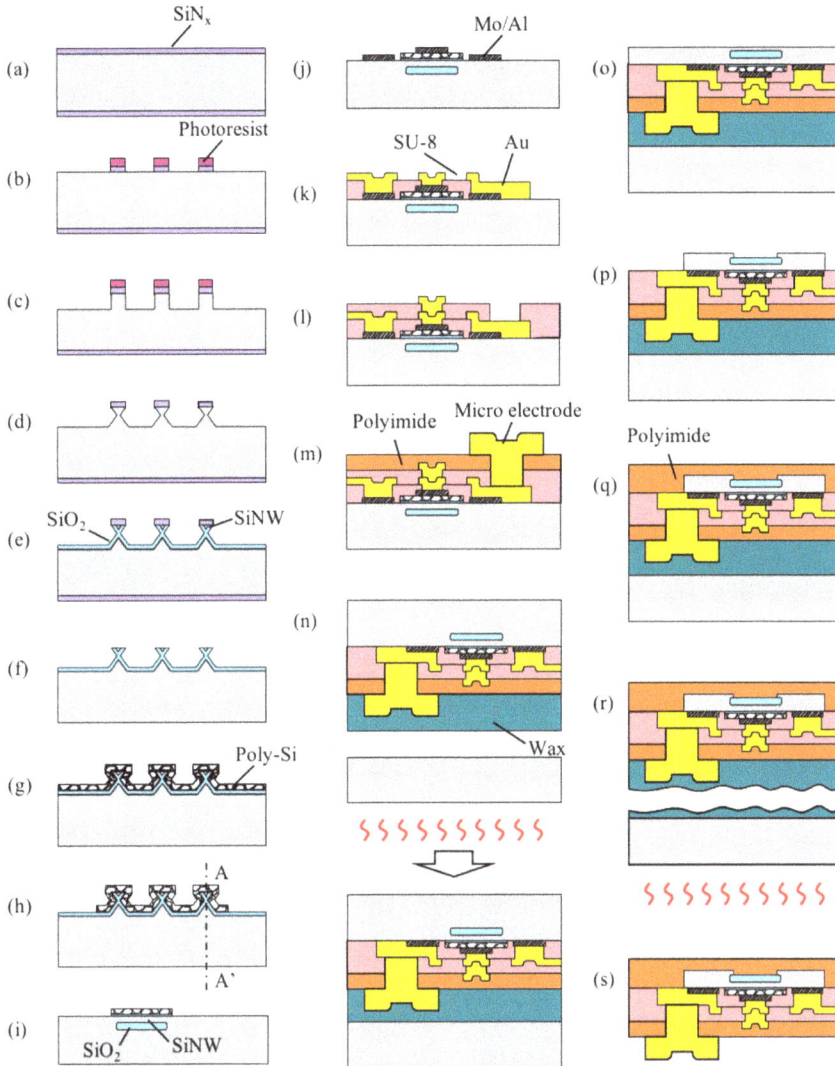

Figure 2. Fabrication process of the proposed high resolution neural stimulation devices integrated with SiNW-based photodetection circuit. (**a**) SiN deposition by low pressure chemical vapor deposition (LPCVD); (**b**) SiN dry etch; (**c**) Si dry etch; (**d**) Si wet etch using tetra-methyl-ammonium-hydroxide (TMAH) solution; (**e**) SiNW formation by wet oxidation process; (**f**) SiN strip by the use of H_3PO_4 solution; (**g**) Gate oxide and Poly-Si formation; (**h**) Poly-Si dry etch; (**i**) Cross-sectional view of A-A' of Figure 2h; (**j**) Source, drain, gate electrodes formation; (**k**) First dielectric layer (SU-8) and electrical lines (V_{DD}, GND) formation; (**l**) Second dielectric layer and electrical lines (V_c, v_p) formation; (**m**) Third dielectric layer (polyimide) and micro electrodes formation; (**n**) Device wafer bonding on a dummy wafer; (**o**) Device wafer thinning by chemical-mechanical polishing (CMP); (**p**) Si dry etch; (**q**) Cover polyimide coating; (**r**) Separating fabricated devices from the dummy wafer; (**s**) Device cleaning by residual wax removal.

Figure 3a shows the shape of the column structure after the dry etching of silicon in Figure 2c: scallops formed on the sidewall of the structure are seen, as the Si DRIE process is used. As seen in Figure 3b, following wet etching using tetra-methyl-ammonium-hydroxide (TMAH) solution, the scallops disappear as the sidewall of the column structure is etched. Figure 3c shows the triangular shape of a silicon nanowire formed following the wet oxidation process. It is seen that the top of the silicon nanowire has formed with a width of approximately 450 nm. Figure 4 shows the 32 × 32 neural stimulation device fabricated using the process in Figure 2. Figure 4a–c show the device after the Si DRIE process in Figure 2p has been completed. The size of the unit cell is 110 × 110 μm and it used 10 SiNWs with a length of 20 μm each to compose NWFET1, NWFEET2, and NWPD. A center microelectrode 30 μm in diameter with a surrounding ground electrode is also present. Figure 4d shows the neural stimulation device separated from the substrate after the process has been completed. The device is approximately 50 μm thick and it is very flexible.

The characteristics of NWPD and NWFET depend on the thickness and doping concentration of the silicon nanowires. In this paper, the thickness of silicon nanowires is controlled by a photolithography process, RIE processes, a Si TMAH wet etching process, and an oxidation process. In the case of TMAH silicon wet etching process, even though there is a slight difference in the wet etching time, an etch stop condition is formed by the hourglass silicon structure so that the deviation of the top width of the silicon structure is insignificant. In the remaining processes, the process deviations are controlled to within approximately 5%, and therefore, the effects on the thickness of the nanowire are not significant. The doping concentration of the silicon nanowires can also be precisely controlled by an ion implantation process. Therefore, the influences of the process variation on the characteristics of NWPD and NWFET are not significant.

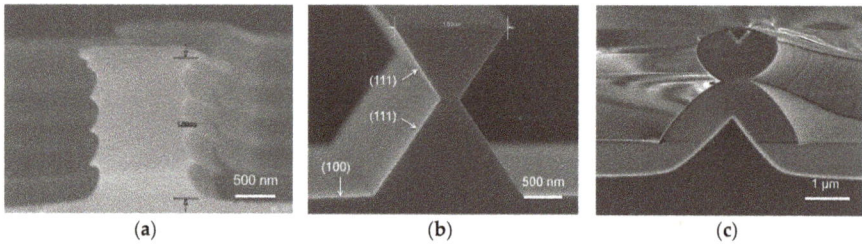

Figure 3. Fabricated SiNWs. (**a**) Formation of column structures by Si deep RIE process; (**b**) Formation of hourglass shaped structures by Si anisotropic wet etch process; (**c**) SiNW formation by wet oxidation process.

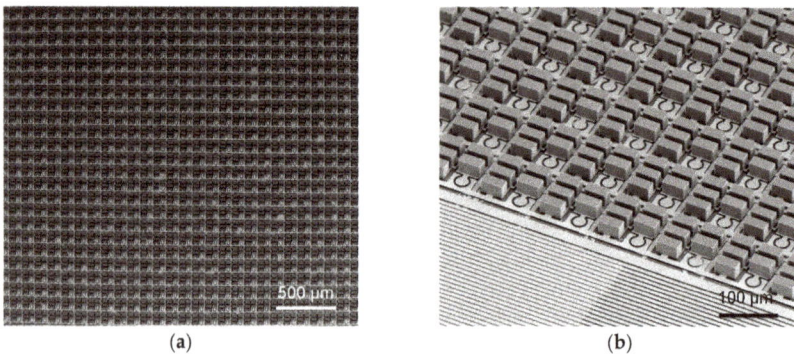

Figure 4. *Cont.*

(c)

(d)

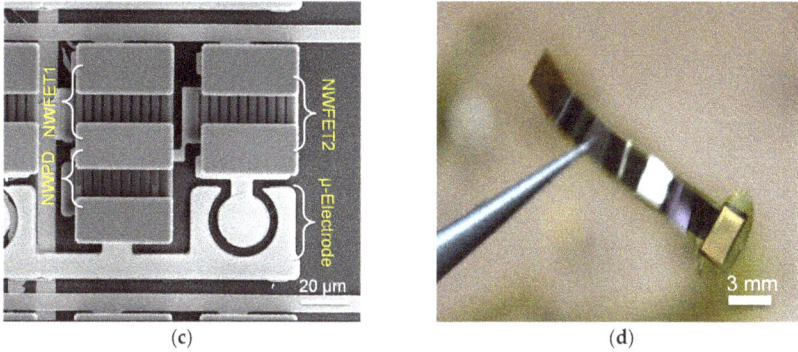

Figure 4. Fabricated high-resolution neural stimulation device. (**a**) Top view of the fabricated device after Si deep RIE process of Figure 2p; (**b**) Perspective view of Figure 4a; (**c**) Unit cell of the device; (**d**) Flexible neural stimulation device with 32 × 32 resolution.

3. Results and Discussions

3.1. Device Characterization

SiNW PDs and SiNW FETs, the basic devices composing the neural stimulation device, were fabricated using the process shown in Figure 2, following which the characteristics of each device were examined. To investigate the resistance variation of an SiNW PD as a function of light intensity, the photo-induced output ($I_{ds} \sim V_{ds}$) characteristics of the SiNW PD were measured at varying halogen lamp-produced light intensities (I_{light}), as shown in Figure 5a. Figure 5b shows the results of calculating the photocurrent (I_{ph}) and resistance (R_{NWPD}) of the SiNW PD against light intensity for $V_{ds} = 1$ V using the *I–V* graph in Figure 5a. The graph shows that both I_{ph} and R_{NWPD} abruptly change within an illuminance range of low light intensity, above which the change is more gradual. R_{NWPD} shows a high value of approximately 5.6 GΩ in a dark environment and approximately 2.9 MΩ in a bright environment of 4040 lux. Thus, the resistance change rate is so great that the ratio between the two resistance values, $R_{NWPD(dark)} / R_{NWPD(bright)}$, goes as high as 1930. In particular, it is apparent from the graph that the SiNW PD shows high sensitivity in a low illuminance range.

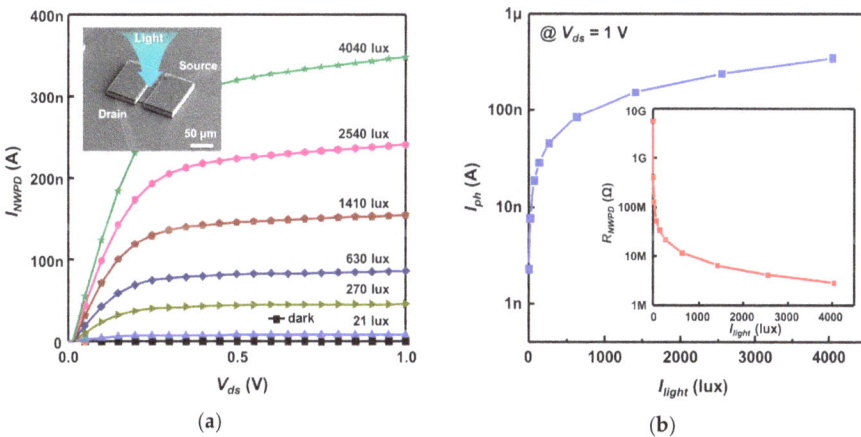

(a)

(b)

Figure 5. *Cont.*

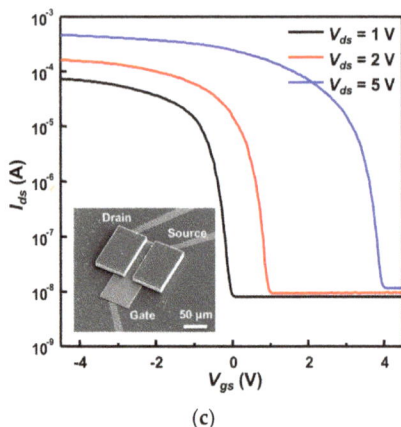

(c)

Figure 5. (a) *I-V* curves of the fabricated SiNW PD against varying light illumination intensity; (b) Photocurrent and resistance values of the SiNW PD against light intensity; (c) V_{gs}-I_{ds} curves of the SiNW FET for several bias voltages.

The relative resistance of the SiNW FET used in the voltage divider circuit to that of the SiNW PD is important. The resistance of the SiNW FET (R_{NWFET}) is controlled by the gate-source voltage (V_{gs}), and the value that it can obtain is shown in Figure 5c, which shows the transfer ($I_{ds} \sim V_{gs}$) characteristics of a fabricated SiNW FET. If the conditions of $R_{NWPD(dark)} \gg R_{NWFET}$ in a dark environment and $R_{NWPD(bright)} \ll R_{NWFET}$ in a bright environment are satisfied, the voltage range V_o of the voltage divider is found according to Equation (1) to be V_{DD} (dark)–0 V (bright), resulting in the maximum swing range. For this, V_{gs} must be set so that $R_{NWPD(dark)} \gg R_{NWFET} \gg R_{NWPD(bright)}$. On the other hand, the threshold voltage (V_{th}), maximum on-current (I_{ON_max}), and on–off ratio are important parameters for the SiNW FET used in the current driver circuit. In Figure 5c, the threshold voltage moves from approximately 0 V (when V_{ds} is 1 V) to 4 V (when V_{ds} is 5 V). I_{ON_max} is approximately 480 µA when V_{ds} is 5 V, and the on–off ratio of SiNW FET is approximately 5×10^4 when V_{ds} is 5 V. Thus, it is found that the SiNW FET has sufficient on-current level and on–off characteristics for use as the current driver circuit.

Figure 6 shows the results of an experiment evaluating the characteristics of both the voltage divider and current driver (which together form the proposed neural stimulation device) and verifying the previously discussed process of stimulation signal modulation. Figure 6a shows the fabricated neural stimulation device. Figure 6b shows the measurement results obtained from the voltage divider, in which V_o was measured against V_c by varying the intensity of light irradiated onto the SiNW PD. In Figure 6b, it is seen that if $V_c < 3.4$ V (Region I in Figure 6b), V_o remains at close to $V_{DD} = 5$ V despite the variations in R_{NWPD} induced by variations in light intensity. This occurs because the value of V_c that determines that R_{NWFET1} always remains much smaller than R_{NWFET1} even though R_{NWPD} is lowered under a bright environment: that is, $R_{NWFET1} \ll R_{NWPD}$. Under this condition, Equation (1) gives $V_o \approx V_{DD}$ regardless of the light intensity. By contrast, if $V_c > 4.1$ V (Region III in Figure 6b), V_o remains in the very low range of 0–0.6 V despite variations in light intensity. This is a case that falls under the condition in which $R_{NWFET1} \gg R_{NWPD}$, under which Equation (1) gives $V_o \approx 0$ V regardless of the light intensity. For the region 3.4 V $< V_c < 4.1$ V (Region II in Figure 6b), the output characteristics of V_o are shown in the graph in Figure 6c, in which the x-axis is replaced by light intensity. If V_c is set close to 3.8 V, the ideal condition of the voltage divider, $R_{NWPD(dark)} \gg R_{NWFET} \gg R_{NWPD(bright)}$, is satisfied. Therefore, when V_c is 3.8 V, V_o has the maximum output range of 4.8 V (dark) to 0.1 V (10,000 lux). From the graph, it is apparent that for $V_c = 3.8$ V and above, the voltage divider works sensitively in the range of low illuminance below 100 lux and is increasingly insensitive as illuminance increases.

By contrast, for $V_c = 3.8$ V and below, it is seen that the voltage divider is rather insensitive in the range of low illuminance and works sensitively in the range of high illuminance above 100 lux. In addition, as V_o acts as the gate voltage of the NWFET2 of the current driver circuit that determines the output current level, it is necessary to consider the light intensity range and the level of concomitant output current in the selection of the value of V_c. Figure 6d shows an experimental setup for investigating the output characteristics of the current driver circuit. The drain of NWFET2 is connected to a reference stimulation signal generated by a function generator having an amplitude of 5 V and a duration of 20 ms. The reference stimulation signal used in the experiment is monophasic, but a biphasic pulse signal can also be used. The drain of NWFET2 is connected to the reference stimulation signal generated by a function generator. The reference stimulation signal has an amplitude of 5 V and a duration of 20 ms. The source of NWFET2 is connected to the Au test electrode, and the test electrode is immersed in phosphate buffered saline (PBS) solution. Figure 6e shows the waveform of current transmitted to the micro electrode measured against gate voltage (V_o). The maximum peak current for V_o is approximately 123 μA when V_o is 0 V, and when $V_o > 4$ V, NWFET2 is off and therefore the current signal is no longer transmitted. Figure 6f shows the waveform of a stimulation current signal (i_{st}) transmitted to test electrodes after randomly varying the intensity of light illuminated onto a neural stimulation device employing a voltage divider and a current driver. The illuminance waveform (I_{light}) and the concomitant stimulation current waveform are simultaneously depicted on the graph. It is seen that each pulse of the reference stimulation signal is modulated to have an amplitude that is relatively proportional to light intensity. The above results show that the proposed neural stimulation device detects light intensity and can perform stimulation signal modulation in proportion to the light intensity.

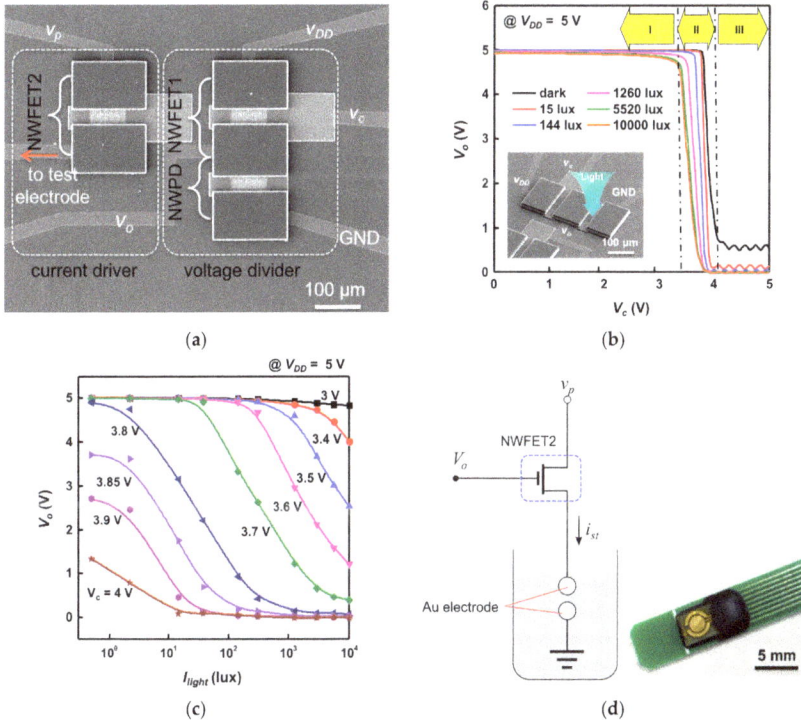

Figure 6. *Cont.*

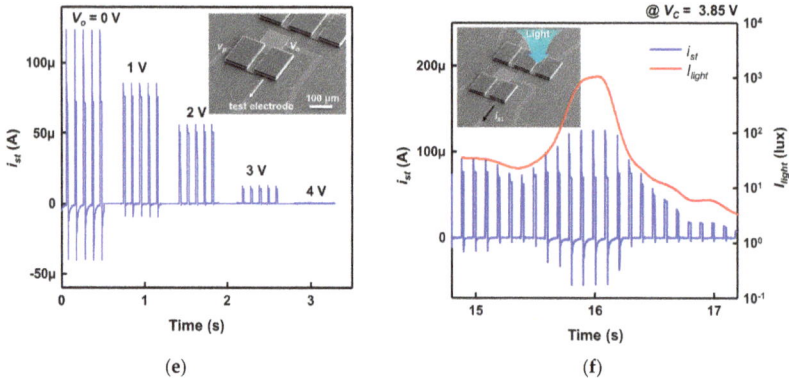

Figure 6. (**a**) Fabricated neural stimulation device; (**b**) Output voltage curve of the voltage divider against control voltage by light intensity; (**c**) Output voltage curve of the voltage divider against light intensity by control voltage; (**d**) Measurement setup of the current driver; (**e**) Waveform of current is transmitted to the micro electrode against gate voltage V_o when V_c = 3.85 V; (**f**) Modulation waveform of stimulation signal for the neural stimulation device, which is proportional to light intensity.

3.2. In Vitro Experiment

An in vitro animal experiment was performed in order to evaluate the effectiveness of activating neurons using the fabricated neural stimulation device. The experimental setup was configured as shown in Figure 7a. A drain voltage (V_{DD}) of 10 V was applied to the voltage divider of the neural stimulation device, and a uniform rectangular pulse v_{st}, with amplitude 12 V, pulse width (duration) 1 ms, and frequency 1 Hz, was generated using a field programmable gate array (FPGA). The source side of NWFET2 was connected to one of the MEA electrodes, as shown in Figure 7a. The MEA, which is shown in Figure 7b, comprised 60 micro electrodes and a reference electrode. The micro electrode was a circular electrode 50 μm in diameter and was fabricated by forming an Au (~2 μm) layer and a Pt-black layer (~4 μm) via successive electroforming processes. The Pt-black layer of the micro electrode had a wide surface area owing to its nano-porous structure and had the effects of lowering the interface impedance between the micro electrodes and the retinal cells and enlarging the injection charge capacity [24]. One MEA electrode connected to the current driver was used to stimulate the retinal nerve, and the remaining electrodes were used to record neural response signals. The retinal cell for the in vitro experiment was extirpated from an *rd1* mouse. As shown in Figure 7c, the separated retinal cell was stuck closely to the MEA chip so that the ganglion cell could come into contact with the MEA. A well structure was formed around the retinal cell and then filled with cerebrospinal fluid (CSF) so that the retinal cell could maintain its function for a long time.

Figure 8a–d shows the neural response signals produced in the in vitro experiment using the neural stimulation device. Figure 8a shows an example of the neural response signals at 60 channels and represents the locations of a stimulating electrode and of a reference electrode. The effectiveness of stimulation can be evaluated by observing significant changes in the number of spikes after the stimulation signal is applied. Figure 8b shows the results of analyzing the neural response signals of two channels. The histogram graph represents the total number of spikes in neural signals in an interval of 10 ms before and after the application of 100 stimulation pulses. In Figure 8b, a distinctive increase in the number of spikes can be identified within about 0.2 s after application of the stimulation pulses. Figure 8c is a color map that represents the number of spikes per pulse (spikes/pulse) obtained from the histogram of Figure 8b against light intensity for 60 channels. As is seen in Figure 8c, the number of spikes increase prominently as the light intensity increases. The neural response against intensity of stimulus can be quantified using the normalized response defined by Equation (2).

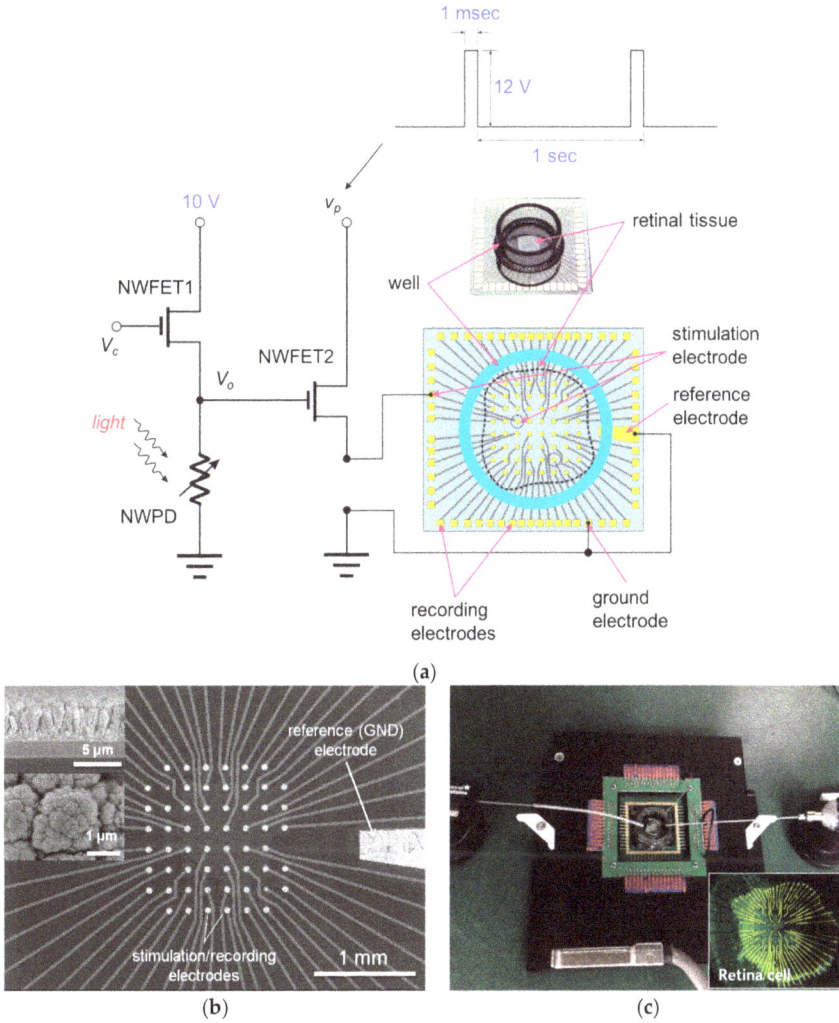

Figure 7. (**a**) Circuit diagram of in vitro animal experimental setup; (**b**) Micro electrode array for recording multi-channel neural signals; (**c**) Arrangement of micro electrode array and retinal tissue using multi-channel probing system (in vitro MEA-Systems of Multi Channel Systems).

$$\text{normalized response} = \frac{\Sigma_{ch} \text{ spikes per pulse after stimulation}}{\Sigma_{ch} \text{ spikes per pulse before stimulation}}, \qquad (2)$$

Figure 8d shows the normalized response curves for four patches of retinal tissue extirpated from *rd1* mice. It is seen that the retinal neurons tend to respond in proportion to the amplitude of the stimulation pulse (i.e., the intensity of light) although there exist some differences in level and shape among the normalized response curves.

(a)

(b)

(c)

(d)

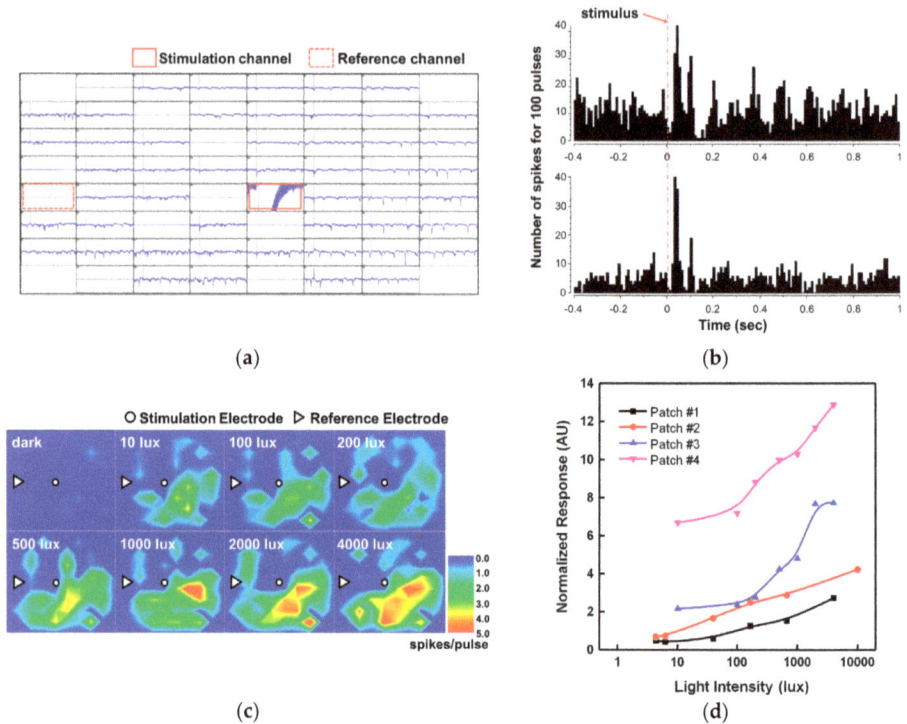

Figure 8. (**a**) Neural response signals recorded at 60 channels; (**b**) Changes in the number of spikes during, before, and after the application of stimulation signals; (**c**) Number of spikes per pulse at each channel against light intensity; (**d**) Normalized response by light intensity as a result of stimulation experiment using four retinal tissues.

4. Conclusions

This paper proposed a method for neural stimulation and a neural stimulation device integrated with an SiNW-based photodetection circuit. The SiNW-based photodetection circuit is designed to have the functions of detecting light and generating a stimulation signal in proportion to light intensity that is then transmitted to a micro electrode. Large resistance variation in the SiNW PD of the voltage divider circuit of a neuron stimulation device is desirable, and the fabricated SiNW PD produces a very large ratio $R_{NWPD(dark)}/R_{NWPD(bright)}$ of 1930. Owing to the large resistance variation of the SiNW PD, the voltage divider exhibits a very large swing range of output voltage. In the current driver circuit of the neuron stimulation device, the SiNW FET, which is driven by the output voltage of the voltage divider, produces a maximum on-current of approximately 480 µA and an on–off ratio of 5×10^4. It was determined that the current driver has a high enough current value and sufficient on–off characteristics to stimulate neurons via micro electrodes. The proposed neuron stimulation device can be applied to a high-resolution retinal prosthesis system, as was demonstrated by fabricating a high-density neural stimulation device with a unit cell size of 110×110 µm and a resolution of 32×32 in the form of a flexible film about 50 µm thick. Its effectiveness as a retinal stimulation device was evaluated by utilizing a unit cell of the neural stimulation device in an in vitro animal experiment involving the retinal tissue of *rd1* mice. A reference stimulation signal of uniform rectangular pulses modulated by the neural stimulation device into a stimulation signal proportional to light intensity was produced and transmitted into micro electrodes to stimulate the retinal nerve. Application of the retinal stimulation pulses to the retinal tissues demonstrated that the number of spikes in neural response signals increase in proportion to light intensity. These results address new challenges in developing neuron stimulation devices using SiNW-based circuits and are a promising step in the development of high-resolution retinal prosthetic systems.

Acknowledgments: This research was partially supported by a grant to Bio-Mimetic Robot Research Center Funded by Defense Acquisition Program Administration and by Agency for Defense Development (UD160027ID). In addition, this research was partially supported by the Public Welfare and Safety Research Program through the National Research Foundation of Korea (NRF) funded by the Ministry of Education, Science and Technology (2012-0008611). The English proofreading service was also supported by the Brain Korea 21 Plus Project in 2016.

Author Contributions: S.W. Jung fabricated SiNW devices and analyzed experimental results. J.Y. Shin and K. Pi conducted in vitro experiments and analyzed the experimental results. Y.S. Goo enucleated the eye from the *rd1* mice, detached retinal tissues from the eye, and set up the in vitro experiments. D.D. Cho supervised all of the SiNW fabrication and experiments.

Conflicts of Interest: The authors declare no conflict of interest.

References

1. Laxton, A.W.; Tang-Wai, D.F.; Mcandrews, M.P.; Zumsteg, D.; Wennberg, R.; Keren, R.; Wherrett, J.; Naglie, G.; Hamani, C.; Smith, G.S.; et al. A phase I trial of deep brain stimulation of memory circuits in Alzheimer's disease. *Ann. Neurol.* **2010**, *68*, 521–534. [CrossRef] [PubMed]
2. Jackson, A.; Zimmermann, J.B. Neural interfaces for the brain and spinal cord-restoring motor function. *Nat. Rev. Neurol.* **2012**, *8*, 690–699. [CrossRef] [PubMed]
3. O'Brien, E.E.; Greferath, U.; Vessey, K.A.; Jobling, A.I.; Fletcher, E.L. Electronic restoration of vision in those with photoreceptor degenerations. *Clin. Exp. Optim.* **2012**, *95*, 473–483. [CrossRef] [PubMed]
4. Koo, K.I.; Lee, S.M.; Yee, J.H.; Ryu, S.B.; Kim, K.H.; Goo, Y.S.; Cho, D.I. A novel in vitro sensing configuration for retinal physiology analysis of a sub-retinal prosthesis. *Sensors* **2012**, *12*, 3131–3144. [CrossRef] [PubMed]
5. Koo, K.I.; Lee, S.M.; Bae, S.H.; Seo, J.M.; Chung, H.; Cho, D.I. Arrowhead-shaped microelectrodes fabricated on a flexible substrate for enhancing the spherical conformity of retinal prostheses. *J. Microelectromech. Syst.* **2011**, *20*, 251–259. [CrossRef]
6. Seo, J.M.; Kim, K.H.; Goo, Y.S.; Park, K.S.; Kim, S.J.; Cho, D.I.; Chung, H. Vision rehabilitation by electrical retinal stimulation: Review of microelectrode approaches. *Sens. Mater.* **2012**, *24*, 153–164.
7. Lee, S.M.; Ahn, J.H.; Seo, S.M.; Chung, H.; Cho, D.I. Electrical characterization of 3D Au microelectrodes for use in retinal prostheses. *Sensors* **2015**, *15*, 14345–14355. [CrossRef] [PubMed]
8. Hirase, H.; Nikolenko, V.; Goldberg, J.H.; Yuste, R. Multiphoton stimulation of neurons. *J. Neurobiol.* **2002**, *51*, 237–247. [CrossRef] [PubMed]
9. Zemelman, B.V.; Lee, G.A.; Ng, M.; Miesenböck, G. Selective photostimulation of genetically ChARGed neurons. *Neuron* **2002**, *33*, 15–22. [CrossRef]
10. Oh, S.J.; Ahn, J.H.; Lee, S.M.; Ko, H.H.; Seo, J.M.; Goo, Y.S.; Cho, D.I. Light-controlled biphasic current stimulator IC using CMOS image sensors for high-resolution retinal prosthesis and in vitro experimental results with rd1 mouse. *IEEE Trans. Biomed.* **2015**, *62*, 70–79. [CrossRef] [PubMed]
11. Wilke, R.; Gabel, V.P.; Sachs, H.; Schmidt, K.U.B.; Gekeler, F.; Besch, D.; Szurman, P.; Stett, A.; Wilhelm, B.; Peters, T.; et al. Spatial resolution and perception of patterns mediated by a subretinal 16-electrode array in patients blinded by hereditary retinal dystrophies. *Investig. Ophthalmol. Vis. Sci.* **2011**, *52*, 5995–6003. [CrossRef] [PubMed]
12. Fujikado, T.; Kamei, M.; Sakaguchi, H.; Kanda, H.; Morimoto, T.; Ikuno, Y.; Nishida, K.; Kishima, H.; Maruo, T.; Konoma, K.; et al. Testing of semichronically implanted retinal prosthesis by suprachoroidal-transretinal stimulation in patients with retinitis pigmentosa. *Investig. Ophthalmol. Vis. Sci.* **2011**, *52*, 4726–4733. [CrossRef] [PubMed]
13. Klauke, S.; Goertz, M.; Rein, S.; Hoehl, D.; Thomas, U.; Eckhorn, R.; Bremmer, F.; Wachtler, T. Stimulation with a wireless intraocular epiretinal implant elicits visual percepts in blind humans. *Investig. Ophthalmol. Vis. Sci.* **2011**, *52*, 449–455. [CrossRef] [PubMed]

14. Humayun, M.S.; Dorn, J.D.; da Cruz, L.; Gagnelle, G.; Sahel, J.A.; Stanga, P.E.; Cideciyan, A.V.; Duncan, J.L.; Eliott, D.; Filley, E.; et al. Interim results from the international trial of Second Sight's visual prosthesis. *Ophthalmology* **2012**, *119*, 779–788. [CrossRef] [PubMed]

15. Zrenner, E.; Bartz-Schmidt, K.U.; Benav, H.; Besch, D.; Bruckmann, A.; Gabel, V.P.; Gekeler, F.; Greppmaier, U.; Harscher, A.; Kibbel, S.; et al. Subretinal electronic chips allow blind patients to read letters and combine them to words. *Proc. Biol. Sci.* **2011**, *278*, 1489–1497. [CrossRef] [PubMed]

16. Palanker, D.; Vankov, A.; Huie, P.; Baccus, S. Design of a high-resolution optoelectronic retinal prosthesis. *J. Neural Eng.* **2005**, *2*, S105–S120. [CrossRef] [PubMed]

17. DeMarco, P.J.; Yarbrough, G.L.; Yee, C.W.; McLean, G.Y.; Sagdullaev, B.T.; Ball, S.L.; McCall, M.A. Stimulation via a subretinally placed prosthetic elicits central activity and induces a trophic effect on visual responses. *Investig. Ophthalmol. Vis. Sci.* **2007**, *48*, 916–926. [CrossRef] [PubMed]

18. Chow, A.Y.; Bittner, A.K. The artificial silicon retina in retinitis pigmentosa aatients (An American Ophthalmological Association Thesis). *Trans. Am. Ophthalmol. Soc.* **2010**, *108*, 120–154. [PubMed]

19. Lee, S.M.; Jung, S.W.; Ahn, J.H.; Yoo, H.J.; Oh, S.J.; Cho, D.I. Microelectrode array with integrated nanowire FET switches for high-resolution retinal prosthetic systems. *J. Microelectromech. Syst.* **2014**, *24*, 075018. [CrossRef]

20. Ahn, J.H.; Lee, S.M.; Hong, S.J.; Yoo, H.J.; Jung, S.W.; Park, S.K.; Ko, H.H.; Cho, D.I. Multi-channel stimulator IC using a channel sharing method for retinal prosthesis. *J. Biomed. Nanotechnol.* **2013**, *9*, 621–625. [CrossRef] [PubMed]

21. Bae, S.H.; Che, J.H.; Seo, J.M.; Jeong, J.; Kim, E.T.; Lee, S.W.; Koo, K.I.; Suaing, G.J.; Lovell, N.H.; Cho, D.I.; et al. In vitro biocompatibility of various polymer-based microelectrode arrays for retinal prosthesis. *Investig. Ophthalmol. Vis. Sci.* **2012**, *53*, 2653–2657. [CrossRef] [PubMed]

22. Lee, S.M.; Jung, S.W.; Park, S.K.; Ahn, J.H.; Hong, S.J.; Yoo, H.J.; Lee, M.H.; Cho, D.I. Fabrication and evaluation of silicon nanowire photodetectors on a flexible substrate for retinal prosthetic system. *Sens. Mater.* **2012**, *24*, 205–220.

23. Lee, K.N.; Jung, S.W.; Shin, K.S.; Kim, W.H.; Lee, M.H.; Seong, W.K. Fabrication of suspended silicon nanowire arrays. *Small* **2008**, *4*, 642–648. [CrossRef] [PubMed]

24. Pi, K.; Shin, J.Y.; Jung, S.W.; Lee, S.; Cho, D.I. Electrical characterization of nanostructured 3D microelectrodes for retinal neuron stimulation. In Proceedings of the 2015 IEEE Sensors, Busan, Korea, 1–4 November 2015.

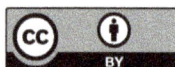

sensors

MDPI

Article

Micro-Droplet Detection Method for Measuring the Concentration of Alkaline Phosphatase-Labeled Nanoparticles in Fluorescence Microscopy

Rufeng Li [1], Yibei Wang [1], Hong Xu [1], Baowei Fei [2] and Binjie Qin [1,*]

[1]   School of Biomedical Engineering, Shanghai Jiao Tong University, Shanghai 200240, China;
      brave_lee@sjtu.edu.cn (R.L.); wangyibei@sjtu.edu.cn (Y.W.); xuhong@sjtu.edu.cn (H.X.)
[2]   Emory University School of Medicine, Georgia Institute of Technology, Atlanta, GA 30329 USA;
      bfei@emory.edu
*   Correspondence: bjqin@sjtu.edu.cn

Received: 1 October 2017; Accepted: 19 November 2017; Published: 21 November 2017

Abstract: This paper developed and evaluated a quantitative image analysis method to measure the concentration of the nanoparticles on which alkaline phosphatase (AP) was immobilized. These AP-labeled nanoparticles are widely used as signal markers for tagging biomolecules at nanometer and sub-nanometer scales. The AP-labeled nanoparticle concentration measurement can then be directly used to quantitatively analyze the biomolecular concentration. Micro-droplets are mono-dispersed micro-reactors that can be used to encapsulate and detect AP-labeled nanoparticles. Micro-droplets include both empty micro-droplets and fluorescent micro-droplets, while fluorescent micro-droplets are generated from the fluorescence reaction between the APs adhering to a single nanoparticle and corresponding fluorogenic substrates within droplets. By detecting micro-droplets and calculating the proportion of fluorescent micro-droplets to the overall micro-droplets, we can calculate the AP-labeled nanoparticle concentration. The proposed micro-droplet detection method includes the following steps: (1) Gaussian filtering to remove the noise of overall fluorescent targets, (2) a contrast-limited, adaptive histogram equalization processing to enhance the contrast of weakly luminescent micro-droplets, (3) an red maximizing inter-class variance thresholding method (OTSU) to segment the enhanced image for getting the binary map of the overall micro-droplets, (4) a circular Hough transform (CHT) method to detect overall micro-droplets and (5) an intensity-mean-based thresholding segmentation method to extract the fluorescent micro-droplets. The experimental results of fluorescent micro-droplet images show that the average accuracy of our micro-droplet detection method is 0.9586; the average true positive rate is 0.9502; and the average false positive rate is 0.0073. The detection method can be successfully applied to measure AP-labeled nanoparticle concentration in fluorescence microscopy.

Keywords: fluorescence microscopy; micro-droplet; spot detection; alkaline phosphatase (AP); nanoparticles

1. Introduction

Advances in microscopy and fluorescence tools have pushed the quantitative biological research for biomolecules at nanometer and sub-nanometer scales [1–3]. Among these fluorescence tools, nanoparticles on which alkaline phosphatase (AP) was immobilized (AP-labeled nanoparticles for short) [4] are widely used as signal markers for tagging biomolecules of interest due to their stabilization and convenience for operation. Covered with a specific antibody, the AP-labeled nanoparticle can label one target biomolecule and emit a fluorescent signal by catalyzing the corresponding substrates. Therefore, the biomolecular concentration can be directly obtained by measuring the AP-labeled nanoparticle concentration. Traditional methods for AP-labeled nanoparticle concentration measurement are to divide the amount of total fluorescent signals from the AP-labeled nanoparticles by the volume of solution in the fluorescence microscopy image. However, it is difficult to count AP-labeled nanoparticles directly from fluorescent images since AP-labeled nanoparticles are too small to detect and are closely clustered. To solve this problem, a widely-used technology called the droplet microfluidics technique has been used to encapsulate the individual AP-labeled nanoparticle in monodispersed micro-droplets [5]. Micro-droplets with a similar size are water-in-oil droplets, which can be used as micro-reactors to encapsulate and detect AP-labeled nanoparticles [6]. All the micro-droplets encapsulate fluorogenic substrates, but only a small portion of micro-droplets would carry AP-labeled nanoparticles. Only the micro-droplets encapsulating AP-labeled nanoparticles will emit remarkable fluorescent signals via the enzymatic reaction between the APs and the corresponding fluorogenic substrates within droplets. We call these micro-droplets fluorescent micro-droplets and the others empty micro-droplets. However, empty micro-droplets may emit weak fluorescent signals that result from a few APs scattered within the micro-droplet in practice. Since the process of encapsulating AP-labeled nanoparticles in micro-droplets follows a random Poisson distribution [6,7], the probability of occurrence of the micro-droplets encapsulating AP-labeled nanoparticles can be obtained via the percentage of the fluorescent micro-droplets. Therefore, we can detect the proportion of fluorescent micro-droplets to the overall micro-droplets to measure the AP-labeled nanoparticle concentration. To achieve this purpose, micro-droplet detection is necessary to analyze the AP-labeled nanoparticle concentration.

The micro-droplet detection usually consists of two steps: detection of the overall micro-droplets and detection of fluorescent micro-droplets. There are certain problems involved in the detection of the overall micro-droplets. The empty micro-droplets with weak luminance are hard to detect due to the weak difference between empty micro-droplets and their surroundings. The complex noise environment in the fluorescence images may also increase the difficulties of micro-droplet detection. There are two important types of noises: the intrinsic photon noises resulting from the random nature of photon emission and the background noises caused by the detector's electronics [8]. Moreover, the additional noises like small bright speckles and vesicles could also impede subsequent droplet detection. Furthermore, there is still a tough issue that most micro-droplets are closely connected in the fluorescence images.

Traditional fluorescent target detection methods have been reported in the literature [9–11]. In [12], the authors provide a thorough comparative evaluation of the most frequently-used spot detection methods. The study shows the superiority of the multiscale variance-stabilizing transform (MSVST) detector method [13] and the H-dome-based detector (HD) method [14]. The MSVST method combines the red variance stabilizing transform (VST) with the isotropic undecimated wavelet transform [13,15] and performs well in filtering mixed-Poisson-Gaussian noises and in detecting fluorescent particles. However, the bright speckles and vesicles in the image may lead to the false detection of micro-droplets. Being different from MSVST, the HD method detects spots by extracting peaks with an amplitude higher than a given height, called domes, in a Laplace-of-Gaussian (LoG) filtered or Gaussian-filtered image. Because the amplitude of the peaks in micro-droplets varies in a large range, the HD method may not work well in micro-droplet detection. To overcome this drawback, Rezatofighi et al. [16] proposed an improved method called the maximum possible height-dome method (MPHD) to adaptively extract the dome. However, it may not perform well when both the bright speckles and closely-connected micro-droplets appear in the image. To further improve the detection performance, Jaiswal et al. [17] proposed a multi-scale spot-enhancing filter method (MSSEF) to calculate the binary map, which is obtained by iteratively applying a threshold to the LoG filtered image with scale changing. This method can significantly improve the detection performance on multiple closely-connected particles. However, since the selected threshold with respect to the mean and variance of the image may be inaccurate, it may not perform well on the micro-droplet detection. Besides, Basset et al. [18–20] proposed methods to select the optimal LoG scale or multiple scales corresponding to the different spot sizes in the image, but test results on fluorescent micro-droplet images proved the ineffectiveness of this method for the micro-droplet detection. As explained by Smal et al. [12], most current methods follow a common detection scheme, which consists of denoising the image, enhancing the spots and, finally, extracting the target spots in a binary map to further count the micro-droplets or estimate the positions. In addition, these methods perform ineffectively for the detection of closely-connected micro-droplets by implementing a connect-component analysis method. Recently, an automatic hotspots detection framework [21] was proposed to successfully detect active areas inside cells that show changes in their calcium concentration. However, this automatic segmentation of intracellular calcium concentration in individual video frames is about 80% accurate and may not be suitable for precisely detecting a single active cell in the highly accurate concentration measurement. Therefore, there is a need to develop new approaches in order to improve the accuracy and robustness for detecting the micro-droplets.

To address these difficulties, we propose an overall micro-droplet detection method for fluorescent micro-droplet images (FMIs).

2. Methods

The proposed method includes the following steps: (1) The Gaussian filter first removes the noise in the red fluorescent micro-droplet image. (2) The contrast-limited adaptive histogram equalization (CLAHE) [22] method divides the whole filtered image into different blocks and adaptively adjusts the local histogram of each block to enhance the contrasts of the weak luminance regions of overall micro-droplets. (3) The red maximizing inter-class variance thresholding [23–25] method (OTSU) segments the enhanced image to get the binary map of the overall micro-droplets. (4) By performing on the segmented binary map, the circular Hough transform method (CHT) [26,27] perfectly detects the overall micro-droplets due to its advantage in detecting the micro-droplets that are closely connected with each other. With the combined strengths of CLAHE, OTSU thresholding and the CHT methods, our method shows significant performances on the overall micro-droplet detection. Finally, the fluorescent micro-droplet can be easily extracted via an intensity-mean-based thresholding segmentation method and be counted with the CHT method again. We have compared the performance of our method on FMIs with the performances of the state-of-the-art methods including MSVST [13], MPHD [16] and MSSEF [17]. The comparative results demonstrate that our method outperforms these state-of-the-art methods.

2.1. Overall Micro-Droplet Detection

Figure 1 shows the overview of the proposed method for overall micro-droplet detection. We begin by preprocessing an input image with a Gaussian filter. Then, CLAHE is performed on the local histogram of the filtered image to enhance the contrast of micro-droplets. After this image enhancement, the difference between micro-droplets and background increases, and an OTSU thresholding-based segmentation method is applied to obtain a binary map of the overall micro-droplets. Finally, the CHT method precisely detects the circular contour of the overall micro-droplets.

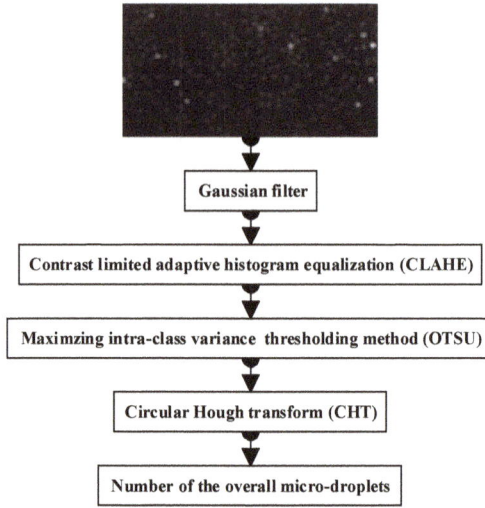

Figure 1. The framework of the proposed method for the overall micro-droplet detection.

2.1.1. Noise Reduction with the Gaussian Filter

The main noise sources in fluorescence microscopy images are the shot noise occurring in the photon counting in the imaging process and the additive Gaussian noise created by the electron characteristics of detectors [8,12]. The shot noise of the photons results from the random nature of photon emission and can be modeled as Poisson noise [8,28] when there is only a handful of photons emitted, whereas the noise can be considered as Gaussian noise when the number of photons is sufficient.

In most situations, the noise in fluorescent micro-droplet images can be approximately considered as Gaussian noise. Therefore, we simply use a normal Gaussian filter to remove the noise. In Figure 2, the signal-to-noise radio (SNR) of the denoised image is enhanced compared to that of the original images. We can see that the noises are eliminated effectively in the zoomed version of filtered image *I*.

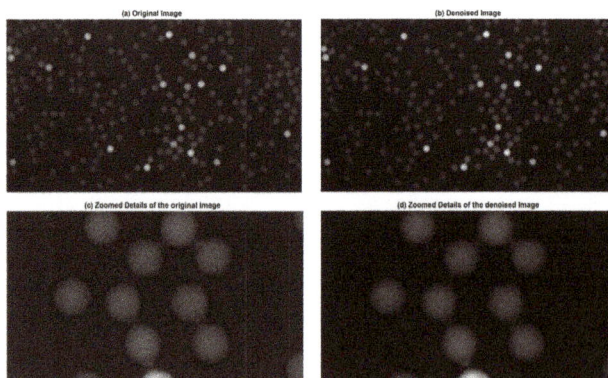

Figure 2. Original fluorescent image with SNR (signal-to-noise radio) of 7.1789 and the denoised image with SNR of 7.7489. (**a**) Original image. (**b**) Denoised image (*I*). (**c**) Zoomed details of the original image. (**d**) Zoomed details of the denoised image.

2.1.2. Contrast Limited Adaptive Histogram Equalization

In the filtered image, there are many micro-droplets with weak luminance. We then use the CLAHE [22] method to enhance the contrast of micro-droplets.

Firstly, the image I is divided into $N * N$ blocks (N is a user-defined constant, and N is by default set to 8) and local histogram of every block is calculated. Since the contrast amplification in the vicinity of a given pixel value is proportional to the histogram value at that pixel value, the local histogram is clipped at a predefined value T to limit the over-amplification of noise. The part of the histogram exceeding T is redistributed among all histogram bins to keep the area of the histogram unvarying. Then, histogram equalization uses the same transformation derived from the local histogram to transform all pixels in the block and enhance local contrasts. With these operations finished, we combine all the blocks together and apply bilinear interpolation to eliminate the block effect of images. Finally, the micro-droplets at low intensities are prominently enhanced. The output of this step is an enhanced image J, which is shown in Figure 3.

2.1.3. Maximizing inter-class Variance Thresholding Method

In Figure 3, the pixels in the enhanced image J can be grouped into two classes including background and micro-droplet pixels in terms of histogram distribution. Therefore, OTSU thresholding [23–25] is the most suited method to extract micro-droplets via histogram thresholding. The optimal threshold of this method is chosen by maximizing inter-class variance. The segmented binary map by the OTSU method effectively highlights the desired micro-droplets. However, there may be several falsely detected spots in the binary map due to the bright specks having a far smaller size than the micro-droplets in image J. In order to obtain accurate detection results, the morphological opening operation is used for post-processing to eliminate the influence of these abnormal spots. The output of this step is denoted as image K.

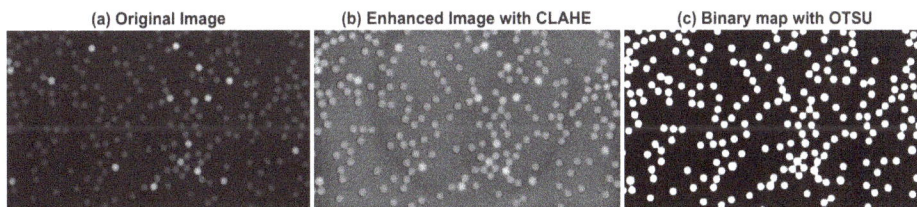

Figure 3. Intermediate results of contrast-limited adaptive histogram equalization (CLAHE) and OTSU on the overall micro-droplet detection: (**a**) Original image. (**b**) Enhanced image with CLAHE (J). (**c**) Binary map with OTSU (K).

2.1.4. Circle Detection via Circular Hough Transform

After getting the segmented binary map, we must count the number of overall micro-droplets to achieve a final detection result. The traditional fluorescent spot detection algorithms are usually based on connected component analysis (CCA). CCA-based methods perform well on detecting isolated micro-droplets, but poorly on detecting closely-connected micro-droplets. With further observation of micro-droplets, we found that all the micro-droplets appear as round spots with a similar radius. Therefore, we can employ CHT [26,27] to detect the spots with radii in a certain range. Moreover, CHT is insensitive to deformation, rotation and scaling of the circle in the image such that it can perfectly detect the incomplete round micro-droplets and closely-connected micro-droplets with lower false detection and higher accuracy. Furthermore, it has a low computational complexity, and the only parameter we need to set is the radius range of micro-droplets.

The CHT algorithm contains the following two essential steps:

- Accumulator array computation:

  The edge detection is carried out on the binary map to get an edge image (L). The edge pixels of L are designated as candidate pixels and are allowed to cast 'votes' in the accumulator array $A(a)$, which represents the weight of the circle with a fixed radius and the center of the circle. Here, $a = \{a, b, r\}$. (a, b) represents the space location of pixels, and r is the radius of the expected circle. At the beginning, all the elements of $A(a)$ are set to 0.

- Center and radius estimation:

  For every pixel x of the fluorescence image, we accumulate all the units of $A(a)$ that satisfy the function $f(x, a) = 0$. $f(x, a)$ is the analytical expression of circle:

$$f(x, a) = (x_1 - a)^2 + (x_2 - b)^2 - r^2 \tag{1}$$

Finally, the circular centers and radii are estimated by detecting the peaks in the accumulator array. We can get the number of micro-droplets by counting the centers of detected circles.

The overall micro-droplets can be detected with the method mentioned above. This method can accurately extract and count the overall micro-droplets on FMIs.

2.2. Fluorescent Micro-Droplet Detection

The fluorescent micro-droplets can be extracted by directly thresholding segmentation due to their high intensity and round shape. However, it is difficult to choose the segmental threshold (D) since the fluorescent micro-droplets in different images can appear to be very different in the fluorescence intensities. We collected the manually-segmented threshold of fluorescent micro-droplets and the intensity mean of the images. By analyzing the relationship of the manually-segmented threshold and the intensity mean of the image, we found that the segmental threshold has a significant linear correlation with the intensity mean of the image. Therefore, we model the relationship mentioned above with a linear fitting method and set up a linear function corresponding to the threshold D of the images:

$$D(m) = 1.3717 * m + 0.0126 \tag{2}$$

where m denotes the intensity mean of the image. After the binary map is obtained, the circular Hough transform (CHT) method (see the details in Section 2.1.4) is applied to count the fluorescent micro-droplets precisely. Figure 4 shows the detected result of this method.

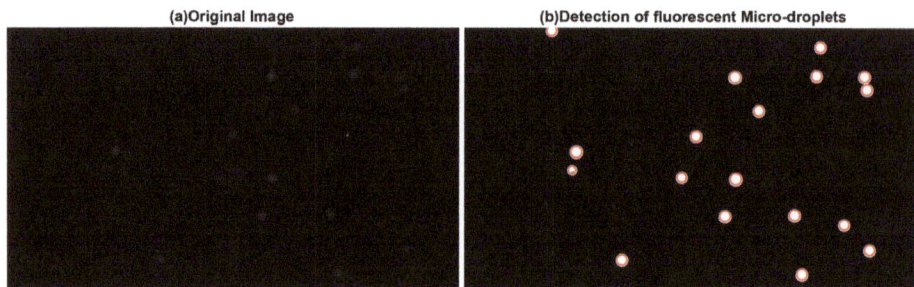

Figure 4. Detection of fluorescent micro-droplets. (**a**) Original image. (**b**) Detection of fluorescent micro-droplets.

2.3. Measurement of AP-Labeled Nanoparticle Concentration

Encapsulating AP-labeled nanoparticles delivered to the droplet-generation nozzle at random is a Poisson process. The probability of encapsulating k AP-labeled nanoparticles in a micro-droplet is then given by equation:

$$P(k) = e^{-\lambda} \frac{\lambda^k}{k!} \tag{3}$$

where λ is the average number of AP-nanoparticles per micro-droplet, e is the base of the natural logarithms, k is from natural numbers and $k!$ is the factorial of k.

After detecting the numbers of fluorescent and overall micro-droplets, we can obtain the probability $P(k \geq 1)$ by directly computing the proportion of the fluorescent micro-droplets to the overall micro-droplets. Then, the average number of AP-nanoparticles per micro-droplet λ can be calculated according to Equations (3) and (4):

$$P(k = 0) + P(k \geq 1) = 1 \tag{4}$$

Finally, λ is converted to the average amount of substance n (in moles) of a single micro-droplet; the AP-labeled nanoparticle concentration c is then measured by dividing the average amount of substance n (in moles) by the average volume V of a single micro-droplet. The concentration unit is given by fM, which corresponds to 10^{-15} mol/L.

2.4. Evaluation

The performance of the overall micro-droplet detection method can be evaluated in the following aspects: (1) Visual evaluations: The visual evaluations firstly give an intuitive performance comparison overview for all the detection methods. (2) TPR and FPR: The true positive rate (TPR) represents the number of true positives (TP) divided by the number of targets in ground truth data, and the false positive rate (FPR) represents the number of the false positives (FP) divided by the number of backgrounds in ground truth data. These two metrics can reflect the detection capability of an algorithm from different perspectives. (3) ROC and F-measure: For the overall evaluation of the detection method, the receiver operating characteristic (ROC curve) is used as a graph metric to uncover the detection power with different TPRs. The area under ROC (AUC) is an estimate of the area under ROC, which indicates the predictive power of the detector. Detectors with higher AUC have better detection power. Furthermore, we computed the F-measure defined by the harmonic mean of precision and recall $F = 2 * Prec * Rec/(Prec + Rec)$. The precision metric $Prec$ is defined as $Prec = TP/(TP + FP)$, and Rec is the index of recall defined as $Rec = TP/(TP + FN)$, where FN is the number of false negatives. The F-measure is a widely-used metric to measure the accuracy of the detection method. The higher F-measure score is related to the higher accuracy. (4) Overall number of micro-droplets detected: The purpose of our work is to precisely count micro-droplets. Therefore, the comparative results on the number of overall micro-droplets detected can directly reflect the superiority of our method.

The fluorescent micro-droplet detection method is evaluated by counting the number of fluorescent micro-droplets detected. We demonstrate the accuracy of this work via the relative error that is defined as the proportion of counting error to the true number counted manually. The counting error is the absolute value of the difference between the true number and the detected number. Low relative errors demonstrate high detection performances.

Finally, we calculate a test AP-labeled nanoparticle concentration with the results of micro-droplet detection and compute a reference concentration with the ground truth data. Then, we use the relative error again to compute the accuracy of our method for the AP-labeled nanoparticle concentration measurement. The comparative results of the test and the reference AP-labeled nanoparticle concentration further demonstrate the performance of our method.

2.5. Code

The source code for the proposed algorithm and associated MATLAB-based GUI are freely available on the author's website, along with instructions for installation and use: http://www.escience.cn/people/bjqin/research.html.

3. Results

This section gives the evaluation of the proposed method on the FMIs acquired from the Nano Biomedical Research Center (NBRC) in Shanghai Jiao Tong University, China. All the FMIs are acquired using an inverted fluorescence microscope (Olympus IX73, Olympus Ltd., Tokyo, Japan) at 100-times magnification when the fluorescence is fully developed. The size of FMI in pixels is 1080×1920, and the diameter of the micro-droplets in the image is approximately 30 µm. The relative experiment details are demonstrated as below. The APs encapsulated in the micro-droplet are obtained from calf intestine. Both APs and AP-labeled nanoparticles were synthesized by NBRC. The substrate concentration employed was 5 mM, where mM represents 10^{-3} mol/L.

3.1. Overall Micro-Droplet Detection

Quantitative evaluations of our method and the state-of-the-art methods mentioned above were carried out on the FMIs. The FMI data consist of a total of fifteen test images. The ground-truth of the overall micro-droplets on the FMIs was manually segmented by two experts at NBRC.

The three methods' parameters are set with the default parameters for achieving the best performances of these methods. As for our method, we set the stand variance σ of Gaussian filtering to one. The contrast enhancement threshold T is set to 0.05, and N is set to eight by default to make the CLAHE achieve the best performances. The search radius of circular Hough transform is set from 16 to 32. All the parameters of our method are set to make our method perform best.

3.1.1. Visual Evaluation

The visual evaluation of different methods is shown in Figure 5. We can see that the proposed method (Figure 5f) perfectly detects all the micro-droplets. Figure 5c also shows that MSVST may detect false micro-droplets. Moreover, Figure 5d,e demonstrates that MSSEF and MPHD may perform poorly on the overall micro-droplet detection.

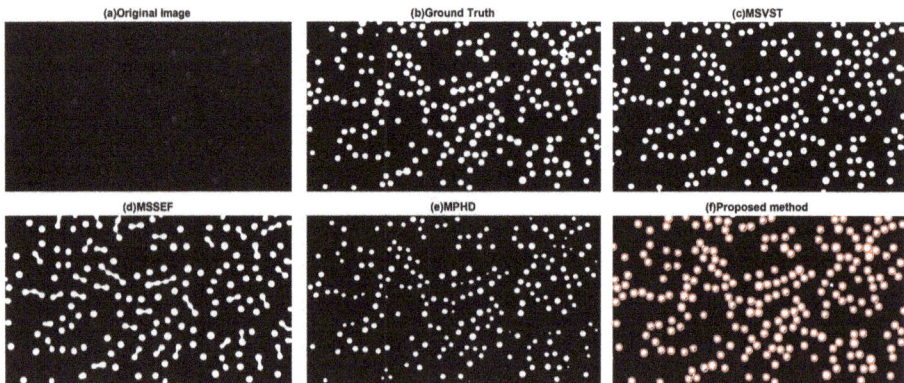

Figure 5. Comparative results of segmented binary maps of different methods: (**a**) Original image. (**b**) Ground truth. (**c**) Multiscale variance-stabilizing transform (MSVST). (**d**) Multiscale spot-enhancing filter method (MSSEF). (**e**) Maximum possible height-dome method (MPHD). (**f**) The proposed method.

3.1.2. TPR and FPR

The comparative evaluations of TPR and FPR are displayed in Figure 6. The TPR of our method is the highest TPR for all the test images, and the highest average TPR achieved by our method is 0.9502. The average FPR of our method is 0.0073. These performance metrics prove that the proposed method has achieved a satisfying micro-droplet detection compared with other methods.

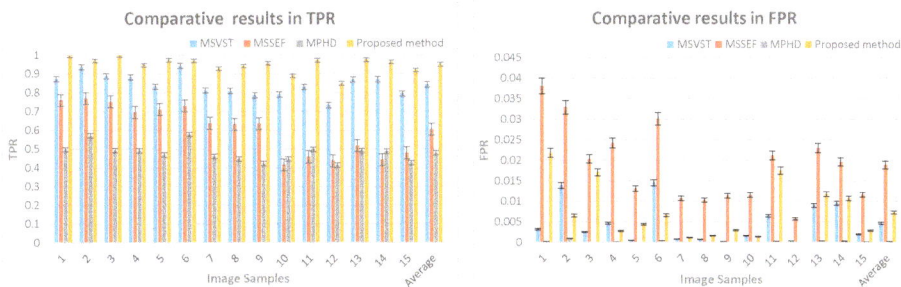

Figure 6. Comparison of TPR and FPR obtained with MSVST, MSSEF, MPHD and the proposed methods on fluorescent micro-droplet images (FMIs).

3.1.3. ROC and F-Measure

The ROC curve in Figure 7 is created by plotting the TPR against the FPR at various threshold settings. Since the AUC is used to evaluate the detecting power of the method, we can use this metric to further reveal the advantage of our method. As shown in Figure 7, the AUC of the proposed method is the highest in all comparative methods. Therefore, we conclude that the proposed method has achieved the best micro-droplet detection performance.

The F-measure is usually used as a detection accuracy metric to evaluate the comprehensive performance of the detector. The higher F-measure corresponds to the better detection. The evaluation results of the F-measure are listed in Table 1. The best average detection accuracy 0.9586 is achieved by our micro-droplet detection method. This highest F-measure score verifies the superiority of the proposed method over other methods.

Table 1. Comparison evaluation of the F-measure obtained with MSVST, MSSEF, MPHD and the proposed methods on FMIs.

Samples	MSVST	MSSEF	MPHD	The Proposed Method
Image1	0.9204	0.7414	0.6640	**0.9231**
Image 2	0.9306	0.7889	0.7250	**0.9674**
Image 3	0.9348	0.8127	0.6610	**0.9597**
Image 4	0.9260	0.7678	0.6591	**0.9656**
Image 5	0.9075	0.8038	0.6392	**0.9770**
Image 6	0.9343	0.7737	0.7318	**0.9677**
Image 7	0.8945	0.7607	0.6311	**0.9604**
Image 8	0.8931	0.7564	0.6183	**0.9663**
Image 9	0.8792	0.7569	0.5946	**0.9721**
Image 10	0.8810	0.5775	0.6183	**0.9402**
Image 11	0.8999	0.6082	0.6653	**0.9655**
Image 12	0.8462	0.6044	0.5859	**0.9186**
Image 13	0.9177	0.6545	0.6586	**0.9707**
Image 14	0.9202	0.5954	0.6555	**0.9692**
Image 15	0.8831	0.6368	0.5987	**0.9551**
Average	0.9046	0.7093	0.6471	**0.9586**

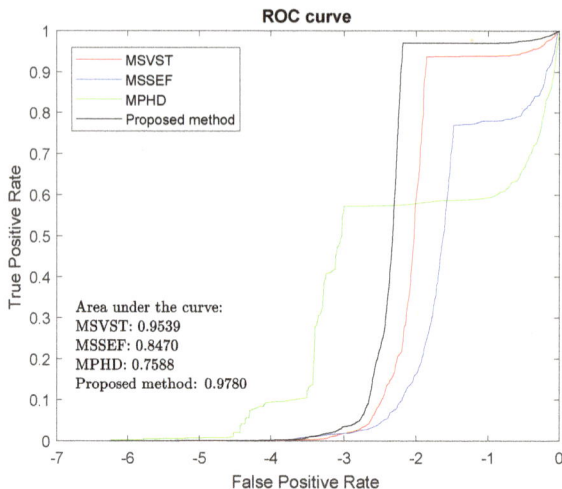

Figure 7. Comparison of the ROC curve obtained with MSVST, MPHD, MSSEF and the proposed methods.

3.1.4. Detected Number of Overall Micro-Droplets

Table 2 shows the final number of micro-droplets detected with different methods. The true number of overall micro-droplets is acquired manually by two experts. Compared with other methods, the proposed method performs stably in detecting capability of the overall micro-droplets in all 15 images, and the detected error is less than two for all the images.

Table 2. Comparison evaluation of the overall number of detected micro-droplets.

Samples	True Number	MSVST	MSSEF	MPHD	The Proposed Method
Image1	161	163	93	152	161
Image 2	222	232	142	202	222
Image 3	221	223	142	202	221
Image 4	223	227	135	198	222
Image 5	219	224	149	202	218
Image 6	229	235	152	210	229
Image 7	250	255	150	236	249
Image 8	239	245	149	224	240
Image 9	245	246	141	224	245
Image 10	381	393	155	350	381
Image 11	372	383	159	348	372
Image 12	381	386	175	345	381
Image 13	347	356	166	320	349
Image 14	414	422	175	371	412
Image 15	358	365	164	325	357

3.2. Fluorescent Micro-Droplet Detection

The detected results of fluorescent micro-droplets are shown in Table 3. The true number of fluorescent micro-droplets is obtained manually by two experts. For the total test images, the proposed method has obtained 100 percent detection accuracy for the thirteen test images with the relative errors in detecting the remaining two images achieving 6.25% and 6.06%. These detected results demonstrate the proposed method's capability in accurately detecting the fluorescent micro-droplets.

Table 3. Comparison evaluation of the number of detected fluorescent micro-droplets.

Samples	True Number	Detected Number of Fluorescent Micro-Droplets	Relative Error
Image1	21	21	0.00%
Image 2	18	18	0.00%
Image 3	18	18	0.00%
Image 4	16	17	6.25%
Image 5	13	13	0.00%
Image 6	24	24	0.00%
Image 7	27	27	0.00%
Image 8	26	26	0.00%
Image 9	9	9	0.00%
Image 10	36	36	0.00%
Image 11	28	28	0.00%
Image 12	30	30	0.00%
Image 13	33	35	6.06%
Image 14	32	32	0.00%
Image 15	31	31	0.00%

3.3. AP-Labeled Nanoparticle Concentration Measurement

Compared with the reference concentration (Table 4), the test AP-labeled nanoparticle concentration calculated with the detected results of micro-droplets has been measured with high accuracy in most samples. The low relative errors in Table 4 further demonstrate the high performance of our method in the measurement of AP-labeled nanoparticle concentration. fM in Table 4 corresponds to 10^{-15} mol/L.

Table 4. Comparison evaluation of the alkaline phosphatase (AP)-labeled nanoparticle concentration measurement.

Samples	True AP-Labeled Nanoparticle Concentration (fM)	Test AP-Labeled Nanoparticle Concentration (fM)	Relative Error
Image1	16.4222	16.4222	0.00%
Image 2	9.9356	9.9356	0.00%
Image 3	9.9825	9.9825	0.00%
Image 4	8.7483	9.3610	7.00%
Image 5	7.1905	7.2246	0.47%
Image 6	13.0088	13.0088	0.00%
Image 7	13.4291	13.4862	0.43%
Image 8	13.5327	13.4730	0.44%
Image 9	4.3976	4.3976	0.00%
Image 10	11.6625	11.6625	0.00%
Image 11	9.1947	9.1947	0.00%
Image 12	9.6366	9.6366	0.00%
Image 13	11.7421	12.4174	5.75%
Image 14	9.4524	9.5002	0.51%
Image 15	10.6424	10.6736	0.29%

4. Discussion

The comparative evaluations demonstrated in Section 3 reveal the effectiveness of the proposed method for micro-droplet detection. With the precise micro-droplet detection, the AP-labeled nanoparticle concentration for the experimental analysis can be calculated accurately. However, it should be noted that the AP-labeled nanoparticle concentration measurement is sensitive to the results of micro-droplet detection. The results in Tables 2 to 4 show that a very slight micro-droplet

Sensors **2017**, *17*, 2685

detecting error may significantly increase the AP-labeled nanoparticle concentration measurement error. Therefore, there is certainly room for further improvement of the proposed method.

5. Conclusions

AP-labeled nanoparticle concentration measurement is of great importance for quantitative biomolecular analysis and measurement. Because the micro-droplet can encapsulate a single AP-labeled nanoparticle and be imaged in fluorescence microscope, the AP-labeled nanoparticle concentration measurement is usually calculated by accurately counting the fluorescent micro-droplets and the overall micro-droplets. This work proposes a micro-droplet detection method for high accuracy AP-labeled nanoparticle concentration measurement by precisely and robustly detecting the weakly luminescent empty micro-droplets that are closely clustered in the complex background noises. The comparative evaluations using the state-of-the-art methods have demonstrated that the proposed method has the best accuracy for micro-droplet detection and AP-labeled nanoparticle concentration measurement.

Acknowledgments: This work was supported by the National Natural Science Foundation of China (21075082 and 61271320) and Medical Engineering Cross Fund of Shanghai Jiao Tong University (YG2014MS29). Baowei Fei was partially supported by NIH Grants CA156775, CA176684 and CA204254 and the Georgia Research Alliance Distinguished Scientists Award. The authors would like to thank all authors for opening source codes used in the experimental comparison in this work. We are thankful to the anonymous reviewers for their valuable comments that greatly helped to improve this paper.

Author Contributions: Rufeng Li and Binjie Qin conceived of and designed the experiments. Rufeng Li and Yibei Wang performed the experiments. Yibei Wang and Hong Xu analyzed the data. Rufeng Li, Baowei Fei and Binjie Qin wrote the paper. Hong Xu and Binjie Qin supervised the experiments.

Conflicts of Interest: The authors declare no conflict of interest.

References

1. Nketia, T.; Sailem, H.; Rohde, G.; Machiraju, R.; Rittscher, J. Analysis of live cell images: Methods, tools and opportunities. *Methods* **2017**, *115*, 65–79.
2. Specht, E.A.; Braselmann, E.; Palmer, A.E. A Critical and Comparative Review of Fluorescent Tools for Live-Cell Imaging. *Annu. Rev. Physiol.* **2017**, *79*, 93–117.
3. Qiang, Y.; Lee, J.Y.; Bartenschlager, R.; Rohr, K. Colocalization analysis and particle tracking in multi-channel fluorescence microscopy images. In Proceedings of the 2017 IEEE 14th International Symposium on Biomedical Imaging (ISBI 2017), Melbourne, Australia, 18–21 April 2017; pp. 646–649.
4. Rissin, D.M.; Kan, C.W.; Campbell, T.G.; Howes, S.C.; Fournier, D.R.; Song, L.; Piech, T.; Patel, P.P.; Chang, L.; Rivnak, A.J.; et al. Single-molecule enzyme-linked immunosorbent assay detects serum proteins at subfemtomolar concentrations. *Nat. Biotechnol.* **2010**, *28*, 595–599.
5. Basova, E.Y.; Foret, F. Droplet microfluidics in (bio)chemical analysis. *Analyst* **2015**, *140*, 22–38.
6. Joensson, H.N.; Andersson Svahn, H. Droplet Microfluidics—A Tool for Single-Cell Analysis. *Angew. Chem. Int. Ed.* **2012**, *51*, 12176–12192.
7. Rissin, D.M.; Walt, D.R. Digital concentration readout of single enzyme molecules using femtoliter arrays and Poisson statistics. *Nano Lett.* **2006**, *6*, 520–523.
8. Thompson, R.E.; Larson, D.R.; Webb, W.W. Precise nanometer localization analysis for individual fluorescent probes. *Biophys. J.* **2002**, *82*, 2775–2783.
9. Kervrann, C.; Sorzano, C.o.S.; Acton, S.T.; Olivo-Marin, J.C.; Unser, M. A guided tour of selected image processing and analysis methods for fluorescence and electron microscopy. *IEEE J. Sel. Top. Signal Process.* **2016**, *10*, 6–30.
10. Wiesmann, V.; Franz, D.; Held, C.; Munzenmayer, C.; Palmisano, R.; Wittenberg, T. Review of free software tools for image analysis of fluorescence cell micrographs. *J. Microsc.* **2015**, *257*, 39–53.
11. Arena, E.T.; Rueden, C.T.; Hiner, M.C.; Wang, S.; Yuan, M.; Eliceiri, K.W. Quantitating the cell: Turning images into numbers with ImageJ. *Wiley Interdiscip. Rev.: Dev. Biol.* **2017**, *6*, doi:10.1002/wdev.260.
12. Smal, I.; Loog, M.; Niessen, W.; Meijering, E. Quantitative comparison of spot detection methods in fluorescence microscopy. *IEEE Trans. Med. Imaging* **2010**, *29*, 282–301.

13. Zhang, B.; Fadili, M.J.; Starck, J.L.; Olivo-Marin, J.C. Multiscale variance-stabilizing transform for mixed-Poisson-Gaussian processes and its applications in bioimaging. In Proceedings of the 2007 14th IEEE International Conference on Image Processing (ICIP 2007), San Antonio, TX, USA, 16–19 September 2007; Volume 6, p. VI-233.
14. Smal, I.; Niessen, W.; Meijering, E. A new detection scheme for multiple object tracking in fluorescence microscopy by joint probabilistic data association filtering. In Proceedings of the 2008 5th IEEE International Symposium on Biomedical Imaging: From Nano to Macro (ISBI 2008), Paris, France, 14–17 May 2008; pp. 264–267.
15. Mallat, S.G. A theory for multiresolution signal decomposition: The wavelet representation. *IEEE Trans. Pattern Anal. Mach. Intell.* **1989**, *11*, 674–693.
16. Rezatofighi, S.H.; Hartley, R.; Hughes, W.E. A new approach for spot detection in total internal reflection fluorescence microscopy. In Proceedings of the 2012 9th IEEE International Symposium on Biomedical Imaging (ISBI 2012), Barcelona, Spain, 2–5 May 2012; pp. 860–863.
17. Jaiswal, A.; Godinez, W.J.; Eils, R.; Lehmann, M.J.; Rohr, K. Tracking virus particles in fluorescence microscopy images using multi-scale detection and multi-frame association. *IEEE Trans. Image Process.* **2015**, *24*, 4122–4136.
18. Basset, A.; Boulanger, J.; Bouthemy, P.; Kervrann, C.; Salamero, J. SLT-LoG: A vesicle segmentation method with automatic scale selection and local thresholding applied to TIRF microscopy. In Proceedings of the 2014 IEEE 11th International Symposium on Biomedical Imaging(ISBI), Beijing, China, 29 April–2 May 2014; pp. 533–536.
19. Basset, A.; Boulanger, J.; Salamero, J.; Bouthemy, P.; Kervrann, C. Adaptive spot detection with optimal scale selection in fluorescence microscopy images. *IEEE Trans. Image Process.* **2015**, *24*, 4512–4527.
20. Acosta, B.M.T.; Basset, A.; Bouthemy, P.; Kervrann, C. Multi-scale spot segmentation with selection of image scales. In Proceedings of the 2017 IEEE International Conference on Acoustics, Speech and Signal Processing (ICASSP), New Orleans, LA, USA, 5–9 March 2017; pp. 1912–1916.
21. Traore, D.; Rietdorf, K.; Al-Jawad, N.; Al-Assam, H. Automatic Hotspots Detection for Intracellular Calcium Analysis in Fluorescence Microscopic Videos. In *Annual Conference on Medical Image Understanding and Analysis*; Springer: Cham, The Netherlands, 2017; pp. 862–873.
22. Zuiderveld, K. Contrast limited adaptive histogram equalization. In *Graphics Gems IV*; Academic Press Professional, Inc.: New York, NY, USA, 1994; pp. 474–485.
23. Otsu, N. A threshold selection method from gray-level histograms. *IEEE Trans. Syst. Man Cybern.* **1979**, *9*, 62–66.
24. Ghaye, J.; Kamat, M.A.; Corbino-Giunta, L.; Silacci, P.; Vergeres, G.; Micheli, G.; Carrara, S. Image thresholding techniques for localization of sub-resolution fluorescent biomarkers. *Cytom. Part A* **2013**, *83*, 1001–1016.
25. Bartell, L.R.; Bonassar, L.J.; Cohen, I. A watershed-based algorithm to segment and classify cells in fluorescence microscopy images. *arXiv* **2017**, arXiv:1706.00815.
26. Acharya, V.; Kumar, P. Identification and Red Blood Cell Automated Counting from Blood Smear Images using Computer Aided System. *Med. Biol. Eng. Comput.* **2017**, doi:10.1007/s11517-017-1708-9.
27. Jain, R.; Kasturi, R.; Schunck, B.G. *Machine Vision*; McGraw-Hill: New York, NY, USA, 1995; Volume 5.
28. Zhu, F.; Qin, B.; Feng, W.; Wang, H.; Huang, S.; Lv, Y.; Chen, Y. Reducing Poisson noise and baseline drift in X-ray spectral images with bootstrap Poisson regression and robust nonparametric regression. *Phys. Med. Biol.* **2013**, *58*, 1739.

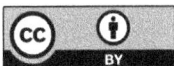

![sensors logo] *sensors*

MDPI

Article

Performance Characterization of a Switchable Acoustic Resolution and Optical Resolution Photoacoustic Microscopy System

Mohesh Moothanchery and Manojit Pramanik *

School of Chemical and Biomedical Engineering, Nanyang Technological University, 62 Nanyang Drive, Singapore 637459, Singapore; mmohesh@ntu.edu.sg
* Correspondence: manojit@ntu.edu.sg; Tel.: +65-6790-5835

Academic Editors: Dragan Indjin, Željka Cvejić and Małgorzata Jędrzejewska-Szczerska
Received: 4 January 2017; Accepted: 9 February 2017; Published: 12 February 2017

Abstract: Photoacoustic microscopy (PAM) is a scalable bioimaging modality; one can choose low acoustic resolution with deep penetration depth or high optical resolution with shallow imaging depth. High spatial resolution and deep penetration depth is rather difficult to achieve using a single system. Here we report a switchable acoustic resolution and optical resolution photoacoustic microscopy (AR-OR-PAM) system in a single imaging system capable of both high resolution and low resolution on the same sample. Lateral resolution of 4.2 μm (with ~1.4 mm imaging depth) and lateral resolution of 45 μm (with ~7.6 mm imaging depth) was successfully demonstrated using a switchable system. In vivo blood vasculature imaging was also performed for its biological application.

Keywords: photoacoustic imaging; AR-PAM; OR-PAM; microscopy; deep tissue imaging

1. Introduction

Photoacoustic microscopy (PAM) is an emerging hybrid in vivo imaging modality, combining optics and ultrasound, which can provide penetration beyond the optical diffusion limit with high resolution. This approach can provide deeper imaging than other optical modalities and has been successfully applied to in vivo structural, functional, molecular, and cell imaging [1–9]. PAM overcomes the limitations of other existing optical modalities combining optical contrast with ultrasound resolution. In PAM, the contrast is related to the optical properties of the tissue, but the resolution is not limited by optical diffusion due to multiple photon scattering. Unlike optical coherence tomography (OCT), PAM does not rely on ballistic or backscattered light. Any light, including both singly and multiply scattered photons, contributes to the imaging signal. As a result, the imaging depth in PAM is relatively large. The key advantages of PAM include (1) combination of high optical contrast and high ultrasonic resolution; (2) good imaging depth; (3) no speckle artifacts; (4) scalable resolution and imaging depth with the ultrasonic frequency; (5) use of non-ionizing radiation (both laser and ultrasound pose no known hazards to humans); and (6) relatively inexpensive.

In PAM, a short laser pulse irradiates the tissue/sample. Due to absorption of light by the tissue chromophores (such as melanin, hemoglobin, and water), there is a temperature rise, which in turn produces pressure waves emitted in the form of acoustics waves. A wideband ultrasonic transducer receives the acoustic signal (known as photoacoustic (PA) waves) outside the tissue/sample boundary. In acoustic resolution photoacoustic microscopy (AR-PAM) deep tissue imaging can be achieved with weak optical and tight acoustic focusing [10–12]. Since AR-PAM lateral resolution is dependent on the ultrasound focus, one can achieve high lateral resolution (~45 μm with 50 MHz focused ultrasound transducer with numerical aperture (NA) 0.44) with an imaging depth of up to 3 mm, as the PA signal in AR-PAM does not depend on the ballistic photons. Resolving single capillaries acoustically need ultrasonic transducers greater than 400 MHz central frequency; however, at this frequency the penetration depth will be less than 100 µm. In optical resolution photoacoustic microscopy (OR-PAM), the lateral resolution can be improved by a tight optical focus; one can achieve a lateral resolution of up to 0.5 µm in the reflection mode and up to 0.2 µm lateral resolution in the transmission mode [13–20]. There were other techniques employed to attain super resolution imaging capability including nonlinear enhancement [17,21], use of double excitation process [22], and use of a photonic nanojet [23,24]. OR-PAM can clearly resolve single capillaries or even a single cell [25]. However, the penetration depth is rather limited due to light focusing and it can image up to ~1.2 mm inside the biological tissue [19]. Therefore, in summary AR-PAM can image deeper, but with lower resolution and OR-PAM can image with very high resolution but limited imaging depth. The imaging speed of the AR- and OR-PAM system mainly depends on the pulse repetition rate of the laser source [26].

Not many efforts have been put to integrate both these systems together. Mostly, two different imaging scanners are used for imaging. However, hybrid imaging with both optical and acoustic resolution PAM enables imaging with scalable resolution and depth. In one approach, the optical and ultrasound focus have been shifted for doing both AR- and OR-PAM. However, since the light focus and ultrasound focus are not aligned, the image quality and resolution was not optimal [27]. In another approach, an optical fiber bundle was used to deliver light for OR- and AR-PAM [28]. In this approach, they have used two separate lasers (high energy laser at 532 nm for the AR and a low energy high repetition rate laser at 570 nm for the OR), making the system inconvenient, expensive, and not suitable for applications including oxygen saturation measurements [29]. In any of these techniques, AR-PAM was not having dark field illumination and hence there were strong photoacoustic signals from the tissue surface. The use of dark field illumination can reduce the generation of strong photoacoustic signals from the skin surface hence deep tissue imaging can be performed using ring-shaped illumination as the detection sensitivity of deep photoacoustic signals will be higher compared to brightfield illumination [12]. Here, we report a switchable AR- and OR-PAM (AR-OR-PAM) imaging system capable of both high-resolution imaging as well as low resolution deep tissue imaging on the same sample utilizing dark field illumination. We use the same laser for both systems. The AR-OR-PAM system was characterized in terms of spatial resolution and imaging depth using phantom experiments. In vivo blood vasculature imaging was performed on mouse ear for demonstrating its biological application.

2. System Description

2.1. The Switchable Acoustic Resolution-Optical Resolution-Photoacoustic Microscopy (AR-OR-PAM) System

The schematic of the AR-OR-PAM system is shown in Figure 1a. Figure 1b shows the photograph of the switchable AR-OR-PAM scanning head. This AR-OR-PAM system employs a nanosecond tunable laser system, consisting of a diode-pumped solid-state Nd-YAG laser (INNOSLAB, Edgewave, Wurselen, Germany) and a dye laser (Credo-DYE-N, Sirah dye laser, Spectra Physics, Santa Clara, CA, USA). The laser system was tunable between 559–576 nm using Rhodamine 6G dye. The wavelength range can be changed depending on the dye used. For example, using DCM dye, the wavelength range can be changed to 602–660 nm. For AR-PAM scanning, the laser beam was diverted using a right angle prism, RAP1 (PS915H-A, Thorlabs, Newton, NJ, USA), placed on a computer controlled motorized stage (CR1/M-Z7, Thorlabs). The diverted beam passed through another right angle prism, RAP2 (PS915H-A, Tholabs), and a variable neutral density filter, NDF2 (NDC-50C-4M, Thorlabs), and coupled on to a multimode fiber, MMF (M29L01, Thorlabs) using a combination of objective (M-10X, Newport, Irvine, CA, USA) and XY translator (CXY1, Thorlabs), which acts as the fiber coupler (FC). The fiber out was fixed on the stage using a translator (TS) (CXY1, Thorlabs). The beam out from the fiber passed through a collimating lens, L1 (LA1951, Thorlabs), and then passed through a conical lens (Con.L), having an apex angle of 130° (1-APX-2-B254, Altechna, Vilnius, Lithuania) to provide a ring-shaped beam. The conical lens was placed on a translating mount, TM1 (CT1, Thorlabs). The ring shaped beam was allowed to focus weakly onto the subject with the focal region coaxially overlapping the ultrasonic focus inside the tissue using a homemade optical condenser (OC) (cone angles: 70°, 110°), having a 50 MHz ultrasonic transducer (UST) (V214-BB-RM, Olympus-NDT, Waltham, MA, USA) in the center. An acoustic lens (AL) (LC4573, Thorlabs) having a radius of curvature of 4.6 mm and a 6 mm diameter was attached using a UV curing optical adhesive (NOA61, Thorlabs) to the bottom of the transducer, which provided an acoustic focal diameter of ~46 μm. In an optically clear medium, the optical focus was around 2 mm in diameter, which was wider than the ultrasonic focus. This type of dark field illumination is beneficial for deep tissue imaging where there are no strong signals from the tissue surface. The laser repetition rate (LRR) was set to be 1 kHz, and the laser energy at focus can be varied up to 30 μJ per pulse. The optical illumination on the object surface was donut shaped with a dark center so that no strong photoacoustic signals were produced from the surface on the object within the ultrasonic field of view. In our setup, all components were integrated and assembled in an optical cage setup. For AR, both 30 mm and 60 mm optical cages (OC connected in 60 mm cage) were used. The use of the cage system made the AR setup compact and easier to assemble and align.

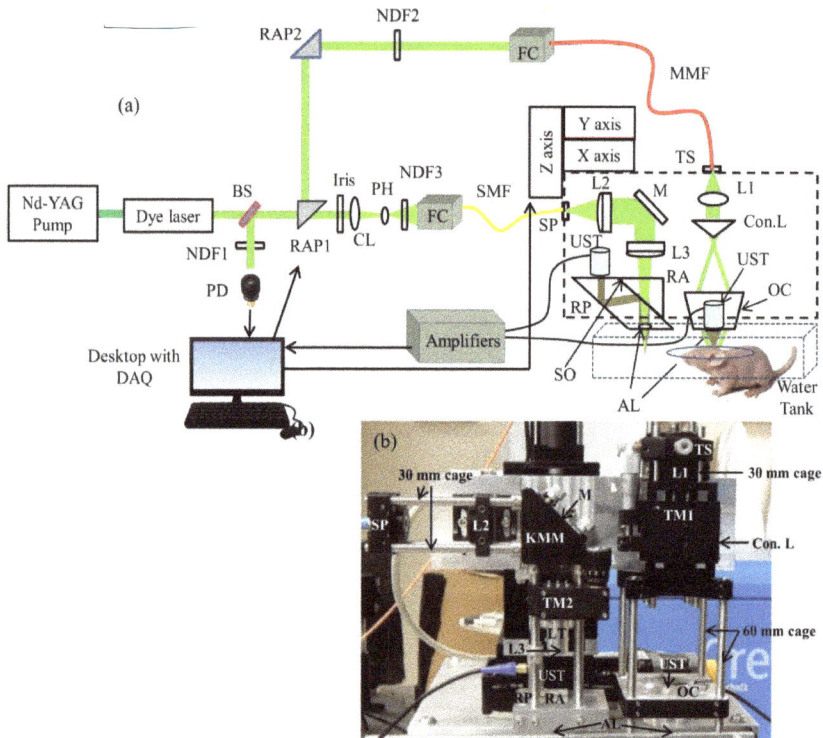

Figure 1. (a) Schematic of the Acoustic Resolution—Optical Resolution—Photoacoustic Microscopy (AR-OR-PAM) imaging system. BS: beam sampler; NDF: neutral density filter; RAP: right angle prism; PD: photodiode; CL: condenser lens; PH: pinhole; FC: fiber coupler; UST: ultrasound transducer; MMF: multimode fiber; SMF: single mode fiber; DAQ: data acquisition card; TS: translation stage; Con.L: conical lens; L1: convex lens; L2 & L3: achromatic lens; RA: right angle prism; RP: rhomboid prism; OC: optical condenser; M: mirror; SP: slip plate; LT: lens tube; TM: translation mount; KMM: kinematic mirror mount; AL: acoustic lens; **(b)** Photograph of the prototype AR-OR-PAM system.

For the OR-PAM setup, the rotational stage (holding the RAP1) would rotate at 90° so that the laser beam went straight and was reshaped by an iris (ID12/M, Thorlabs) and then focused by a condenser lens, CL (LA4327, Thorlabs), and passed through a 50 μm pinhole, PH (P50S, Thorlabs), for spatial filtering. The filtered beam was attenuated by a variable neutral density filter, NDF3 (NDC-50C-4M, Thorlabs), and launched on to a single-mode fiber, SMF (P1-460B-FC-1, Thorlabs), using a single mode fiber coupler, FC (F-91-C1, Newport). The output port of the single-mode fiber was placed on a slip plate positioner, SP (SPT1, Thorlabs). The output beam from the SMF was then collimated by an achromatic lens, L2 (32-317, Edmund Optics, Barrington, New Jersey, United States) was reflected by a stationary elliptical mirror, M (PFE10-P01, Thorlabs), was fixed on a Kinematic mirror mount, KMM (KCB1, Thorlabs), and filled the back aperture of another identical achromatic lens, L3, placed on a translation mount, TM2 (SM1Z, Thorlabs). The achromatic lens was placed on the translation mount with the help of a lens tube, LT (SM05L10, Thorlabs). The effective clear aperture of the achromatic lens through the tube was 10.9 mm, which makes the effective numerical aperture (NA) of the achromatic lens as 0.11. The beam then passed through an optoacoustic beam combiner consisting of a right angled prism, RA (PS615, Thorlabs) and a rhomboid prism, RP (47-214, Edmund optics) with a layer of silicon oil, SO (DMPS1M, Sigma Aldrich, St. Louis, MI, USA) in between. The silicon oil layer acts as optically transparent and acoustically reflective film. An acoustic lens, AL (LC4573, Thorlabs) provided acoustic focusing (a focal diameter of ~46 μm), was attached at the bottom of the rhomboid prism. The ultrasonic transducer, a 50 MHz center frequency (V214-BB-RM, Olympus-NDT), was placed on top of the rhomboid with an epoxy layer from a single part of a two part epoxy (G14250, Thorlabs) for effective coupling. To maximize the detection sensitivity, the optical and acoustic foci were aligned confocally. The laser repetition rate for the OR-PAM was set to 5 kHz and the laser energy at focus could be varied up to 200 nJ per pulse. Like AR, the OR systems components were also integrated and assembled in a 30 mm optical cage system.

The AR-OR combined system was attached to a homemade plate that helps in switching between AR and OR scanhead easily by sliding the scanhead on top of the imaging area. At present, the *y*-axis translation stage used has a range of 5 cm; therefore, the switching between the AR and OR systems was done by manual sliding. However, if one uses the *y*-axis translation stage with a 10 cm range, manual transition can be avoided. The AR-OR combined scanner head was attached to a 3-axis motorized stage (PLS 85 for *X* and *Y* axis, VT 80 for *Z* axis, PI—Physik Instrumente, Karlsruhe, Germany). All three stages were controlled by a 3-axis controller (SMC corvus eco, PI micos) connected to the computer. For photoacoustic imaging, the bottom of the AR-OR-PAM scanner head was submerged in a water-filled tank (13 cm × 30 cm) for acoustic coupling. An imaging window of 7 cm × 7 cm was opened at the bottom of the tank and sealed with a polyethylene membrane for optical and acoustic transmission. The PA signal acquired by the UST was amplified by two amplifiers (ZFL-500LN, Mini Circuits, Brooklyn, NY, USA) each having a 24 dB gain, and was recorded using a data acquisition (DAQ) card, (M4i.4420, Spectrum, Grosshansdorf, Germany) in a desktop computer (Intel xeon E5-1630 3.7 GHz processor, 16 GB RAM, 64 bit windows 10 operating system). The DAQ card had a 16 bit analog-to-digital converter (ADC), a 250 Ms/s sampling rate, 2 channels, and a 4 GB on-board memory. The same desktop computer was used for both AR and OR-PAM systems. The scanning and data acquisition was controlled using Labview software (National Instrument). Two-dimensional continuous raster scanning of the imaging head was used during image acquisition. The time-resolved PA signals were multiplied by the speed of sound, 1540 m/s in soft tissue [30] to obtain an A-line. Multiple A-lines were captured during the continuous motion of the Y stage to produce a two-dimensional B-scan. Multiple B-scans of the imaging area were captured and stored in the computer. MATLAB (MathWorks, Natick, MA, USA) was used to process and obtain the maximum amplitude projection (MAP) photoacoustic images.

The synchronization of the data acquisition and the stage motion was controlled by the signal from a photodiode (PD) (SM05PD1A, Thorlabs). A beamsampler, BS (BF10-A, Thorlabs), was placed in front of the laser beam diverted a small portion of the beam (5%) to the PD. A neutral density filter,

NDF 1 (NDC-50C-4M, Thorlabs), was placed in front of the PD to control the energy falling on the PD. The PD signal can also used for compensating pulse-to-pulse laser energy variations during data acquisition. All experiments were done at a laser wavelength of 570 nm in this work.

2.2. Laser Safety

For in vivo imaging, the maximum permissible pulse energy is governed by American National Standards Institute (ANSI) laser safety standards [31]. The safety limit varies with illumination wavelength, pulse duration, exposure duration, and exposure area. The maximum pulse energy by a single laser pulse (MPE_{SP}) on the skin surface should not exceed $MPE_{SP} = 2C_A 10^{-2}$ J/cm^2, where C_A the wavelength correction factor, is unity for visible wavelength range (400–700 nm). The irradiance should not exceed 200 mW/cm^2 if a point on skin is exposed to more than 10 s. In the case of raster scanning, a point on the skin will not be exposed for 10 s; hence, the maximum permissible exposure (MPE_{AVE}) is limited by 1.1 $C_A t^{0.25}$ mJ/cm^2, where t denotes the exposure duration in seconds.

For AR-PAM, the diameter of the optical focus at the ultrasound focus was 2 mm. Having a minimum pixel separation of 15 μm, an average of 133 (N) adjacent laser pulses overlap at the ultrasound focus. At 1 kHz LRR, the exposure time was 133 ms, so the maximum pulse energy for the pulse train (MPE_{TRAIN}) was 664 mJ/cm^2 (1.1 $C_A t^{0.25}$). The MPE_{SP} for the pulse train was $MPE_{AVG} = MPE_{TRAIN}/N = 664/133 = 5$ mJ/cm^2. The current AR-PAM system can deliver per pulse energy of 0.32 mJ/cm^2 (30 μJ/pulse, 2 mm diameter focus), which is well below the MPE_{SP} safety limit. For AR-PAM experiments, we used a pulse energy of 30 μJ/pulse for imaging depth and 6 μJ/pulse for the resolution test and in vivo ear blood vasculature imaging.

For OR-PAM, we believe the effect of optical aberrations at the prism surface and acoustic lens might have reduced the objective NA from 0.11 to 0.075, which will give a spot size diameter of 3.9 μm (which agrees with our lateral resolution). Assuming the optical focus is 150 micron below the skin surface for in vivo imaging, the surface spot size was 22.5 μm in diameter. Having a minimum pixel separation of 2 μm, an average of 11 (N) adjacent laser pulses overlaps on the skin surface. At 5 kHz LRR, the exposure time was 2.4 ms. Therefore, the MPE_{TRAIN} was 238 mJ/cm^2. The MPE_{SP} for the pulse train was $MPE_{AVG} = MPE_{TRAIN}/N = 238/11 = 21.6$ mJ/cm^2. The current OR-PAM system can deliver an MPE_{SP} of 20.4 mJ/cm^2 (90 nJ/pulse, 0.075 NA) at the skin surface (close to the safety limit). For OR-PAM experiments, we used a pulse energy of 20 nJ/pulse for the resolution test and 90 nJ/pulse for imaging depth and in vivo ear blood vasculature imaging.

3. Experimental Methods

In order to evaluate the system performance of the switchable AR-OR-PAM system, a series of experiments were conducted to determine the spatial resolution and the maximum imaging depths for both AR- and OR-PAM. In vivo imaging was also done using the switchable system to show the biological imaging capability of the system.

3.1. Spatial Resolution Quantification

The lateral resolution of the AR and OR system was determined by imaging a 100 nm gold nanoparticle (742031, Sigma Aldrich). To determine the resolution of the AR-PAM system, a single nanoparticle was scanned with a step size of 5 microns. Similarly, the nanoparticle was scanned with a step size of 0.5 microns in order to find the resolution of the OR-PAM system. The photoacoustic amplitude along the central lateral direction of the nanoparticle image was fitted to a Gaussian function. The full width at half maximum (FWHM) of the Gaussian fit was considered the lateral resolution. Theoretically, the optical diffraction-limited lateral resolution for the OR-PAM was calculated from 0.51 λ/NA, where λ was the laser wavelength, and NA was the numerical aperture of the objective. Similarly, the theoretical lateral resolution for the AR-PAM was determined using the equation 0.72 λ/NA, where λ was the central acoustic wavelength, and NA was the numerical aperture of the ultrasonic transducer. The photoacoustic axial spread profile from the nanoparticle was used to determine the axial resolution of the system. Both OR-PAM and AR-PAM share the same axial resolution since the same ultrasound transducer (and the focusing lens) was used in both systems. The axial resolution was determined by acoustic parameters according to 0.88 c/Δf, where c is the speed of sound in soft tissue, and Δf is the frequency bandwidth of the ultrasonic transducer. Since the size of the nanoparticle was much smaller than the axial resolution, the axial spread profile can be considered as axial point spread function of the imaging system. The FWHM of the envelope gives the axial resolution. The axial resolution was also calculated by numerically shifting and summing two A-line signals and by checking whether the two peaks could be differentiated in the envelope with a contrast-to-noise ratio (CNR) greater than 2. The CNR was plotted against the shift between the two impulse responses. The contrast was defined as the difference between the smaller of the two peaks in the photoacoustic envelope and the valley between the peaks. The noise was the standard deviation in the background photoacoustic signal.

3.2. USAF Resolution Test Target Imaging

The lateral resolution of the AR and OR system was further validated imaging a USAF 1951 test target (R1DS1P, Thorlabs). Initially, a 5 mm × 5 mm area (Group numbers 2 to 7) were scanned using AR-PAM. The scan step size was 10 μm in both X and Y directions. Similarly, a 1.3 mm × 1.3 mm area (Group numbers 4 to 7) was scanned using OR-PAM with a step size of 0.5 μm in both X and Y directions. Finally, a 0.3 mm × 0.3 mm area consisting of the smallest groups (Group Numbers 6 and 7) were scanned using OR-PAM imaging with a step size of 0.5 μm in both X and Y directions.

3.3. Imaging Depth

To determine the maximum imaging depth of both AR-PAM and OR-PAM, a black tape was inserted obliquely on a chicken tissue. A single B-scan image was captured using both AR-PAM and OR-PAM. The signal-to-noise ratio (SNR) was also determined at the maximum imaging depth. SNR is defined as V/n, where V is the peak-to-peak PA signal amplitude, and n is the standard deviation of the background noise.

3.4. In Vivo Imaging of Mouse Ear Blood Vasculature

To demonstrate in vivo imaging using the combined system, the ears of 4-week-old female mice with body weights of 25 g, procured from InVivos Pte. Ltd. (Singapore), were used. Animal experiments were performed according to the approved guidelines and regulations by the institutional Animal Care and Use committee of Nanyang Technological University, Singapore (Animal Protocol Number ARF-SBS/NIE-A0263). The animal was anesthetized using a cocktail of ketamine (120 mg/kg) and xylazine (16 mg/kg) injected intraperitoneally (dosage of 0.1 mL/10 g, body weight). After removing hair from the ear, the mouse was positioned on a platform that also has a miniature plate to position the ear. The animal was further anesthetized with vaporized isoflurane system (1 L/min oxygen and 0.75% isoflurane) during the imaging period. The imaging region was placed into contact with the polyethylene membrane using ultrasound gel. Using AR-PAM, a large area (9 mm × 7 mm) of the ear was first imaged, using a step size of 15 μm in the Y direction and 30 μm in the X direction. The same area (4.5 mm × 5 mm) was scanned using OR-PAM with a step size of 2 μm in the Y direction and 3 μm in the X direction.

4. Results and Discussion

4.1. Spatial Resolution of the Imaging System

The lateral resolution of the AR-PAM is shown in Figure 2a. The measured lateral resolution is 45 μm determined by FWHM. Similarly, lateral resolution of OR-PAM is shown in Figure 2b. The measured lateral resolution determined from the FWHM is 4.2 μm. The inset of the figures shows the corresponding PAM image of the gold nanoparticle.

Figure 2c shows the axial spread profile of the averaged PA signal from the gold nanoparticle and its envelope. The axial resolution was measured to be 33 μm. The experimentally determined axial resolution matches closely to the theoretical axial resolution of 29 μm. The simulated results in Figure 2d show that we can distinguish the two absorbers separated by 16.5 μm with a CNR of 2. Figure 2e shows the plot of CNR versus axial shift.

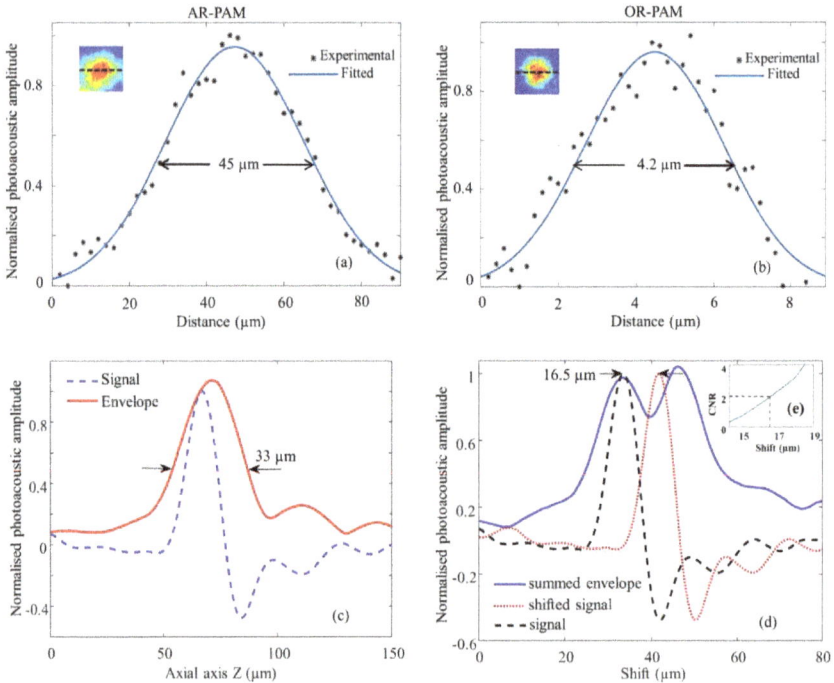

Figure 2. Spatial resolution test of the AR-OR-PAM system: Lateral resolution estimated by imaging gold nanoparticles ~100 nm diameter, Black (*) dots: photoacoustic signal; blue line: Gaussian-fitted curve; (**a**) AR-PAM; (**b**) OR-PAM. The inset shows the representative AR-PAM image in (**a**) and OR-PAM image in (**b**) of the single gold nanoparticle; (**c**) Photoacoustic axial spread profile and its envelope; (**d**) Simulated photoacoustic shift-and-sum A-line signals. The dashed line and dotted line indicate two photoacoustic signals 16.5 μm apart. The solid line indicates the summed envelope of the two shifted signals; (**e**) Contrast-to-noise ratio (CNR) versus the shift distance between the two signals.

4.2. USAF Resolution Test Target Imaging

MAP AR-PAM image of a USAF resolution test target is shown in Figure 3a. From Figure 3a,d, we can see that the AR-PAM system is capable of resolving 49.61 μm line pairs (Group 3, Element 3) with a modulation transfer function (MTF) of 0.28. Figure 3b is a MAP OR-PAM image done on the red dotted area shown in Figure 3a.

Figure 3c shows the MAP OR-PAM image done on the yellow dotted area on Figure 3b. From Figure 3c,d, we can see that the OR-PAM system can clearly resolve 3.91 μm line pairs (Group 7, Element 1) with an MTF of 0.64. Theoretically, the optical diffraction-limited lateral resolution for the OR-PAM is 2.6 μm. The experimentally measured lateral resolution was poorer than the diffraction-limit estimate, which might be due to wavefront aberrations. Similarly, the theoretical lateral resolution for the AR-PAM is 46 μm. The theoretical resolution agrees well with our experimental data.

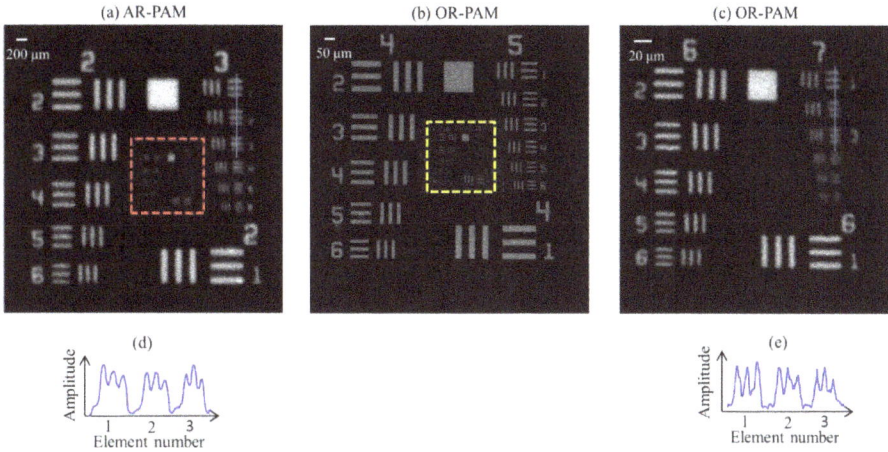

Figure 3. Lateral resolution test of the AR-OR-PAM system: (**a**) AR-PAM image of an air force resolution test target; (**b**) OR-PAM image of the red dotted area; (**c**) OR-PAM image of the yellow dotted region of the test target; (**d**) The cross-sectional profile of the first two elements in Group 3 of the resolution target, blue line in (**a**); (**e**) The cross-sectional profile of the first three elements in Group 7 of the resolution target, blue line in (**c**).

4.3. Imaging Depth

Figure 4a shows the schematic of a black tape obliquely inserted on chicken tissue. Figure 4b shows the B-scan PA image from AR-PAM. It is evident that the AR-PAM system can clearly image the black tape down to ~7.6 mm beneath the tissue surface. Similarly, using the OR-PAM system, we can clearly image the black tape down to ~1.4 mm beneath the tissue surface. For AR-PAM, the SNR at 4.6 mm and 7.6 mm imaging depth were 2.5 and 1.4, respectively. In case of OR-PAM, the SNR of the target object (black tape) at 1.4 mm imaging depth was 1.5.

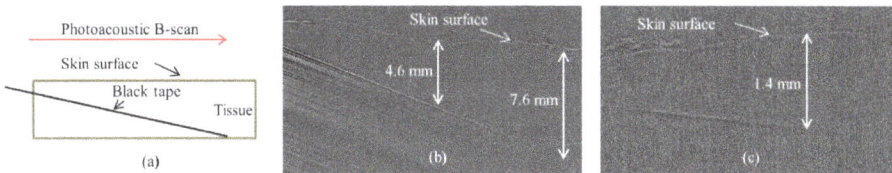

Figure 4. Single B-scan PA image of a black tape inserted obliquely in a chicken tissue. (**a**) Schematic diagram; (**b**) AR-PAM image; (**c**) OR-PAM image.

4.4. In Vivo Imaging of Mouse Ear Blood Vasculature

Figure 5a shows the photograph of the mouse ear vasculature. A unidirectional B-scan imaging of 9 mm × 7 mm area using AR-PAM took 10 min to complete. The MAP image of AR-PAM is show in Figure 5b. Figure 5c shows the zoomed out image of the white dotted region in Figure 5b. The same area as in Figure 5b (4.5 mm × 5 mm) was scanned using OR-PAM (imaging time 50 min). The MAP image of the OR-PAM is shown in Figure 5d. Figure 5c,d are the same region scanned with AR-PAM and OR-PAM. We can see OR-PAM can clearly resolve single capillaries that AR-PAM cannot resolve. AR-PAM can resolve deep vessels thicker than 45 μm. Figure 5e shows the zoomed out area (white dotted region in Figure 5d). Due to the high resolution of the OR-PAM, the region appears clearer, and smaller structures are also visible.

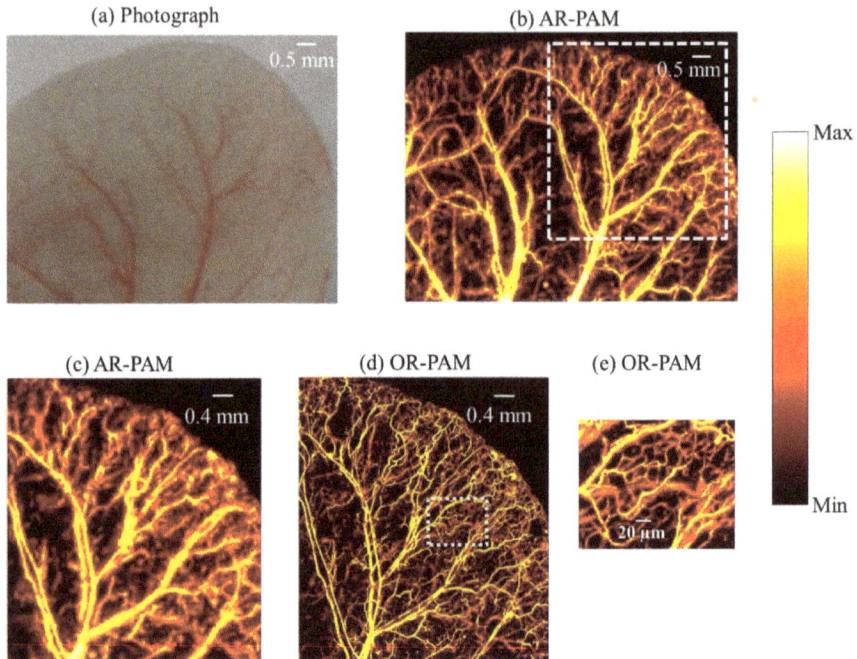

(a) Photograph
(b) AR-PAM
0.5 mm
0.5 mm
Max
(c) AR-PAM
0.4 mm
(d) OR-PAM
0.4 mm
(e) OR-PAM
20 µm
Min

Figure 5. In vivo photoacoustic image of mouse ear: (**a**) photograph of the mouse ear vasculature; (**b**) AR-PAM image; (**c**) close up of the region of interest (ROI) in (**b**) as shown by white dash line; (**d**) OR-PAM image of the same ROI; (**e**) close up of the region of interest in (**d**) as shown by white dotted line.

In summary, a switchable AR-OR-PAM system that can achieve high-resolution imaging utilizing optical focusing as well as deep tissue imaging using dark field illumination and acoustic focusing was developed. This combined photoacoustic microscopy system can provide high spatial resolution, which makes the system important for applications including imaging of angiogenesis and drug response, where imaging single capillaries as well as deep vasculatures will be important. Further improvement in the system can be done by replacing the switchable plate with a 10 cm traveling motorized stage (*y*-axis). Wavefront aberration corrections for the OR-PAM will improve the lateral resolution further. Delivering higher pulse energy to the AR-PAM will improve the SNR and imaging depths as well. The limitations of the proposed technique include the scanning speed. Currently longer scanning time is required, which can be further reduced by acquiring data in both directions during imaging. High speed imaging using OR-PAM was reported by the use of a high repetition rate laser and a water immersible MEMS (microelectromechanical system) mirror [32]. Simultaneous image acquisition using both AR-PAM and OR-PAM is not possible at the moment. Developing a system that can do simultaneous data acquisition using OR-PAM and dark field AR-PAM would have been more advantageous.

5. Conclusions

A switchable acoustic resolution and optical resolution photoacoustic microscopy system that can achieve both high-resolution imaging at lower imaging depth and lower resolution imaging at higher imaging depth was developed. This is the first combined system using the same laser, which can be easily switched between OR-PAM and dark field AR-PAM. The combined system will have a 4.2 µm resolution with a 1.4 mm imaging depth, as well as a 45 µm resolution with a 7.6 mm imaging depth.

Sensors **2017**, *17*, 357

The system is made of minimal homemade components, making it easier to assemble, align, and build. Using the combined system, in vivo imaging was successfully demonstrated. The developed system can be used for pre-clinical imaging. Major preclinical applications include imaging of angiogenesis, microcirculation, tumor microenvironments, drug response, brain functions, biomarkers, and gene activities.

Acknowledgments: The authors would like to acknowledge the financial support from Tier 2 grant funded by the Ministry of Education in Singapore (ARC2/15: M4020238). The authors would like to thank Benjamin Tay Wee Ann for Labview programming and Chow Wai Hoong Bobby for machine shop help. The authors would also like to thank Lidai Wang (City University of Hong Kong), Liang Song (Shenzhen Institute of Advanced Technology, Chinese Academy of Science), Junjie Yao (Duke University), and Song Hu (University of Virginia) for useful discussions.

Author Contributions: M.M. and M.P. conceived and designed the system and experiments. M.M. developed the system; performed the experiments; analyzed the data; wrote the paper. M.P. supervised the project. All authors contributed to critical reading of the manuscript.

Conflicts of Interest: The authors declare no conflict of interest.

References

1. Wang, L.V.; Yao, J. A practical guide to photoacoustic tomography in the life sciences. *Nat. Methods* **2016**, *13*, 627–638. [CrossRef] [PubMed]
2. Zhou, Y.; Yao, J.; Wang, L.V. Tutorial on photoacoustic tomography. *J. Biomed. Opt.* **2016**, *21*, 061007. [CrossRef] [PubMed]
3. Yao, J.; Wang, L.V. Photoacoustic Brain Imaging: From Microscopic to Macroscopic Scales. *Neurophotonics* **2014**, *1*, 011003. [CrossRef] [PubMed]
4. Wang, L.V.; Hu, S. Photoacoustic Tomography: In Vivo Imaging from Organelles to Organs. *Science* **2012**, *335*, 1458–1462. [CrossRef] [PubMed]
5. Beard, P. Biomedical photoacoustic imaging. *Interface Focus* **2011**, *1*, 602–631. [CrossRef] [PubMed]
6. Pan, D.; Pramanik, M.; Senpan, A.; Allen, J.S.; Zhang, H.; Wickline, S.A.; Wang, L.V.; Lanza, G.M. Molecular photoacoustic imaging of angiogenesis with integrin-targeted gold nanobeacons. *FASEB J.* **2011**, *25*, 875–882. [CrossRef] [PubMed]
7. Pan, D.; Pramanik, M.; Senpan, A.; Ghosh, S.; Wickline, S.A.; Wang, L.V.; Lanza, G.M. Near infrared photoacoustic detection of sentinel lymph nodes with gold nanobeacons. *Biomaterials* **2010**, *31*, 4088–4093. [CrossRef] [PubMed]
8. Wang, L.V. Multiscale photoacoustic microscopy and computed tomography. *Nat. Photonics* **2009**, *3*, 503–509. [CrossRef] [PubMed]
9. Zhang, E.Z.; Laufer, J.G.; Pedley, R.B.; Beard, P.C. In vivo high-resolution 3D photoacoustic imaging of superficial vascular anatomy. *Phys. Med. Biol.* **2009**, *54*, 1035–1046. [CrossRef] [PubMed]
10. Park, S.; Lee, C.; Kim, J.; Kim, C. Acoustic resolution photoacoustic microscopy. *Biom. Eng. Lett.* **2014**, *4*, 213–222. [CrossRef]
11. Zhang, H.F.; Maslov, K.; Stoica, G.; Wang, L.V. Functional photoacoustic microscopy for high-resolution and noninvasive in vivo imaging. *Nat. Biotechnol.* **2006**, *24*, 848–851. [CrossRef] [PubMed]
12. Maslov, K.; Stoica, G.; Wang, L.V. In vivo dark-field reflection-mode photoacoustic microscopy. *Opt. Lett.* **2005**, *30*, 625–627. [CrossRef] [PubMed]
13. Zhang, C.; Maslov, K.; Wang, L.V. Subwavelength-resolution label-free photoacoustic microscopy of optical absorption in vivo. *Opt. Lett.* **2010**, *35*, 3195–3197. [CrossRef] [PubMed]
14. Kim, J.Y.; Lee, C.; Park, K.; Lim, G.; Kim, C. Fast optical-resolution photoacoustic microscopy using a 2-axis water-proofing MEMS scanner. *Sci. Rep.* **2015**, *5*, 07932. [CrossRef] [PubMed]
15. Matthews, T.P.; Zhang, C.; Yao, D.K.; Maslov, K.; Wang, L.V. Label-free photoacoustic microscopy of peripheral nerves. *J. Biomed. Opt.* **2014**, *19*, 016004. [CrossRef] [PubMed]
16. Hai, P.; Yao, J.; Maslov, K.I.; Zhou, Y.; Wang, L.V. Near-infrared optical-resolution photoacoustic microscopy. *Opt. Lett.* **2014**, *39*, 5192–5195. [CrossRef] [PubMed]
17. Danielli, A.; Maslov, K.; Garcia-Uribe, A.; Winkler, A.M.; Li, C.; Wang, L.; Chen, Y.; Dorn, G.W., 2nd; Wang, L.V. Label-free photoacoustic nanoscopy. *J. Biomed. Opt.* **2014**, *19*, 086006. [CrossRef] [PubMed]

18. Zhang, C.; Maslov, K.; Hu, S.; Chen, R.; Zhou, Q.; Shung, K.K.; Wang, L.V. Reflection-mode submicron-resolution in vivo photoacoustic microscopy. *J. Biomed. Opt.* **2012**, *17*, 020501. [CrossRef] [PubMed]

19. Hu, S.; Maslov, K.; Wang, L.V. Second-generation optical-resolution photoacoustic microscopy with improved sensitivity and speed. *Opt. Lett.* **2011**, *36*, 1134–1136. [CrossRef] [PubMed]

20. Maslov, K.; Zhang, H.F.; Song, H.; Wang, L.V. Optical-resolution photoacoustic microscopy for in vivo imaging of single capillaries. *Opt. Lett.* **2008**, *33*, 929–931. [CrossRef] [PubMed]

21. Nedosekin, D.A.; Galanzha, E.I.; Dervishi, E.; Biris, A.S.; Zharov, V.P. Super-resolution nonlinear photothermal microscopy. *Small* **2014**, *10*, 135–142. [CrossRef] [PubMed]

22. Yao, J.; Wang, L.; Li, C.; Zhang, C.; Wang, L.V. Photoimprint Photoacoustic Microscopy for Three-Dimensional Label-Free Subdiffraction Imaging. *Phys. Rev. Lett.* **2014**, *112*, 014302. [CrossRef] [PubMed]

23. Upputuri, P.K.; Krishnan, M.; Pramanik, M. Microsphere enabled sub-diffraction limited optical resolution photoacoustic microscopy: A simulation study. *J. Biomed. Opt.* **2017**, *22*, 045001. [CrossRef] [PubMed]

24. Upputuri, P.K.; Wen, Z.-B.; Wu, Z.; Pramanik, M. Super-resolution photoacoustic microscopy using photonic nanojets: A simulation study. *J. Biomed. Opt.* **2014**, *19*, 116003. [CrossRef] [PubMed]

25. Strohm, E.M.; Moore, M.J.; Kolios, M.C. Single Cell Photoacoustic Microscopy: A Review. *IEEE J. Sel. Top. Quant. Electron.* **2016**, *22*, 6801215. [CrossRef]

26. Allen, T.J.; Berendt, M.O.; Spurrell, J.; Alam, S.U.; Zhang, E.Z.; Richardson, D.J.; Beard, P.C. Novel Fibre Lasers as Excitation Sources for Photoacoustic Tomography and Microscopy. *Proc. SPIE* **2016**, *9708*, 97080W-1.

27. Estrada, H.; Turner, J.; Kneipp, M.; Razansky, D. Real-time optoacoustic brain microscopy with hybrid optical and acoustic resolution. *Laser Phys. Lett.* **2014**, *11*, 045601. [CrossRef]

28. Xing, W.; Wang, L.; Maslov, K.; Wang, L.V. Integrated optical- and acoustic-resolution photoacoustic microscopy based on an optical fiber bundle. *Opt. Lett.* **2013**, *38*, 52–54. [CrossRef] [PubMed]

29. Jeon, S.; Kim, J.; Kim, C. In Vivo Switchable Optical- and Acoustic-Resolution Photoacoustic Microscopy. *Proc. SPIE* **2016**, *9708*. [CrossRef]

30. Madsen, E.L.; Zagzebski, J.A.; Banjavie, R.A.; Jutila, R.E. Tissue mimicking materials for ultrasound phantoms. *Med. Phys.* **1978**, *5*, 391–394. [CrossRef] [PubMed]

31. American National Standard for Safe Use of Lasers. *ANSI Standard Z136.1–2000*; Laser Institute of America: Orlando, FL, USA, 2000.

32. Yao, J.; Wang, L.; Yang, J.M.; Maslov, K.I.; Wong, T.T.W.; Li, L.; Huang, C.H.; Zou, J.; Wang, L.V. High-speed label-free functional photoacoustic microscopy of mouse brain in action. *Nat. Methods* **2015**, *12*, 407–410. [CrossRef] [PubMed]

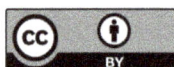

sensors

MDPI

Article

Biomechanical Modeling of Pterygium Radiation Surgery: A Retrospective Case Study

Bojan Pajic [1,2,3,4], Daniel M. Aebersold [5], Andreas Eggspuehler [6], Frederik R. Theler [7] and Harald P. Studer [1,8,*]

1   Eye Clinic Orasis, Swiss Eye Research Foundation, CH-5734 Reinach, Switzerland; bpajic@datacomm.ch
2   Department of Physics, Faculty of Sciences, University of Novi Sad, 21000 Novi Sad, Serbia
3   Division of Ophthalmology, Department of Clinical Neurosciences, Geneva University Hospitals, CH-1205 Geneva, Switzerland
4   Faculty of Medicine of the Military Medical Academy, University of Defence, 11000 Belgrade, Serbia
5   Department of Radiation Oncology, Inselspital, Bern University Hospital, University of Bern, CH-3010 Bern, Switzerland; daniel.aebersold@insel.ch
6   Department of Neurology, Schulthess Klinik, CH-8008 Zuerich, Switzerland; a.eggspuehler@gmx.net
7   Optimo Medical, CH-2503 Biel, Switzerland; frederik.theler@optimo-medical.com
8   OCTlab, Department of Ophthalmology, University of Basel, CH-4001 Basel, Switzerland
*   Correspondence: harald.studer@gmail.com; Tel.: +41-76-588-4619

Academic Editors: Dragan Indjin and Małgorzata Jędrzejewska-Szczerska
Received: 31 March 2017; Accepted: 19 May 2017; Published: 24 May 2017

Abstract: Pterygium is a vascularized, invasive transformation on the anterior corneal surface that can be treated by Strontium-/Yttrium90 beta irradiation. Finite element modeling was used to analyze the biomechanical effects governing the treatment, and to help understand clinically observed changes in corneal astigmatism. Results suggested that irradiation-induced pulling forces on the anterior corneal surface can cause astigmatism, as well as central corneal flattening. Finite element modeling of corneal biomechanics closely predicted the postoperative corneal surface (astigmatism error −0.01D; central curvature error −0.16D), and can help in understanding beta irradiation treatment. Numerical simulations have the potential to preoperatively predict corneal shape and function changes, and help to improve corneal treatments.

Keywords: pterygium; radiation; cornea surgery; biomechanics; finite element modeling; simulation

1. Introduction

Pterygium, also called Surfer's Eye, is a vascularized, invasive transformation growing on the anterior corneal surface, starting in the conjunctiva near the limbal region and with expanding towards the corneal center. The Bowmann's membrane, underneath the epithelium, thereby serves as a controlling structure for the pterygium. Besides UV light, the following co-factors promoting the development of a pterygium have been reported in literature: chronic exposure to ultraviolet light in combination with hot and dry climate, chronic irritation by dust, and frequent exposure to wind [1]. The in-growth almost exclusively starts nasally (92%) [2], possibly because in that area the rays from the sun pass laterally through the cornea, intensifying the tissues' exposure to UV light.

Even though co-factors are named, the main etiological reason for developing a pterygium is ultraviolet light exposure [3,4], as a recent mathematical model demonstrated that ultraviolet irradiation can lead to limbal stem cell dysfunction [5–7]. The fact that Fibroblast Growth Factor (FGF), Vascular Endothelial Growth Factor (VEGF), Transforming Growth Factor β (TGF β), and Stem Cell Factor (SCM) are increased in pterygial tissue [8–10], while IGFBP3 is decreased, further suggests that growth proliferation is not controlled in the same way as in tumor cells and, as a consequence, that pterygium is not neoplasia. Rather, it is a degenerative alteration [11], as VEGF leads to angiogenesis and SCM to the modulation of mast cells.

Various surgical treatments for pterygium have been suggested in the past and have been frequently employed in the field. However, depending on the technique, the recurrence rate of pterygium used to be relatively high, in a range from 35% to 68% [12–14]. More modern surgical procedures involving the implementation of antimetabolites, such as Mitomycin C, or the introduction of radiotherapy, decrease the recurrence rate down to a level of 1.7% to 12.5% [2,6,15–18]. Furthermore, therapy concepts such as pterygium excision with conjunctival autografts and subconjunctival amniotic membranes also reduce this rate down to a level of ~1% [19].

In their previous research [5–7,10,20], the authors of these papers showed that with the introduction of Strontium-/Yttrium-90 beta-irradiation as an exclusive, non-surgical treatment, no recurrences have occurred to date. Even though the result of beta-irradiation treatment is an inactive pterygium without vessels, the procedure may induce certain amounts of corneal astigmatism [5–7,10,20]. The authors hypothesized that the observed changes in cylinder value may stem from pulling forces placed the cornea by the retracting pterygium. Hence, it is of great importance to understand the underlying biomechanical connection between beta-irradiation and its pterygium reduction, as well as the induction of corneal astigmatism. The goal of this study is to develop a mathematical model to describe the governing biomechanical processes.

2. Materials and Methods

The right eye of a 56-year-old female subject, diagnosed with pterygium, was treated with Strontium-/Yttrium-90 irradiation treatment (see Figure 1a). Preoperative Pentacam (Oculus Optikgeräte GmbH, Wetzlar, Germany) measurements were taken to create a subject-specific finite element model. The model was numerically simulated using the Optimeyes software (Optimo Medical AG, Biel, Switzerland), employing an earlier published [21–25] constitutive material model. Optimeyes is a comprehensive technology platform for the simulation and prediction of corneal shape and function changes, caused by mechanical interferences with the tissue. The software allowed us to create patient-specific finite element models from anterior segment tomography measurement data, compute initial stress-distribution, and run numerical simulations of cornea surgical treatments. Simulation results were then compared to the 25-month postoperative follow-up Pentacam measurements. Comparison included corneal shape and corneal function analysis.

2.1. Pterygium Surgery with Beta Irradiation

A convex plate with a diameter of 12 mm, attached to a pen-like holder, was used as a Strontium-/Yttrium-90 applicator. The radioactive substance was attached to the inner surface of the plate, and softly put onto the eye, well centered over the pterygium. To reduce irradiation exposure of the surrounding tissue, a surround of 0.002 mm stainless steel and 0.01 mm aluminum, fitted to the edge of the applicator plate, filtered the original Strontium-90 irradiation down to 3%, and the Yttrium-90 down to 60%. The irradiation application scheme was as follows: A dosage of 6 gray ($1\ Gy = 1\ J/kg$) of the ionizing radiation was applied twice a week, for three consecutive weeks. Hence, a total dose of 6×6 Gy was administered to the pterygium.

2.2. Constitutive Material Model

Biomechanically, corneal tissue is known for being nearly incompressible, having non-linear elastic characteristics, being highly inhomogeneous in-plane as well as over its thickness, and for revealing a high degree of anisotropy. In this work, we used a previously published biomechanical model [21–25] which used additive terms in a non-linear, hyper elastic strain energy function to describe the tissue characteristics. Generally speaking, strain-energy functions are derived from the laws of thermodynamics, and relate deformation (right-hand side of the equation) to deformation energy (left-hand side of the equation). The formulation used in this work was already available in the Optimeyes software, and is given as:

$$\Psi = U + \overline{\Psi}_m[C_{10}] + \frac{1}{\pi}\int \Phi \cdot \left(\overline{\Psi}_{f1}[\gamma_m, \mu_m] + \overline{\Psi}_{f2}[\gamma_k, \mu_k]\right)d\theta \tag{1}$$

where U is a penalty-term, preventing volume changes and therefore modeling the incompressibility of corneal tissue, $\overline{\Psi}_m$ is a non-linear adaptation of Hooke's law—called neo-hookean—representing the tissue matrix with its proteoglycans and glycosaminoglycans, and $\overline{\Psi}_{f1}$ and $\overline{\Psi}_{f2}$ are anisotropic polynomial material functions [26] modeling the main collagen fibers and the cross-links, respectively. The probability distribution function Φ defines a realistic fiber distribution, as has been assessed through X-ray scattering by Aghamohammadzadeh et al. [27]. The distribution is defined in the model by assigning a weighting to each possible direction (0° to 180°) for any location in the model, and as a function of corneal depth. Material constants (Table 1) were determined using three sets of experimental data: one from button inflation experiments [28] and two (one superior-inferior strip, one superonasal-inferotemporal strip) from strip extensometry [29] experiments. The inverse finite element method was used to fit the above strain energy function to the experimental data from our earlier work [21].

Table 1. Material coefficients, matching the age of the study subjects, that have been used in conjunction with the constitutive material model implementation. C_{10} is the material constant of the neo-hookean hyper elastic material model for tissue matrix (proteoglycans and glycosaminoglycans, etc.), γ_m, μ_m are material constants of the polynomial material function Ψ_{f1}, introduced by Markert et al. [26], which model the main corneal collagen fibers, and γ_k, μ_k are material constants of the polynomial material function Ψ_{f2}, which model the collagen cross-links. Material coefficients were obtained from our earlier work [21].

C_{10}[MPa]	γ_m	μ_m[MPa]	γ_k	μ_k[MPa]
0.06	0.13	24.0	0.08	95.0

2.3. Patient-Specific Radiation Surgery Simulation

A patient-specific finite element model for the patient in the study was obtained with a three-step algorithm, available in the Optimeyes software: (i) The geometrical information obtained from spatial elevation data of the front and back surface of the patient's cornea (acquired with the Scheimpflug tomography system Pentacam HR, Oculus Optikgeräte GmbH, Germany) was used to warp a spherical template cornea model to create a patient-specific finite element mesh containing 35,000 elements and over 44,000 nodes. (ii) The initial stress distribution in the model was then computed with an iterative approach [30,31]. (iii) Finally, the effects of the surgery were simulated. The anterior and posterior surfaces, computed by the finite-element (FE) model, were then compared to the postoperative surfaces to assess the accuracy and reliability of FE modeling. The details of the algorithm steps i–iii are described below:

(i)   Mesh warping: In our earlier work [23], we showed that a model with patient-specific geometry of the human cornea can be obtained by warping a spherical finite element mesh such that its anterior and posterior surfaces match the respective surfaces of the tomography measurements. Thereby, the tomography surfaces are expressed as the coefficients obtained from Zernike expansion (up to the twelfth order, and over the central 8.0 mm optical zone of the cornea), and the inside mesh nodes proportionally follow the deformation of the respective surface nodes. This way, the template mesh was warped to match the patient's cornea, without producing distorted elements (which is crucial for finite element analysis).

(ii) Calculation of initial stress distribution: Since the Pentacam Scheimpflug camera measures corneal geometry in vivo, whereby the corneal tissue is under mechanical stress, the shape in the absence of acting forces is a priori not known. An iterative approach to calculate the initial stress distribution in the model, as was previously published [30,31], was employed in this study.

(iii) Surgery simulation: A specific, three-dimensional, finite element model was created in the finite element software package ANSYS 17.1 (ANSYS Inc., Canonsburg, PA, USA). The model represents the full cornea, plus a 4-mm wide rim of scleral tissue. The model was fixed at the edge of the scleral rim, and a pressure of 15 mmHg on the models inside represented the intraocular pressure. The anterior surface of the model cornea is prepared such that a specific part exactly corresponds to the shape and position of the subject's pterygium (see Figure 1b). Pressure was applied to that specific part, modeling the pulling forces of the retracting pterygium, tangentially to the corneal surface and towards the limbus (see Figure 2). This simulation approach reproduces the pulling effects placed onto the corneal surface when radiation-induced tissue shrinking in pterygium tissue occurs. The pterygium tissue itself was not modelled.

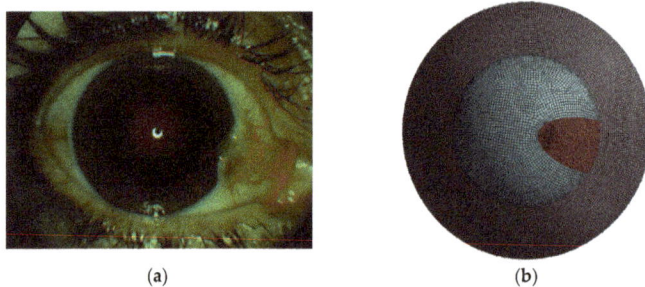

(a) (b)

Figure 1. (a) Top-view image of the study subject with pterygium in-growth in the cornea; (b) Three-dimensional finite element model of the cornea and parts of the sclera, as seen from the top. The specific area (shown in red), representing where the pterygium pulls on the anterior corneal surface.

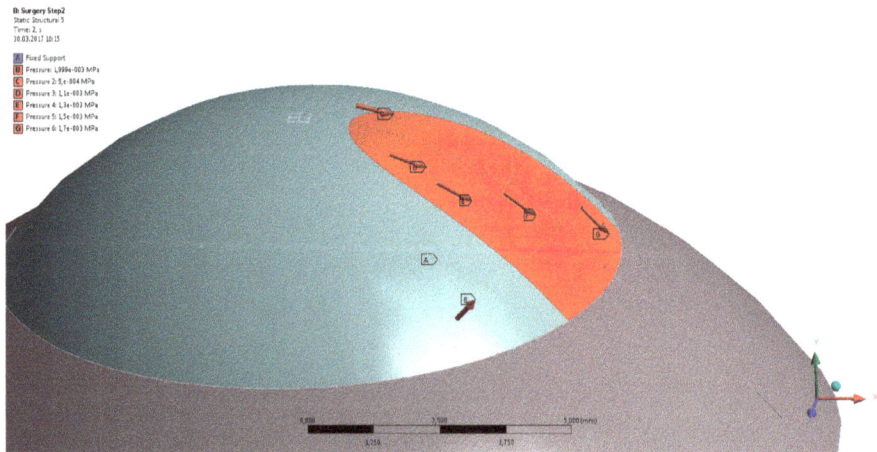

Figure 2. Three-dimensional finite element model of the cornea and the 4-mm scleral rim. The red area represents the specific part of the anterior surface of the cornea model where the tangential pulling forces were applied.

The anterior and posterior surface final geometry after finite element simulation were automatically imported, and then analyzed in the user interface of the Optimeyes software. The software uses an 8.0-mm region of interest for Zernike decomposition of the anterior and posterior corneal surface in the model, and the keratometric index n = 1.3375 for curvature calculation. Thereby, the sagittal curvature was calculated as $C_S = (n-1)/R$, where R is the radius of the curvature, the normal distance between a surface point and the central axis of the cornea. From the sagittal curvatures, corneal astigmatism was calculated as the difference between the steep and flat simulated keratometry values over a central annulus of a 0.5- to 2.0-mm radius. Elevation data were calculated as the normal distance between the cornea and a reference surface, a best-fit sphere fitted over a central 8.0-mm diameter zone.

Corneal shape was compared by analyzing sagittal curvature maps of the anterior corneal surface. Color-coded curvature maps, provided by the Pentacam software as well as by the Optimeyes software, were used to calculate anterior corneal astigmatism, as well as central and paracentral corneal curvatures. Astigmatism was thereby calculated on an apex-centered annulus of 0.5 mm < r < 2.5 mm. Central corneal curvature is the average curvature on an apex-centered disk with a 2.0-mm radius. Paracentral corneal curvature is the average curvature on an apex-centered annulus of 2.0 mm < r < 3.5 mm. Corneal function was compared by analyzing anterior corneal wavefront indices over a central wavefront pupil with a 6-mm diameter.

Besides postoperative geometrical shape, the deformed finite element model also provides full-field biomechanical stress information for every simulation step as part of the software package. The average stress (and standard deviation) was calculated from the simulation within the central 3.0-mm zone.

3. Results

Results from the patient-specific finite element simulations were compared to the actual clinical follow-up anterior segment tomography measurements. The simulation results showed a close match to the clinical data. While the simulation predicted an increase in astigmatism cylinder of +0.32D, in clinics, an increase of +0.31D was observed (see Figure 3a). The astigmatism axis did not change. The central corneal curvature decreased from 44.15D to 43.70D post-surgically. The simulation predicted a decrease to 43.86D. Furthermore, while the paracentral curvature decrease from 43.28D to 43.15D, the simulation predicted a decrease to 43.10D (see Figure 3b).

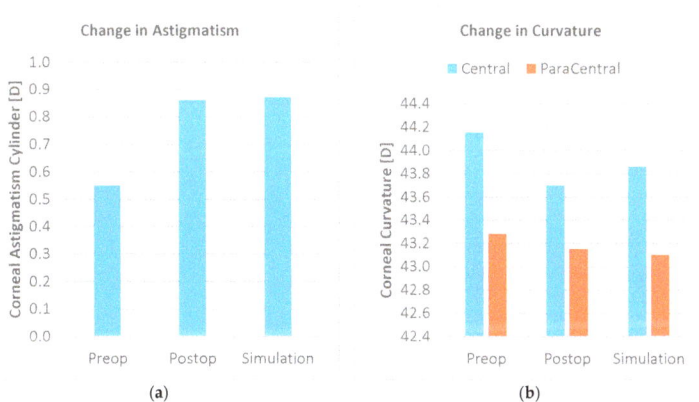

Figure 3. (**a**) Comparison of postoperative astigmatism cylinder and predicted cylinder. The simulation predicted the postoperative cylinder values very closely; (**b**) Comparison of postoperative central and paracentral curvatures and predicted curvature. Postoperative central and paracentral curvatures were well predicted by the simulation model.

While Figure 4 compares the postoperative corneal sagittal curvature map to the predicted curvature map, Figure 5 shows the postoperative corneal pachymetry next to the predicted pachymetry map. Pachymetry slightly increased in clinics, as central corneal thickness went up from 512 to 528 micron, but remained stable in the simulation.

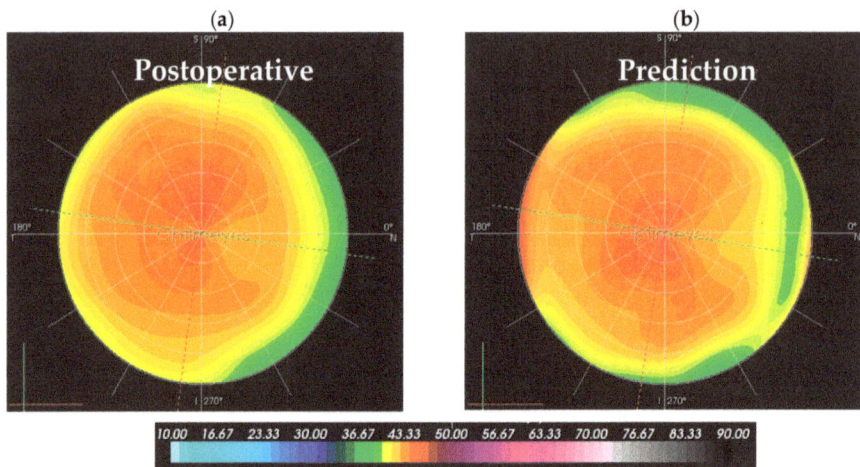

Figure 4. Sagittal anterior corneal curvature maps in Diopters [D] for the central 10.0-mm optical zone. (**a**) The left map is the post-surgical follow-up map, assessed by the Pentacam HR; (**b**) The right map shows the simulated prediction after the numerical simulation of pulling forces.

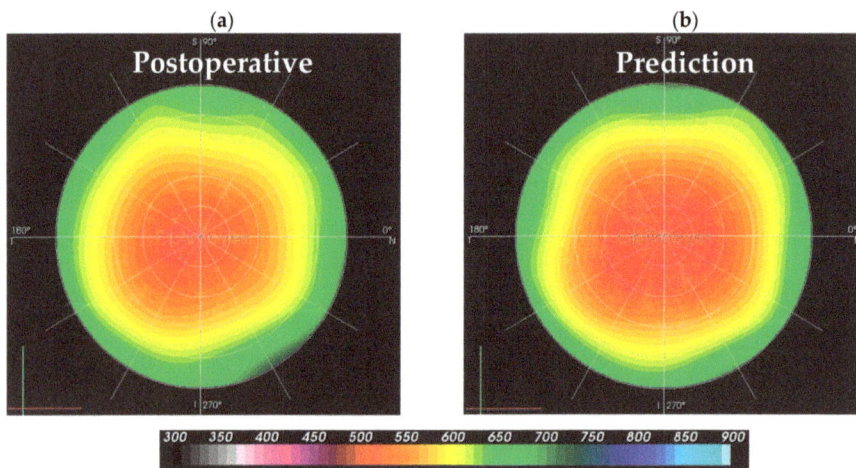

Figure 5. Corneal pachymetry maps, with a scale from 300 to 900 micrometers for the central 10.0-mm optical zone. (**a**) The left-hand side represents the postoperative pachymetry map; (**b**) The right-hand side depicts the simulated prediction of corneal thickness.

3.1. Corneal Function

Corneal function was analyzed by comparison of anterior corneal wavefront coefficients between the postsurgical and the simulated cornea. Figure 6 depicts spherical, astigmatic, coma, trefoil, and tetrafoil aberrations, as well as the root means square of higher order aberrations (Zernike order 4 and higher). Predicted spherical, astigmatic, and coma aberrations were close to the clinical follow-up measurements. The more irregular terms of trefoil and tetrafoil did not show a good match.

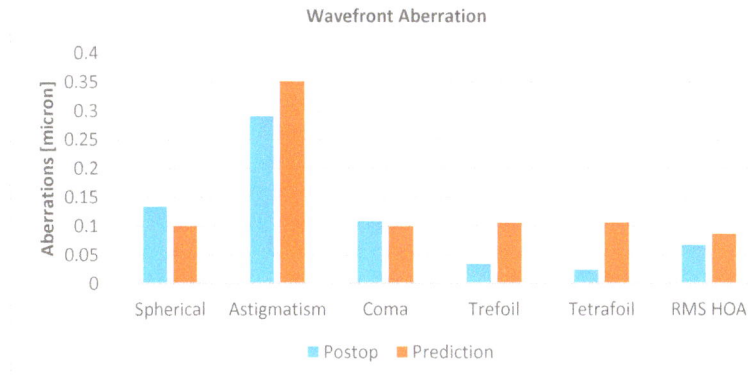

Figure 6. Zernike coefficients, given in micrometers, of spherical, astigmatic, coma, trefoil, tetrafoil, and root means square of higher order (RMS-HOA) wavefront aberrations. While the predicted values were comparable to postoperative wavefront coefficients for spherical (−26%), astigmatic (+21%), coma (−8%), and higher order aberrations (+28%), trefoil (+217%) and tetrafoil (+360%) were not well predicted.

3.2. Corneal Biomechanics

Besides model deformation, finite element modeling allows for the calculation of mechanical stresses and strains. Stresses inside corneal tissue are computed as force over area, and are given in the unit kilo-pascal (kPa). Strain is the deformation relative to the initial dimension, and thus unit-less. Biomechanical simulation results showed an average stress increase in the tissue underneath the pterygium of 5% (from 13.7 kPa to 14.4 kPa). Strains in the area increased from 0.0110 to 0.0120 (4.8%). As Figure 7 shows, on the anterior corneal surface area of the pterygium, stresses increased by 16%, from 9.97 kPa to 11.60 kPa (on the same area on the posterior surface, stress change was negligible with −0.3%). Strains on the anterior corneal surface under the pterygium increased from 0.0083 to 0.0097, but did not change on the posterior surface under the same area (from 0.0147 to 0.0146).

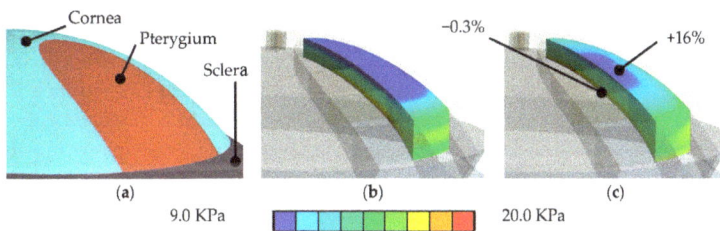

Figure 7. (a) Geometry of a cornea with pterygium. (b) Stress state before and (c) after applying the pulling force of the retracting pterygium. The color scale goes from blue (9 kPa) up to red (20 kPa). Therefore, blueish and greenish colors indicate low stress states, and orange and reddish colors indicate states of high stress. The simulation predicted an overall stress increase in corneal tissue under the pterygium of 2.4%.

4. Discussion and Conclusions

This work focused on numerical simulations of an earlier published beta-irradiation method for corneal pterygium treatment. The goal of the study was to better understand the relationship between Sr-90/Ytt-90 irradiation and clinically observed induction of corneal astigmatism, and to investigate the question of whether the retracting forces of a shrinking pterygium can be the cause of astigmatic changes. Furthermore, the model was intended to reveal the underlying biomechanical processes taking place during the treatment.

It has been shown in literature [6,7,10] that treatment with Sr-90/Ytt-90 irradiation only leads to the devascularization and reduction of the pterygium, without a single case of recurrence. Nevertheless, while corneal pachymetry remained stable after the treatment for all cases, changes in corneal astigmatism cylinder and axis were observed. It was hypothesized that the irradiation-induced retraction of the pterygium places pulling forces onto the anterior corneal surface, which as a consequence causes flattening along the central meridian of the pterygium, and ultimately leads to the induction of corneal astigmatism. Furthermore, clinical findings suggest that the amount of induced astigmatism depends on the preoperative extent of the pterygium. To the best of our knowledge, this is the first time that the mechanisms behind irradiation-induced astigmatic changes in the cornea are investigated with biomechanical simulations.

The results of biomechanical surgery simulation suggest that the clinically observed induction of corneal astigmatism after irradiation treatment might well be caused by pulling forces, exerted onto the anterior corneal surface by the retracting pterygium tissue. The simulation models, based on pre-treatment Pentacam examinations, reproduced pterygium treatment inside the computer and predicted the clinical outcome of a 25-month follow-up well, as compared to the acquired Pentacam data. Consequently, it appears likely that the biomechanical simulation model closely represents the clinical reality, and that it is biomechanical effects that cause the induction of corneal astigmatism. Since the applied pulling force of 30 Millinewton (mN) were chosen to predict postoperative astigmatism best, it remains to be proven clinically that this force corresponds to the actual forces created by pterygium retraction.

Furthermore, simulation results suggest that, in addition to astigmatic changes, the cornea would also experience flattening. Interestingly, the predicted flattening effects in the central and paracentral cornea closely corresponded to the clinical results. On the other hand, predicted wavefront aberrations only partially matched with the clinical follow-up measurements. This might have to do with the fact that the simulation model was passed on the preoperative topography measurement and that because of the pterygium, the preoperative trefoil and tetrafoil aberrations might have been imprecisely assessed prior to the surgery. Still, important aberrations such as spherical, astigmatic, and coma aberrations were well predicted with by the simulation model. The fact that our clinical findings corresponded well with a theoretical model strongly supports the hypothesis that pterygium treatment by Sr-90/Ytt-90 irradiation can induce astigmatism as well as central and paracentral corneal flattening.

Even though the employed simulation model was patient-specific with respect to corneal shape, it has the limitation of assuming non-individualized biomechanical properties. Further limitations of the modeling are the assumed amount of pulling forces, the fact that the modeling only considered the anterior section of the eye and was working with an average intraocular pressure of 15 mmHg, and, most importantly, that modeling neglected potential radiation-induced tissue modifications and multi-physical effects. Nevertheless, the model still demonstrates that forces exerted on the cornea by the contracting pterygium may well be the root cause of induced corneal astigmatism as well as corneal flattening. Finite element modeling might help in the future to further understand the biomechanical effects of pterygium surgery, define improved treatment schemes, and reduce induced corneal shape changes.

Author Contributions: Bojan Pajic provided the treatment indication, developed the study design, acquired clinical data, and contributed to writing the paper. Daniel M Aebersold performed the irradiations/treatments and substantially contributed the study design. Andreas Eggspuehler supplied surgical advice and substantially contributed to the design of the study. Frederik Theler performed finite element simulations and mathematical modeling. Harald Studer performed data analysis and contributed to writing the paper.

Conflicts of Interest: Harald Studer has a commercial interest in the Optimeyes software. Frederik Theler has a commercial interest in the Optimeyes software. All other authors declare no conflict of interest.

References

1. Taylor, H.R. Etiology of climatic droplet keratopathy and pterygium. *Br. J. Ophthalmol.* **1980**, *64*, 154–163. [CrossRef] [PubMed]

2. Cooper, J.S. Postoperative irradiation of pterygia: Ten more years of experience. *Radiology* **1978**, *128*, 753–756. [CrossRef] [PubMed]

3. Coronea, M.T.; Di Girolamo, N.; Wakefield, D. The pathogenesis of pterygia. *Curr. Opin. Ophthalmol.* **1999**, *10*, 282–288. [CrossRef]

4. Moran, D.J.; Hollows, F.C. Pterygium and ultraviolet radiation: A positive correlation. *Br. J. Ophthalmol.* **1984**, *68*, 343–346. [CrossRef] [PubMed]

5. Pajic, B.; Pugnale-Verillotte, N.; Greiner, R.H.; Pajic, D.; Eggspühler, A. Résultat de la thérapie au strontium-yttrium-90 des ptérygions. *J. Fr. Ophthalmol.* **2002**, *25*, 473–479.

6. Pajic, B.; Pallas, A.; Aebersold, D.; Gruber, G.; Greiner, R.H. Prospective Study on Exclusive, Nonsurgical Strontium-/Yttrium-90 Irradiation of Pterygia. *Strahlenther. Onkol.* **2004**, *180*, 510–516. [CrossRef] [PubMed]

7. Pajic, B.; Greiner, R.H. Long term results of non-surgical, exclusive Strontium-/Yttrium-90 Beta-irradiation of pterygia. *Radiother. Oncol.* **2005**, *74*, 25–29. [CrossRef] [PubMed]

8. Kria, L.; Ohira, A.; Amemiya, T. Immunohistochemical localization of basic fibroblast growth factor, platelet derived growth factor, transforming growth factor-β and tumor necrosis factor-α in the pterygium. *Acta Histochem.* **1996**, *98*, 195–201. [CrossRef]

9. Nakagami, T.; Watanabe, I.; Murakami, A.; Okisaka, S.; Ebihara, N. Expression of Stem Cell Factor in Pterygium. *Jpn. J. Ophthalmol.* **2000**, *44*, 193–197. [CrossRef]

10. Vastardis, I.; Pajic, B.; Greiner, R.; Pajic-Eggspuehler, B.; Aebersold, D. Prospective study of exclusive Strontium-/Yttrium-90 β- irradiation of primary and recurrent pterygia with no prior surgical excision: Clinical outcome of long-term follow-up. *Strahlenther. Onkol.* **2009**, *185*, 808–814. [CrossRef] [PubMed]

11. Wong, Y.W.; Chew, J.; Yang, H.; Tan, D.; Beuerman, R. Expression of insulin-like growth factor binding protein- 3 in pterygium tissue. *Br. J. Ophthalmol.* **2006**, *90*, 769–772. [CrossRef] [PubMed]

12. Bahrassa, F.; Datta, R. Postoperative beta radiation treatment of pterygium. *Int. J. Radiat Oncol. Biol. Phys.* **1983**, *9*, 679–684. [CrossRef]

13. Bernstein, M.; Unger, S.M. Experiences with surgery and strontium 90 in the treatment of pterygium. *Am. J. Ophthalmol.* **1960**, *49*, 1024–1029. [CrossRef]

14. De Keizer, R.J.W. Pterygium excision with or without postoperative irradiation, a double blind study. *Doc. Ophthalmol.* **1982**, *52*, 309–315. [CrossRef] [PubMed]

15. Frucht-Perry, J.; Siganos, C.S.; Ilsar, M. Intraoperative application of topical mitomycin C for pterygium surgery. *Ophthalmology* **1996**, *103*, 674–677. [CrossRef]

16. Hayasaka, S.; Noda, S.; Yukari, Y.; Setogawa, T. Postoperative installation of Mitomycin C in the treatment of recurrent pterygium. *Ophthalmic Surg.* **1989**, *20*, 580–583. [PubMed]

17. Paryani, S.B.; Scott, W.P.; Wells, J.W., Jr.; Johnson, D.W.; Chobe, R.J.; Kuruvilla, A.; Schoeppel, S.; Deshmukh, A. Management of pterygium with surgery and radiation therapy. *Int. J. Radiat. Oncol. Biol. Phys.* **1994**, *28*, 101–103. [CrossRef]

18. Rachmiel, R.; Leiba, H.; Levartovsky, S. Results of treatment with topical mitomycin C 0.02% following excision of primary pterygium. *Br. J. Ophthalmol.* **1995**, *79*, 233–236. [CrossRef] [PubMed]

19. Shusko, A.; Hovanesian, J.A. Pterygium excision with conjunctival autograft and subconjunctival amniotic membrane as antirecurrence agents. *Can. J. Ophthalmol.* **2016**, *51*, 412–416. [CrossRef] [PubMed]

20. Pajic, B.; Vastardis, I.; Rajkovic, P.; Pajic-Eggspuehler, B.; Aebersold, DM.; Cvejic, Z. A mathematical approach to human pterygium shape. *Clin. Ophthalmol.* **2016**, *10*, 1343–1349. [CrossRef] [PubMed]

21. Studer, H.P.; Larrea, X.; Riedwyl, H.; Büchler, P. Biomechanical Model of Human Cornea Based on Stromal Microstructure. *J. Biomech.* **2010**, *43*, 836–842. [CrossRef] [PubMed]
22. Studer, H.P.; Büchler, P.; Ridewly, H. Importance of Multiple Loading Scenarios for the Identification of Material Coefficients of the Human Cornea. *CMBBE* **2012**, *15*, 93–99. [CrossRef] [PubMed]
23. Studer, H.P.; Riedwyl, H.; Amstutz, C.A.; Hanson, J.V.; Büchler, P. Patient-specific finite-element simulation of the human cornea: A clinical validation study on cataract surgery. *J. Biomech.* **2013**, *46*, 751–758. [CrossRef] [PubMed]
24. Studer, H.P.; Pradhan, K.R.; Reinstein, D.Z.; Businaro, E.; Archer, T.J.; Gobbe, M.; Roberts, C.J. Biomechanical Modeling of Femtosecond Laser Keyhole Endokeratophakia Surgery. *J. Refract. Surg.* **2015**, *31*, 480–486. [CrossRef] [PubMed]
25. Whitford, C.; Studer, H.; Boote, C.; Meek, K.M.; Elsheikh, A. Biomechanical Model of the Human Cornea: Considering Shear Stiffness and Regional Variation of Collagen Anisotropy and Density. *JMBBM* **2015**, *42*, 76–87. [CrossRef] [PubMed]
26. Markert, B.; Ehlers, W.; Karajan, N. A general polyconvex strain-energy function for fiber-reinforced materials. *Proc. Appl. Math. Mech.* **2005**, *5*, 245–246. [CrossRef]
27. Aghamohammadzadeh, H.; Newton, R.; Meek, K. X-ray scattering used to map the preferred collagen orientation in the human cornea and limbus. *Structure* **2004**, *12*, 249–256. [CrossRef] [PubMed]
28. Elsheikh, A.; Wang, D.; Pye, D. Determination of the modulus of elasticity of the human cornea. *J. Refract. Surg.* **2007**, *23*, 808–818. [PubMed]
29. Elsheikh, A.; Anderson, K. Comparative study of corneal strip extensometry and inflation tests. *J. R. Soc. Interface* **2008**, *2*, 177–185. [CrossRef] [PubMed]
30. Pinsky, P.M.; van der Heide, D.; Chernyak, D. Computational modeling of mechanical anisotropy in the cornea and sclera. *J. Cataract Refract. Surg.* **2005**, *31*, 136–145. [CrossRef] [PubMed]
31. Pandolfi, A.; Manganiello, F. A model for the human cornea: Constitutive formulation and numerical analysis. *Biomech. Model. Mechanobiol.* **2006**, *5*, 237–246. [CrossRef] [PubMed]

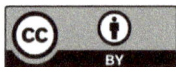

Article

Excimer Laser Surgery: Biometrical Iris Eye Recognition with Cyclorotational Control Eye Tracker System

Bojan Pajic [1,2,3,4], Zeljka Cvejic [2], Zoran Mijatovic [2,*], Dragan Indjin [5] and Joerg Mueller [1]

[1]   Swiss Eye Research Foundation, Eye Clinic ORASIS, 5734 Reinach AG, Switzerland;
      bpajic@datacomm.ch (B.P.); joerg.mueller@nova-optik.ch (J.M.)
[2]   Faculty of Sciences, Department of Physics, University of Novi Sad, Trg Dositeja Obradovica 4,
      Novi Sad 21000, Serbia; zeljkac@uns.ac.rs
[3]   Medical Faculty, Military Medical Academy, University of Defans Belgrade, Belgrade 11000, Serbia
[4]   Division of Ophthalmology, Department of Clinical Neurosciences, Geneva University Hospitals,
      Genève 1205, Switzerland
[5]   School of Electronic and Electrical Engineering, University of Leeds, Leeds LS2 9JT, UK; d.indjin@leeds.ac.uk
[*]   Correspondence: mijat@uns.ac.rs; Tel.: +381-64-2168-375

Academic Editor: Vittorio M. N. Passaro
Received: 26 March 2017; Accepted: 23 May 2017; Published: 25 May 2017

Abstract: A prospective comparative study assessing the importance of the intra-operative dynamic rotational tracking—especially in the treatment of astigmatisms in corneal refractive Excimer laser correction—concerning clinical outcomes is presented. The cyclotorsion from upright to supine position was measured using iris image comparison. The Group 1 of patients was additionally treated with cyclorotational control and Group 2 only with X-Y control. Significant differences were observed between the groups regarding the mean postoperative cylinder refraction ($p < 0.05$). The mean cyclotorsion can be calculated to $3.75°$ with a standard deviation of $3.1°$. The total range of torsion was from $-14.9°$ to $+12.6°$. Re-treatment rate was 2.2% in Group 1 and 8.2% in Group 2, which is highly significant ($p < 0.01$). The investigation confirms that the dynamic rotational tracking system used for LASIK results in highly predictable refraction quality with significantly less postoperative re-treatments.

Keywords: cyclorotation control eye tracker system; Excimer laser; refractive surgery

1. Introduction

In recent years, several improvements in the diagnostic aspects of refractive corneal surgery have been introduced which have contributed to improved precision and the availability of new clinical information such as wavefront aberration maps and three-dimensional corneal maps with high precision elevation data [1,2].

From the indication and algorithm points of view, parallel developments have been started by expanding the treatment ranges for high levels of astigmatism, aspheric ablation profiles, and the correction of high order aberrations [3–6].

These developments have resulted in the therapeutic components of a refractive platform that needs to be equipped with new technologies in order to provide a laser system capable of delivering superior precision and to utilize a new level of available information. It is well known that the eye can rotate several degrees when a person moves from a sitting position to a prone position. Having in mind that wavefront and topographic data are collected in the sitting position and that refractive surgery is performed in supine position, there is a great chance for potential error. Therefore, if the laser is tracking the center of the pupil, it would be most impossible to detect a rotational change because the center of the pupil may not be affected.

One of the essential components required to achieve this goal is a sophisticated eye tracking technology. The automated system that utilizes an eye tracking feature is a part of today's novel refractive laser systems.

Technolas 217z100P eye tracking system is a video-based system that uses infrared (IR) radiation to illuminate and capture the image by combining the advantages of being independent of the surrounding iris color conditions and the illumination level of the surgical field.

The relevance of cyclotorsion and its impact on the effectiveness of the ablation process are well known and several other systems have begun to include compensating technologies into their platforms [7]. As the observed rotational misalignment during the ablation cannot be neglected, the eye tracking system could improve surface ablation results when treating high astigmatism or when being wavefront guided.

2. Materials and Methods

We measured and adjusted the eye tracker system of Technolas 217z100P™ (Technolas, Munich, Germany) in LASIK (LASer-assisted In situ Keratomileusis) treatments on a total of 88 eyes in this study, 44 eyes with rotational tracker in Group 1 and 44 eyes with only X/Y tracker system in Group 2. For patients where bilateral treatment was performed, only data from the right eyes were used. The cyclotorsion from upright to supine position was measured using iris image comparison and it was not necessary to mark the cornea. All flaps created with the LDV high frequency femtosecond laser and energy range in nJ, were designed to deliver equivalent geometric dimensions 110 μm flap thickness, 9.5 mm flap diameter with superior hinge angle. The mean age of patients was: 36 ± 7.9 years (range: 23–61 years) in Group 1 and 36 ± 8.2 years (range: 21–62 years) in Group 2. The preoperative mean refractive spherical equivalent in Group 1 was -3.43 ± 2.61 D (range -10.5 to -0.75 D) and -3.69 ± 2.55 D in Group 2 (range -8.75 to -1.00 D) (the left part of the Figures 1 and 2 marked as before surgery).

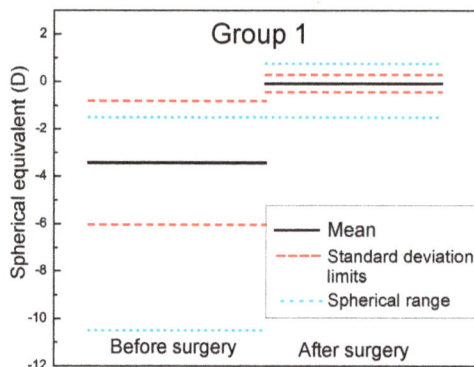

Figure 1. Refractive spherical equivalent pre- and postoperative Group 1.

The mean cylinder was -1.14 ± 1.00 D (range -5.75 to 0.00 D) in Group 1 and -1.12 ± -1.0 D (range -6.00 to -0.00 D) in Group 2 (the left part of the Figures 3 and 4 marked as $-$ before surgery).

There was no significant difference between the groups regarding the mean preoperative spherical equivalent and cylinder refraction ($p > 0.05$).

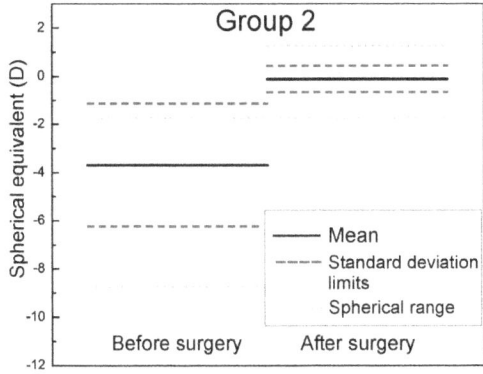

Figure 2. Refractive spherical equivalent pre- and postoperative Group 2.

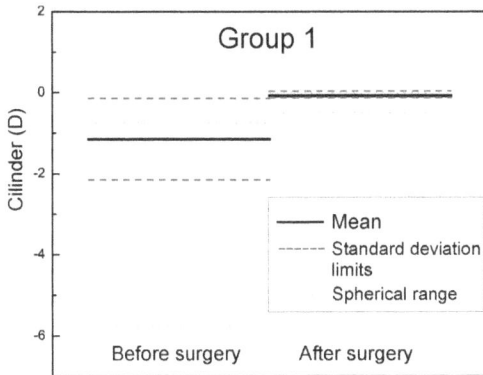

Figure 3. Mean cylinder pre- and postoperative Group 1.

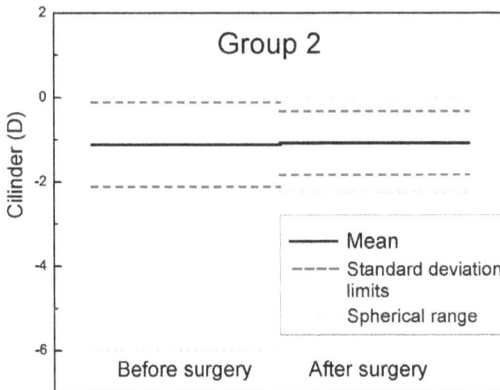

Figure 4. Mean cylinder pre- and postoperative Group 2.

By introducing the rotational eye tracker in the Technolas 217z100P™ the already approved X/Y tracker, which compensates actively for transversal movements of the eye, will be upgraded to compensate for misalignments in rotation. While it uses the acquired iris images only, additional objectively acquired information is needed to provide a rotational tracking capability. The 217z100P rotational tracker module is based on iris pattern recognition technology. It is well known that iris patterns are similar to finger prints with unique biometric properties of the individual. By using the appropriate technology, not only the individual eye can be recognized but also specific match parameters—such as rotational misalignment between two images of the same iris—can be obtained. The basic data used to analyze iris patterns are acquired infrared images of the iris. With special image processing and normalization technologies, the iris images are processed to account for differences in illumination conditions (large and small pupils) or even from different systems (such as Zywave wavefront sensor and laser system). The Zywave wavefront sensor is a diagnostic system which utilizes the same wavelength to acquire an Infrared (IR) image forms, the eye, and the corresponding iris [8]. Finally, the process described above results in a digital code which is created as follows: determine automatically pupil boundary and limbus boundary of the reference image (Figure 5).

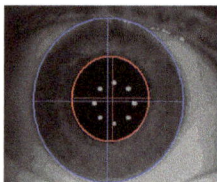

Figure 5. Pupil and limbus boundary recognition of the reference image.

Certain sanity checks are applied to ensure that the automatically identified pupil and limbus geometries are within reasonable measures. The visible iris pattern defined as the structures between the pupil boundary and the limbus edge are used to create a normalized band (Figure 6).

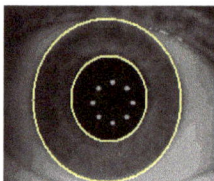

Figure 6. Visible iris pattern definition.

All operations which lead to the final digital iris code are performed within this normalized band (Figure 7).

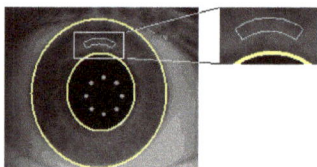

Figure 7. Digital iris code performance.

Within this band of iris image data, a unique digital code is generated. The basic data stream of this digital code consists of information obtained at 980 different iris locations. This iris code is, therefore, a unique code for this specific iris pattern and is used to detect potential torsional deviations between two different images from the same iris. The output parameters of the rotational eye tracker system—such as pupil radius/center and limbus radius/center—are given in resolution less than 30 µm. The rotation angle between images is within ±14.8° and with the resolution of 0.7° (=360°/512). Response time is 40 ms (i.e., 25 Hz).

During the static cyclotorsion compensation, the first step is a diagnostic phase which consists of obtaining IR iris image and deriving digital iris code from this reference iris image. This is followed with a planning phase where obtained data are transferred to the laser system. The next phase is a cyclotorsion compensation phase in which the patient's head is aligned in the supine position. After that, the second IR iris image is acquired for comparison between the reference and actual iris code.

During to intra-operative rotational compensation phase (dynamic cyclotorsion compensation), the referenced image is used as the first image for providing the iris code. Afterwards, a new iris image and code are required, while laser system is treating the patient's eye. The next step is determining rotational angle to achieve maximum overlap of iris code and transferring this info to the laser software. The correct treatment pattern is determined according to the rotational angle.

To observe and track the eye movements of a patient during surgery, the laser is equipped with two different cameras for the eye tracking system. One camera detects eye movements in the x/y direction. It is optimized for the area around the pupil and operational frequency is 240 Hz. The other eye-tracker camera detects the rotational movements of the eye and has a wider display window, so that the iris and limbal region can be observed. Operational frequency of this camera is 25 Hz. The slower frequency of the rotational eye tracker camera is justified with the slow speed of cyclotoric movements of eyes, while the x/y tracker must handle very fast saccadic movements in the x/y direction.

Due to the different observation angles of the two camera systems, it is also possible to detect movements in the height of an eye (also called Z-tracking) by the observation of the pupil centers obtained from the both cameras. The Z-tracking is opposite to the lateral and torsional tracking of a passive tracking system which simply deactivates the laser application if the eye moves outside of a given range of ±0.5 mm of the nominal Z-position. It should also be mentioned that the lateral eye tracker system works independently from the other two systems (rotational and Z-tracking). All mentioned eye tracking modules can block a laser pulse if the position is not accurate. The surgeon is able to deactivate the rotational eye-tracker system (including Z-tracking) at any time of surgery, while the x/y tracker can remain activated. If it is needed, the user can manually deactivate the x/y tracker too.

The system delivers the cyclorotational angle from a supine to horizontal position and additionally the dynamic eye tracker systems records the angle differences during the surgery. This results in an overall angle from the beginning until the end of surgery. This value is taken for the mean calculation of all eyes where the surgeries were undertaken with the cyclorotational eye tracker system, referred to as Group 1.

3. Results

The six-month postoperative mean refractive spherical equivalent was -0.08 ± 0.36 D in Group 1 (range -1.5 to $+0.75$ D) and -0.11 ± 0.55 D in Group 2 (range -1.75 to $+1.25$ D) (the right part of the Figures 1 and 2 marked as after surgery). In Figures 1 and 2, it is very well revealed the refractive clinical outcome: preoperative vs. six months postoperative.

The mean cylinder was -0.08 ± 0.05 D (range -0.5 to 0.0 D) in Group 1 and -1.08 ± 0.75 D (range -2.25 to 0.0 D) in Group 2 (the right part of the Figures 3 and 4 marked as after surgery). In Figure 8, the double angle scatter plot of the cylinder value and angle is shown for the Group 1. Only a small range of astigmatism power and angle can be seen in contrast to the Group 2 where results for a double angle scatter plot analysis are shown in Figure 9.

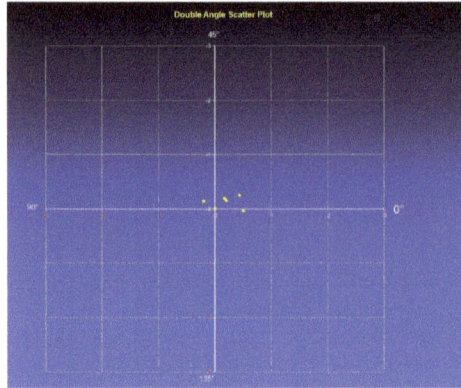

Figure 8. Double angle scatter plot for group 1.

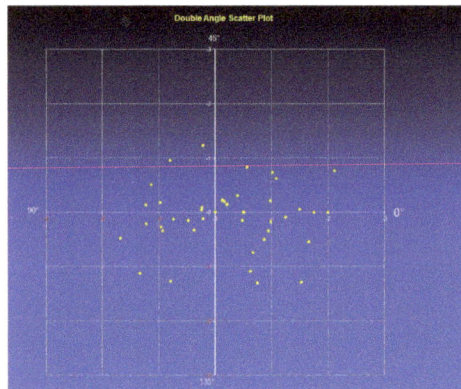

Figure 9. Double angle scatter plot for group 2.

There is no much difference between the groups related to the mean postoperative spherical equivalent ($p > 0.05$) but significant difference in outcomes was observed related to the mean cylinder ($p = 0.0043$). The cylinder range of 2.25 D in Group 2 is remarkably high compared with the results obtained for Group 1, where only a range of 0.5 was measured. From supine to horizontal patient position there was an average static cyclotorsion deviation of $-1.45°$ in Group 1. During the surgery the average cyclotorsion was calculated to be 3.75° with a standard deviation of 3.1°. Torsion was ranged from $-14.9°$ to $+12.6°$.

In the Group 1, the safety of BSCVA (Best Spectacle-Corrected Visual Acuity) remained unchanged in 5 cases, 25 cases gained 1 line, 10 cases gained 2 lines, and 4 cases gained more than 2 lines of visual acuity (Figure 10).

In the Group 2, the safety of BSCVA remained unchanged in 17 cases, 1 case lost 2 lines, 1 case lost 1 line, 22 cases gained 1 line, and 3 cases gained 2 lines of visual acuity (Figure 11).

Re-treatment rate is 2.2% in the Group 1 compared to 8.2% in Group 2. The difference is highly significant ($p < 0.01$).

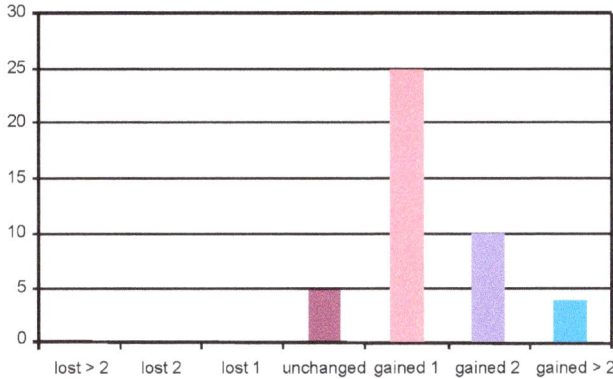

Figure 10. Treatment safety of Group 1.

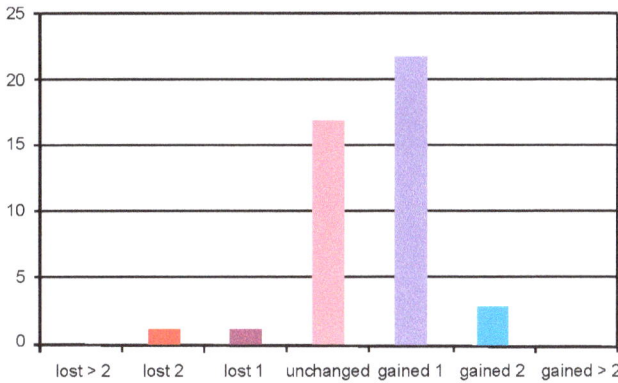

Figure 11. Treatment safety of Group 2.

4. Discussion

The rotational eye-tracker system has the ability not only to correct the rotation of an eye due to a change of the body position but also the ability to correct cyclotoric movements intra-operatively. This intra-operative cyclotorsion can occur, for example, due to a loss of fixation of the patient, excitement, or small head rotations. To ensure accurate pulse position during treatment the recognition process is continuously active during laser ablation. These images are continuously compared to the reference image, which is the last image of the initial recognition process. For each image, the quality factor and rotation angle is calculated and the remaining pulse list is rotated to the actual valid rotation angle. Therefore, even if intra-operative cyclotorsions occur, the dynamic application of the iris recognition process and the following correction ensure accurate pulse positioning during the treatment. During laser treatment, the images of the eye can lose contrast, for example due to dehydrating of the corneal surface, consequently, the difference between the reference image and the actual real time image is increased. In this case, the software is capable of recording a new reference image with the last valid rotation angle and continues to track the rotation angle using the new reference image. In our study, a highly significant difference was observed between the postoperative cylindric correction with and without a cyclotorsion control. The mean cyclotorsion was 3.75° with a standard deviation of 3.1°. The total range of torsion was from −14.9° to +12.6°. If a cylindric refraction of 4 D should be corrected with a cyclorotation of 10° without a cyclotorsion control and a correction error of 1D will be expected calculated mathematically with vector analysis. It has been shown in other studies that 50%—and in some case up to 65%—of the population has a cyclotorsion difference between standing and horizontal positions of more than 2° [7,9,10]. The cyclorotation can increase in individuals even up to 17° [7,11]. This confirms that the cyclotorsion control is a very important tool regarding the clinical outcome. In Group 2 we detected one eye which lost one line and another eye that lost two lines of visual acuity. In our opinion, the higher grade of astigmatism error in Group 2 leads to higher aberrations and, consecutively, to a decrease of the best-corrected visual acuity in these specific cases. Our results show good agreement with other published literature [7,12–14]. Different studies investigated the amount of cyclotorsion of eyes during LASIK treatments. Swami et al. [9] marked 240 eyes preoperatively while the patients were seated. Immediately before beginning the treatment, they measured the rotational misalignment of the eyes on the supine patients and found a mean cyclotorsion of 4.1° (±3.7°) while 8% of the eyes showed a deviation greater than 10°. Ciccio et al. [7] repeated the measurements, marking the horizontal axis of 1019 eyes prior to wavefront measurements, and detected the mark on the supine patient under the laser. The angle of misalignment was measured and analyzed whereby a mean rotational angle of the eyes from seated to supine patient of 4.05° (±2.9°) was observed. Moreover, they found a difference between left eyes and right eyes in the predominant trend of the rotation with 46% of the patients showing bilateral excyclotorsion and only 1.7% displaying bilateral incyclotorsion.

As already mentioned, it is well known that iris patterns are unique properties of an individual (such as finger prints) and the probability of finding two objects with the same iris pattern is extremely low. The challenge is to utilize this fact in a way that the realization provides an accurate determination of the special alignment of the unique pattern when compared to a reference image of the same eye. The strategy to fulfil these criteria is developed by means of using a sophisticated approach to analyze the complex iris structures and to transform this information into a digital code of the iris. This code should be sufficiently unique but still compact enough to provide a realistic processing time according to the desired application.

A central iris recognition and comparison module is used in all the applications mentioned. This module is the main tool in the process of identification of the iris patterns as well as in the determination of the rotational misalignment between two specific images. The initial point for an iris recognition process is always the availability of two iris images that can be compared to each other. Depending on whether or not they belong to the same eye, the key question is whether there is a measurable rotational angle between the two images.

The study was approved by the local institutional review board (Kantonalethikkommission Nr 2006/11, Aargau) and adhered to the tenets of the Declaration of Helsinki.

5. Conclusions

In this study, we present the results of 88 treatment sessions, 44 with and 44 without a cyclorotational eye tracker system. There was no significant difference of clinical outcome regarding the spherical equivalent, however there was a highly significant difference regarding the cylinder treatment. The advantage of iris recognition ensures a much better laser spot position during the surgery while it is not always the case in an only X/Y eyetracker control procedure. The dynamic cyclorotational eye tracker system leads to a high level of cylinder control during corneal refractive surgery with the Excimer laser. Therefore, the proposed system used for LASIK results in highly predictable refraction quality with significantly less postoperative re-treatments.

Acknowledgments: This work was supported by European Cooperation in Science and Technology (COST) Action BM1205.

Author Contributions: Bojan Pajic and Zeljka Cvejic conceived and designed the experiments; Bojan Pajic and Jörg Müller performed the experiments; Zoran Mijatovic and Jörg Müller analyzed the data; Dragan Indjin contributed analysis tools; all authors wrote the paper.

Conflicts of Interest: The authors declare no conflict of interest.

References

1. Taravella, M.J.; Davidson, R.S. Corneal Topography and Wavefront Imaging—IV Chapter. In *Ophthalmology*, 4th ed.; Yanoff, M., Duker, J.S., Eds.; Elsevier Saunders: Philadelphia, PA, USA, 2014; pp. 168–173.
2. Zhon, C.; Chair, X.; Yuan, L.; He, Y.; Ren, Q. Corneal higher-order aberrations after customized aspheric ablation and conventional ablation for myopic correction. *Curr. Eye Res.* **2007**, *32*, 431–438. [CrossRef]
3. Mrochen, M.; Kaemmerer, M.; Seiler, T. Wavefront-guided laser in situ keratomileusis: Early results in three eyes. *J. Refract. Surg.* **2000**, *16*, 116–121. [PubMed]
4. McDonald, M.B. Summit Autonomous custom cornea LASIK outcomes. *J. Refract. Surg.* **2000**, *16*, 617–618.
5. Smolek, K.M. Method for Expressing Clinical and Statistical Signicance of Ocular and Corneal Wavefront Error Aberrations. *Cornea* **2012**, *31*, 212–221. [CrossRef] [PubMed]
6. Seiler, T.; Kaemmerer, M.; Mierdel, P.; Krinke, H.E. Ocular optical aberrations after photorefractive kerarectomy for myopia and myopic astigmatism. *Arch. Ophthalmol.* **2000**, *118*, 17–21. [CrossRef] [PubMed]
7. Ciccio, A.E.; Durrie, D.S.; Stahl, J.E. Ocular cyclotorsion during customized laser ablation. *J. Refract. Surg.* **2005**, *21*, S772–S774. [PubMed]
8. Holladay, J.T.; Dudeja, D.R.; Chang, J. Functional vision and corneal changes after laser in situ keratomileusis determined by contrast sensitivity, glare testing and corneal topography. *J. Cataract. Refract. Surg.* **1999**, *25*, 663–669. [CrossRef]
9. Chernyak, D.A. Cyclotorsion eye motion occurring between wavefront measurement and refractive surgery. *J. Cataract. Refract. Surg.* **2004**, *30*, 633–638. [CrossRef] [PubMed]
10. Tjon-Fo-Sang, M.J.; De Faber, J.T.H.N.; Kingma, C.; Beckhuis, W.H. Cyclotorsion: A possible cause of residual astigmatism in refractive surgery. *J. Cataract. Refract. Surg.* **2002**, *28*, 599–602. [CrossRef]
11. Fea, A.M.; Sciandra, L.; Annetta, F.; Musso, M.; Dal Vecchio, M.; Grignolo, F.M. Cyclotorsional eye movements during a simulated PRK procedure. *Eye* **2006**, *20*, 764–768. [CrossRef] [PubMed]
12. Swami, A.U.; Steinert, R.F.; Osborne, W.E. Rotational malposition during laser in situ keratomileusis. *Am. J. Ophthalmol.* **2002**, *133*, 561–562. [CrossRef]
13. Neuhann, I.M.; Lege, B.A.; Hassel, J.M. Static and Dynamic rotational eye tracking during LASIK treatment of myopic astigmatism with Zyoptix laser platform and Advanced Control Eye Tracker. *J. Refract. Surg.* **2010**, *26*, 17–27. [CrossRef] [PubMed]
14. Prakash, G.; Agarwal, A.; Kumar, D.A. Surface ablation with iris recognition and dynamic rotational eye tracking-based tissue saving treatment with the Technolas 217z excimer laser. *J. Refract. Surg.* **2011**, *27*, 323–331. [CrossRef] [PubMed]

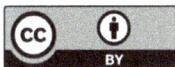

Article

A Novel Laser Refractive Surgical Treatment for Presbyopia: Optics-Based Customization for Improved Clinical Outcome

Bojan Pajic [1,2,3,4], **Brigitte Pajic-Eggspuehler** [1], **Joerg Mueller** [1], **Zeljka Cvejic** [2] and **Harald Studer** [1,5,*]

[1]   Eye Clinic Orasis, Swiss Eye Research Foundation, CH-5734 Reinach, Switzerland; bpajic@datacomm.ch (B.P.); brigitte.pajic@orasis.ch (B.P.-E.); joerg.mueller@nova-optik.ch (J.M.)

[2]   Department of Physics, Faculty of Sciences, University of Novi Sad, Trg Dositeja Obradovica 4, 21000 Novi Sad, Serbia; zeljkac@uns.ac.rs

[3]   Division of Ophthalmology, Department of Clinical Neurosciences, Geneva University Hospitals, CH-1205 Geneva, Switzerland

[4]   Faculty of Medicine of the Military Medical academy, University of Defence, 11000 Belgrade, Serbia

[5]   OCTlab, Department of Ophthalmology, University of Basel, CH-4001 Basel, Switzerland

*   Correspondence: harald.studer@gmail.com; Tel.: +41-76-588-4619

Academic Editor: Dragan Indjin
Received: 31 March 2017; Accepted: 7 June 2017; Published: 13 June 2017

Abstract: Laser Assisted in Situ Keratomileusis (LASIK) is a proven treatment method for corneal refractive surgery. Surgically induced higher order optical aberrations were a major reason why the method was only rarely used to treat presbyopia, an age-related near-vision loss. In this study, a novel customization algorithm for designing multifocal ablation patterns, thereby minimizing induced optical aberrations, was used to treat 36 presbyopic subjects. Results showed that most candidates went from poor visual acuity to uncorrected 20/20 vision or better for near (78%), intermediate (92%), and for distance (86%) vision, six months after surgery. All subjects were at 20/25 or better for distance and intermediate vision, and a majority (94%) were also better for near vision. Even though further studies are necessary, our results suggest that the employed methodology is a safe, reliable, and predictable refractive surgical treatment for presbyopia.

Keywords: presbyopia; LASIK; presbyLASIK; uncorrected visual acuity

---

1. Introduction

Laser Assisted in Situ Keratomileusis (LASIK) is proven to be a safe, fast, and reliable procedure for corneal refractive surgery. The procedure comprises three steps: (i) cutting a thin flap on the outer corneal surface, (ii) ablating tissue underneath the flap with an excimer laser, and (iii) putting the flap back into place on the stromal bed. Only a relatively small number of side effects, such as dry-eye, halos, corneal ectasia, and epithelial ingrowth under the flap, have been reported. Modern excimer laser systems have demonstrated their ability and performance in treating various ametropic conditions, such as nearsightedness (myopia), farsightedness (hyperopia), and astigmatism. By 2009, more than 27 million eyes had successfully been treated with LASIK refractive surgery all around the world.

Even though various approaches—based on diverse technologies and methodologies—for the treatment of age-related far or nearsightedness have been proposed and documented in literature, effective presbyopia treatment remains a challenge in modern eye care. State-of-the-art treatment involves the implantation of multifocal intraocular lenses [1,2], which by nature is a highly invasive surgical procedure, and postoperative refraction planning remains highly complex. Other approaches such as mono-vision corneal procedures [3,4] use excimer lasers and LASIK to treat presbyopia, but these methods are unfortunately not well tolerated by many subjects. Corneal inlay implantation [5,6], intrastromal femtosecond laser corrections [7], or other excimer laser-based presbyopia treatments [8] have been used in clinics with some success over the last few years.

In any such procedure, besides restoring the patients' vision and ability to see far- as well as near-distance objects, the focus should always be that (i) the treatment is reversible and (ii) that postsurgical enhancement, or touch-up, is always possible. Generally speaking, corneal approaches are the least invasive, and are highly accurate and safe procedures. Furthermore, they omit risks that are inherent to the intraocular procedure. It has previously been reported that multifocal LASIK treatments, sometimes also called presbyLASIK treatments, in the cornea showed good refractive results for near, intermediate, and distance vision in hyperopic presbyopia patients [8–10]. The good results of those studies suggest that postoperative refraction was easily predictable, and that presbyLASIK was well tolerated by the study subjects. However, because LASIK ablation patterns for myopic eyes are fundamentally different from those of hyperopic treatments, this prospective study aimed to assess the performance of presbyLASIK customized multifocal procedures for myopic presbyopia patients.

2. Materials and Methods

This prospective, single-surgeon study of myopic presbyopia treatments with a multifocal presbyLASIK procedure included 72 eyes of 36 patients. All eyes underwent pre- and postoperative full clinical biomicroscopical examination, Orbscan IIz corneal topography (BAUSCH + LOMB, TECHNOLAS Perfect Vision GmbH, Munich, Germany) and Zywave II wavefront aberrometry analysis (BAUSCH + LOMB, Rochester, NY, USA). Additionally, monocular and binocular uncorrected near (UNVA), intermediate (UIVA), and distance (UDVA) visual acuity were assessed using a LogMAR chart. For all examinations, the eyes had undilated pupils, and were conducted preoperatively, as well as one week, one month, three months, and six months postoperatively.

All study subjects underwent Supracor refractive surgery, operated with a 217P Excimer laser (BAUSCH + LOMB, TECHNOLAS Perfect Vision GmbH, Munich, Germany). The dominant eye of each individual subject was targeted plano for far vision (0.0 diopters), while the respective non-dominant eye of the same subject was targeted at −0.5 diopters. All LASIK flaps were created with a Ziemer LDV femtosecond laser platform (Ziemer Ophthalmology, Port, Switzerland), and had a superior hinge and a thickness of 110 microns. All treatments were planned and executed in two main steps: first, the normal ablation pattern for the myopic condition of the subject's eyes were applied to the cornea, according to the surgeon's nomogram, and by targeting the mean refractive spherical equivalent (MRSE) to be optimal for distance vision. Second, the aforementioned 3-mm zone near the addition was applied (see Figure 1) to create the extra refractive power in the central cornea. The resulting multifocal shape allowed the patient to have clear vision over a wide range of depth of focus.

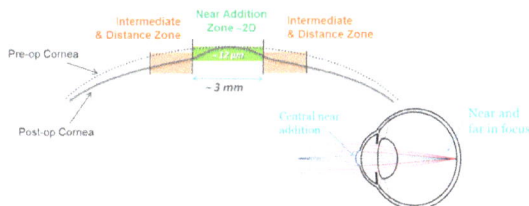

Figure 1. Schematic description of the Supracor treatment. The multifocal ablation pattern combines a regular ablation for the subjects' ametropic condition (shown in orange) with a 3-mm central zone near the vision add-on (shown in green). The add-on typically adds 2 diopters of refractive power to the central cornea.

The treatment planning software of a 217P laser system calculates a multifocal ablation pattern by combining the normal distance vision treatment plan for the ametropic condition of the subject, with a near vision addition in the 3-mm central zone of the treatment (see Figures 2 and 3). On one hand, the normal distance vision treatment thereby uses an adaptation of the original Munnerlyn formula [11] to flatten the overall cornea in the peripheral and paracentral zone. This flattening is customized to the individual eye, to reduce the cornea's refractive power and to bring the focus point of the eyes optical system right onto the retina. The near-vision addition, on the other hand, creates a small central region of higher curvature and hence a higher refractive power. The higher power is customized such that close-by targets are well focused on the retina. The hypothesis of multifocal ablations is that the brain is capable of blending the retinal images, and hence enables the subject to have good near, intermediate, and distance visual acuity. In order to prevent undesired optical side effects from the transition between the small area of high curvature and the flatter corneal region, a proprietary customization algorithm ensures that postoperative spherical aberrations are avoided.

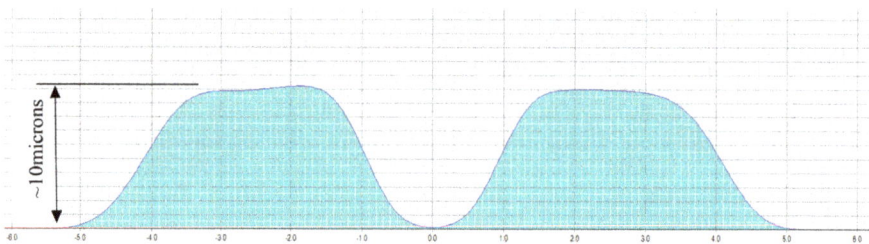

Figure 2. Typical multifocal ablation profile of a presbyopia-only treatment. The schematic indicates the amount of ablated tissue (blue area), with respect to the distance from the center of the cornea. Such a profile creates a steep central zone of 3 mm, providing extra refractive power for near-vision.

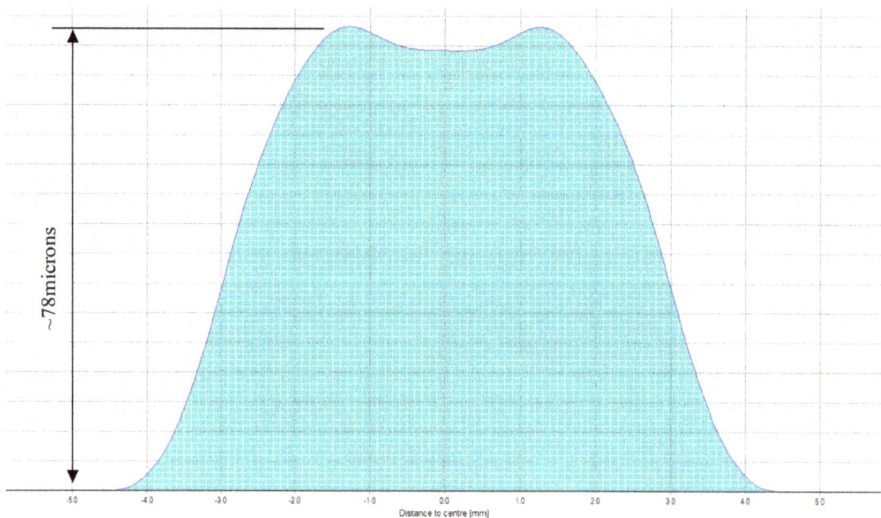

Figure 3. Typical multifocal ablation profile of a combined myopic and presbyopic treatment. The schematic indicates the amount of ablated tissue (blue area), with respect to the distance from the center of the cornea. Such a profile corrects the subjects' nearsightedness, as well as creates a steep central zone of 3 mm, providing extra refractive power for near-vision.

3. Results

All 72 surgical procedures were successfully executed, no side effects were detected, and not a single complication occurred during the study period. Measured on the LogMAR scale with respect to preoperative visual acuity (near: 0.29 ± 0.3, intermediate: 0.38 ± 0.36, distance: 0.75 ± 0.45), the visual acuity of subjects six months after surgery improved significantly, for near $(-0.01 \pm 0.11, p = 5 \times 10^{-6})$, intermediate $(-0.01 \pm 0.07, p = 2 \times 10^{-7})$, and distance vision $(-0.09 \pm 0.09, p = 4 \times 10^{-12})$. Furthermore, the visual acuity of all eyes remained stable postoperatively after six months. The excimer laser system applied the planned ablation patterns at a very high precision, as the differences between the targeted and achieved spherical equivalent (SEQ), given in the unit of refractive power—diopters (D), at six months postoperative were -0.01 ± 0.14 D (standard deviation—SD) with an r-square of $R^2 = 0.997$ and -0.27 ± 0.30 D (SD) with $R^2 = 0.986$, for dominant and non-dominant eyes, respectively (see Figure 4). Moreover, 72% of the dominant eyes had an SEQ accuracy to the target of ± 0.13 D, 17% were between +0.14 D and +0.50 D, and 11% were between -0.14 D and -0.50 D. In the non-dominant eyes, 42% were within ± 0.13 D, 47% were within +0.14 D and +0.50 D, 8% were within -0.14 D and -0.50 D, and 3% were between +0.51 D and 1.00 D.

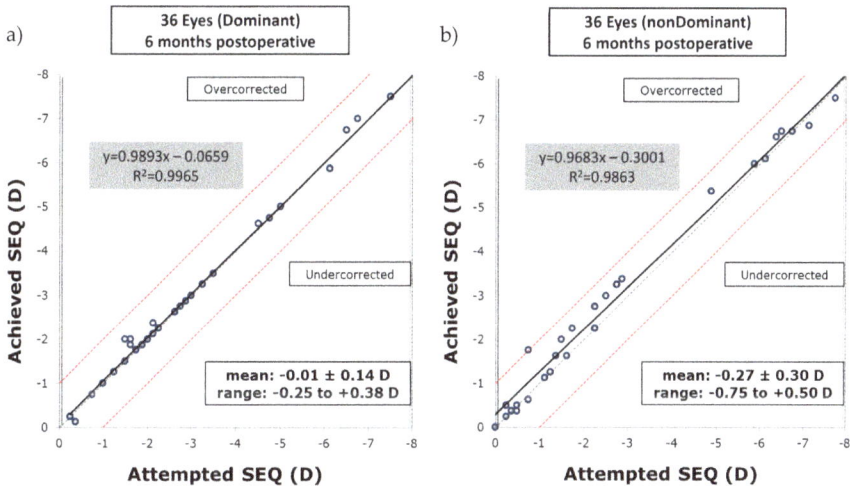

Figure 4. Attempted versus achieved spherical equivalent (SEQ) of (**a**) dominant and (**b**) non-dominant eyes, six months postoperatively. The regression lines in each graph indicate a small undercorrection for low values and a slight overcorrection for high values of spherical equivalent. SEQ: spherical equivalent; D: unit of refractive power, diopters.

The surgical treatment reduced spherical, and quadrafoil aberration in most eyes. Fifty-eight out of the 72 eyes had a decreased spherical aberration between 0.21 to 0.40 microns. Nine eyes had a decrease of quadrafoil aberration between 10 and 20 microns, and 62 eyes had a decrease of more than 20 microns of quadrafoil aberration (see Figure 5).

(a) Spherical aberration (Z400) baseline vs 6M postop (n=72)

(b) Quadrafoil aberration (Z440) baseline vs 6M postop (n=72)

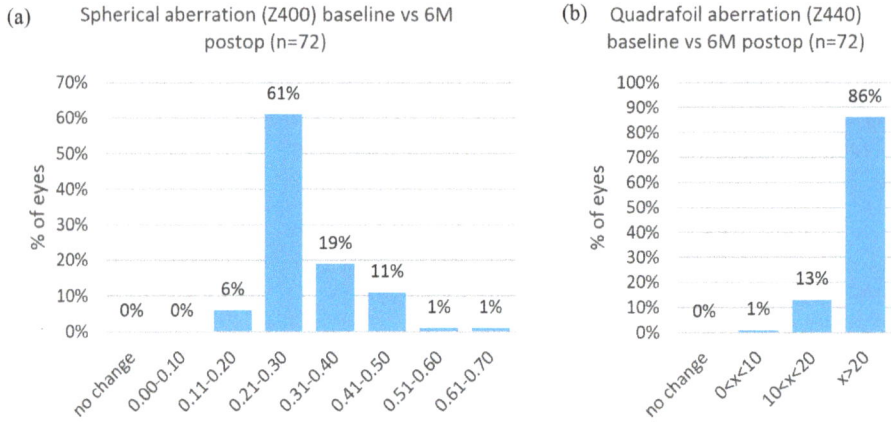

Figure 5. Surgically induced spherical (**a**) and quadrafoil (**b**) aberrations in micrometers, compared preoperatively (baseline) to postoperatively (postop). The treatment induced 0.21 to 0.40 microns of spherical aberration (Z400) and more than 20 microns of quadrafoil aberration (Z440) in most eyes.

Figure 6 presents the monocular mean and standard deviation of visual acuity before and after the surgery, for near, intermediate, and distance vision of all 36 subjects, in the LogMAR scale. At the six-month post-surgical follow-up for the dominant eyes, uncorrected near, intermediate, and distance visual acuity of 0.09 ± 0.11 (SD), 0.02 ± 0.04 (SD), and 0.02 ± 0.07 (SD) were observed, respectively. Meanwhile, for the non-dominant eyes, the six-month follow-up showed 0.04 ± 0.10 (SD), 0.01 ± 0.03 (SD), and 0.08 ± 0.08 (SD), for near, intermediate, and distance uncorrected visual acuity. Figure 7 indicates that while 36% of the dominant eyes had 20/20 uncorrected near visual acuity or better, six months after the intervention, 64% of the non-dominant were at 20/20 for uncorrected near visual acuity. The results in the figure further show that all eyes had 20/40 uncorrected visual acuity or better for distance and intermediate vision, while only 92% of the dominant and 97% of the non-dominant eyes had 20/40 uncorrected visual acuity for near vision. Figure 8 shows that the mean binocular visual acuity was at 0.03 ± 0.1 (SD), 0.01 ± 0.02 (SD), and 0.00 ± 0.05 (SD) for uncorrected near, intermediate, and distance vision, six months after the treatment. Further, the results show that 78% of the subjects had 20/20 uncorrected near visual acuity, 92% had 20/20 uncorrected intermediate visual acuity, and 86% had 20/20 distance visual acuity, at six months after surgery.

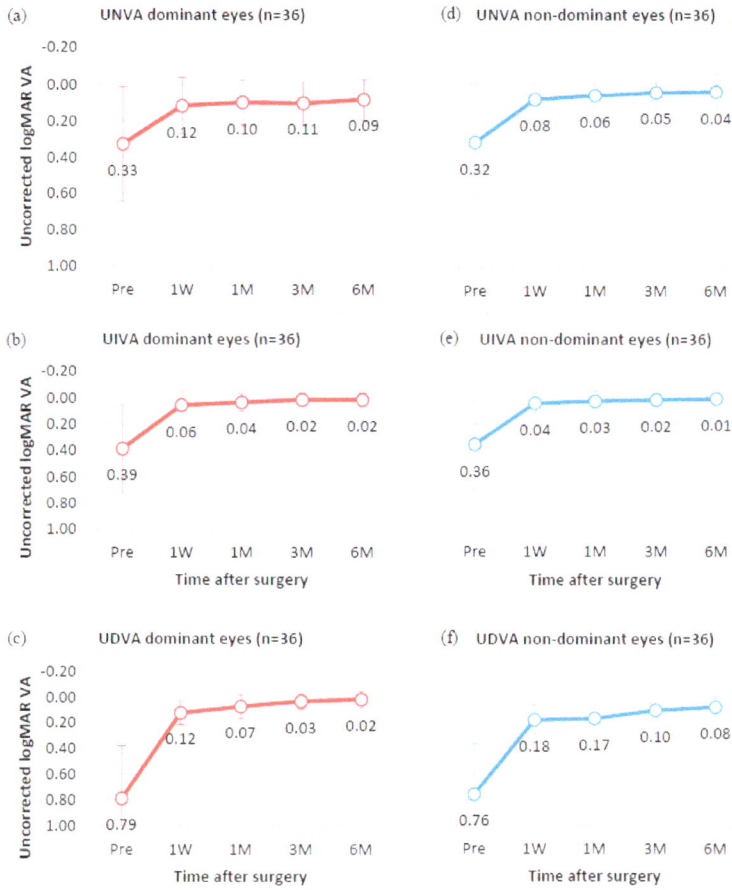

Figure 6. Mean and standard deviation of monocular uncorrected visual acuity for near (UNVA), intermediate (UIVA), and distance vision (UDVA) for 36 dominant (**a–c**) (shown in red), and 36 non-dominant (**d–f**) (shown in blue) eyes. Values are given preoperatively, and at one week (1 W), one month (1 M), three months (3 M), and six months (6 M) postsurgical follow-up.

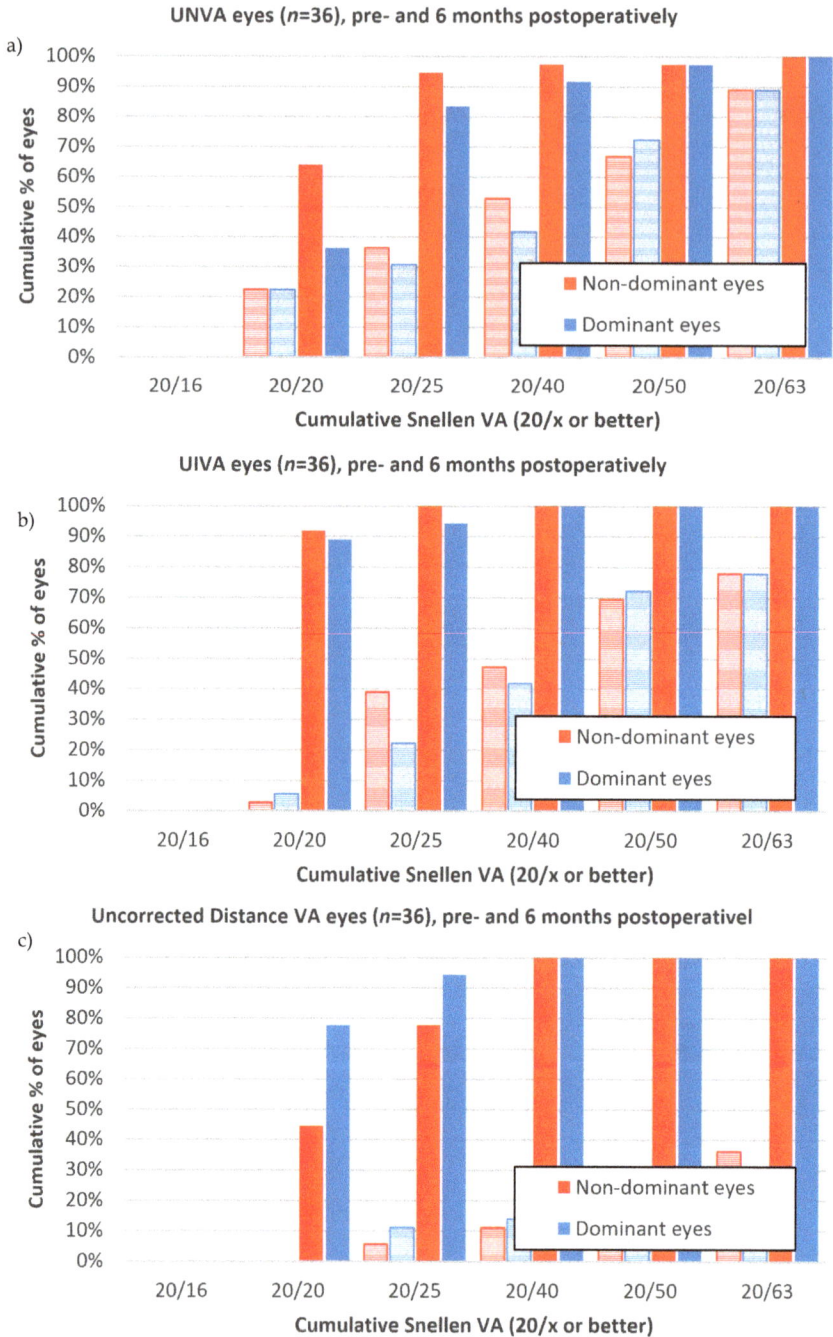

Figure 7. Cumulative percentage of subjects with 20/x dominant and non-dominant near (**a**), intermediate (**b**), and distance (**c**) visual acuity for 36 subjects. Dashed bars are preoperative, and solid bars are six-months postoperative data. Each percentage value is to be interpreted as 20/x vision or better.

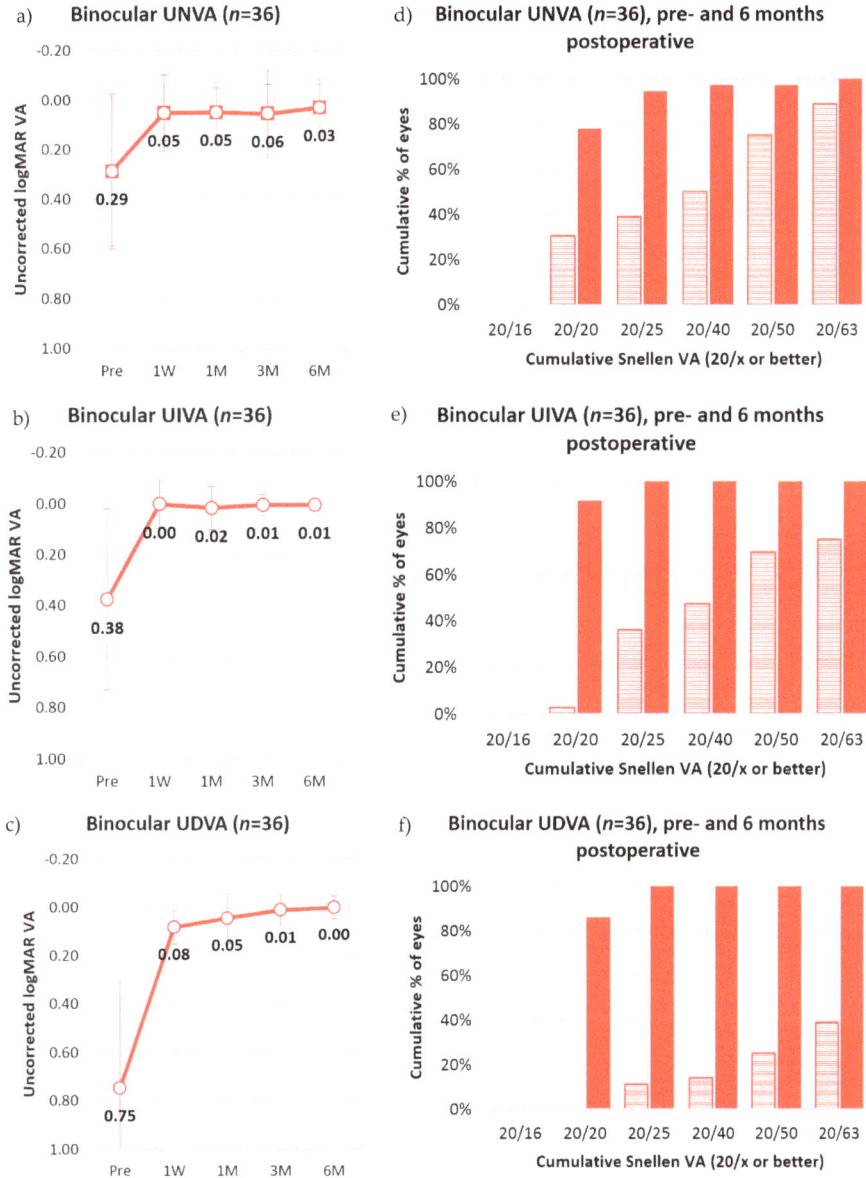

Figure 8. (**a–c**) Mean and standard deviation of binocular uncorrected visual acuity UNVA, UIVA, and UDVA vision for 36 subjects. Values are given preoperatively, and at one week (1 W), one month (1 M), three months (3 M), and six months (6 M) postsurgical follow-up. (**d–f**) Cumulative percentage of subjects with 20/x binocular near (UDVA), intermediate (UIVA), and distance (UDVA) vision for 36 subjects. Each percentage value is to be interpreted as 20/x vision or better.

4. Discussion

A prospective, single-center, single-surgeon clinical study on multifocal, myopic, presbyLASIK treatments, with an excimer laser, was carried out on 36 subjects. The applied treatment targeted the dominant eye to plano and the non-dominant eye to −0.5 diopters, while introducing a near addition of two diopters in the central cornea to increase the depth of focus.

Results suggest that the applied presbyLASIK procedure is an effective treatment for presbyopia. All study subjects had an uncorrected visual acuity of 20/40 or better for near, intermediate, and distance vision. Over 90% of the subjects were at 20/25 (LogMAR ≤ 0.10) or better, and about 80% were even at 20/20 (LogMAR ≤ 0.00) or better, again for the whole range of near, intermediate, and distance vision. In contrast to that, multifocal lens implantation results in the literature showed LogMAR 0.09 ± 0.08, LogMAR 0.10 ± 0.11, and LogMAR 0.07 ± 0.05, for near, intermediate, and distance vision [2], respectively, and in some cases even required spectacle correction for acceptable distance vision [1]. Mono vision treatments only showed 20/20 or better in 36.7% of the subjects for near, and in 31.1% of the subjects for distance visual acuity [3]. Results of intracorneal inlays were comparable for uncorrected near vision [6], and distance vision was not reported.

As expected, while the dominant eyes in this study generally had higher monocular visual acuity for distance vision, the non-dominant eyes performed better in monocular near vision. Presumably, the brains of the study candidates were capable of blending the two distinct monocular images into a binocular image, electively focusing on near, intermediate, and distant targets. This circumstance is supported by the thoroughly high satisfaction of all of the study patients.

Generally speaking, the excimer procedure employed in this study was less invasive compared to other presbyopia methods, such as refractive lens implantation. LASIK is a very well accepted and extensively proven procedure. It features high precision in positioning of the correction, in refractive outcome, as well as in predictability of the result. A key factor for this is the high precision and repeatability of flap quality and thickness [12]. A remaining problem with LASIK-based presbyopia treatments, however, is that the multifocal ablation may induce unwanted optical aberrations. Multifocal ablations usually are composed of a correction for distance vision (myopic or hyperopic), and a near addition. Lower order optical aberrations, specifically spherical aberrations, may be caused by the distance correction ablation. Additional higher order aberrations stemming from the transition between the distance treatment zone and the near addition might be induced, even though they may be outside of the region of the central addition, yet inside the optical zone of the distance vision correction. It seems apparent that the resulting refractive surface might evoke unfavourable optical aberrations [9,13,14]. Our wavefront results suggest that the customization algorithm for aberration reduction works very well. In almost all cases, spherical (Z400) as well as quadrafoil (Z440) aberrations were significantly reduced by the treatment.

The thoroughly positive results with the LASIK-based presbyopia treatment in this study can, at least partially, be attributed to the aspherical customization algorithm. The algorithm utilized the K-readings as well as the conic constant (Q) of the cornea to minimize the induction of adverse optical aberration effects [8,10,12]. In addition, using LASIK provides the option to re-touch the treatment with relative ease, and therefore has the potential to remove or enhance the presbyopic addition [9]. Even though further studies with more surgical cases are necessary to confirm these results, the presbyLASIK treatment employed in this study has great potential to become a gold standard for the treatment of presbyopia, as it safe and shows reliable, predictable, and satisfying outcomes.

Acknowledgments: The study was supported by the Swiss Commission for Technology and Innovation (CTI), through CTI project 13404.1.

Author Contributions: Bojan Pajic provided the treatment indication, developed the study design, acquired clinical data, and contributed to writing the paper. Brigitte Pajic-Eggspuehler performed data analysis and substantially contributed the study design. Joerg Mueller supplied surgical advices and substantially contribute to the design of the study. Zeljka Cvejic contributed substantially to the development of the study design. Harald Studer performed data analysis and contributed to writing the paper.

Conflicts of Interest: All authors declare no conflict of interest.

References

1. Chang, J.S.; Ng, J.C.; Lau, S.Y. Visual outcomes and patient satisfaction after presbyopic lens exchange with a diffractive multifocal intraocular lens. *J. Refract. Surg.* **2012**, *28*, 468–474. [CrossRef] [PubMed]
2. Tsaousis, K.T.; Plainis, S.; Dimitrakos, S.A.; Tsinopoulos, I.T. Binocularity anhances visual acuity of eyes implanted with multifocal intraocular lenses. *J. Refract. Surg.* **2013**, *29*, 246–250. [CrossRef] [PubMed]
3. Braun, E.H.; Lee, J.; Steinert, R.F. Monovision in LASIK. *Ophthalmology* **2008**, *115*, 1196–1202. [CrossRef] [PubMed]
4. Jain, S.; Ou, R.; Azar, D.T. Monovision outcomes in presbyopic individuals after refractive surgery. *Ophthalmology* **2001**, *108*, 1430–1433. [CrossRef]
5. Bouzoukis, D.I.; Kymionis, G.D.; Panagopoulos, S.I.; Diakonis, V.F.; Pallikaris, A.I.; Limnopoulou, A.N.; Portaliou, D.M.; Pallikaris, I.G. Visual outcomes and safety of small diameter intrastromal refractive inlay for the corneal compensation of presbyopia. *J. Refract. Surg.* **2012**, *28*, 168–173. [CrossRef] [PubMed]
6. Yilmaz, O.F.; Alagoz, N.; Pekel, G.; Azman, E.; Aksoy, E.F.; Cakır, H.; Bozkurt, E.; Demirok, A. Intracorneal inlay to correct presbyopia: Long-term results. *J. Cataract Refract. Surg.* **2011**, *37*, 1275–1281. [CrossRef] [PubMed]
7. Menassa, N.; Fitting, A.; Auffarth, G.U.; Holzer, M.P. Visual outcomes and corneal changes after intrastromal femtosecond correction of presbyopia. *J. Cataract Refract. Surg.* **2012**, *28*, 765–773. [CrossRef] [PubMed]
8. Saib, N.; Abrieu-Lacaille, M.; Berguiga, M.; Rambaud, C.; Froussart-Maille, F.; Rigal-Sastourne, J.C. Central PresbyLASIK for Hyperopia and Presbyopia Using Micro-monovision With the Technolas 217P Platform and SUPRACOR Algorithm. *J. Refract. Surg.* **2015**, *31*, 540–546. [CrossRef] [PubMed]
9. Vastardis, I.; Pajic-Eggspuehler, B.; Mueller, J.; Cvejic, Z.; Pajic, B. Femtosecond laser-assisted in situ keratomileusis multifocal ablation profile using a mini-monovision approach for presbyopic patients with hyperopia. *Clin. Ophthalmol.* **2016**, *10*, 1245–1256. [CrossRef] [PubMed]
10. Ryan, A.; O'Keefe, M. Corneal approach to hyperopic presbyopia treatment: Six-month outcomes of a new multifocal excimer laser in situ keratomileusis procedure. *J. Cataract Refract. Surg.* **2013**, *39*, 1226–1233. [CrossRef] [PubMed]
11. Munnerlyn, C.R.; Koons, S.J. Photorefractive keratectomy: A technique for laser refractive surgery. *J. Cataract Refract. Surg.* **1988**, *14*, 46–52. [CrossRef]
12. Pajic, B.; Vastardis, I.; Pajic-Eggspuehler, B.; Gatzioufas, Z.; Hafezi, F. Femtosecond laser versus mechanical microkeratome-assisted flap creation for LASIK: A prospective, randomized, paired-eye study. *Clin. Ophthalmol.* **2014**, *8*, 1883–1889. [CrossRef] [PubMed]
13. Alio, J.L.; Chaubard, J.J.; Caliz, A.; Sala, E.; Patel, S. Correction of Presbyopia by Technovision Central Multifocal LASIK (PresbyLASIK). *J. Refract. Surg.* **2006**, *22*, 453–460. [CrossRef] [PubMed]
14. Eppstein, R.L.; Gurgos, M.A. Presbyopia Treatment by Monocular Peripheral PresbyLASIK. *J. Refract. Surg.* **2009**, *25*, 516–523. [CrossRef]

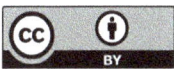

sensors

MDPI

Article

Cataract Surgery Performed by High Frequency LDV Z8 Femtosecond Laser: Safety, Efficacy, and Its Physical Properties

Bojan Pajic [1,2,3,4,*], Zeljka Cvejic [2] and Brigitte Pajic-Eggspuehler [1]

[1]   Eye Clinic Orasis, Swiss Eye Research Foundation, 5734 Reinach AG, Switzerland; brigitte.pajic@orasis.ch
[2]   Department of Physics, Faculty of Sciences, University of Novi Sad, Trg Dositeja Obradovica 4,
      21000 Novi Sad, Serbia; zeljkac@uns.ac.rs
[3]   Division of Ophthalmology, Department of Clinical Neurosciences, Geneva University Hospitals,
      Rue Gabrielle-Perret-Gentil 4, 1205 Genève, Switzerland
[4]   Faculty of Medicine of the Military Medical academy, University of Defense, 11000 Belgrade, Serbia
*   Correspondence: bpajic@datacomm.ch; Tel.: +41-62-765-6080

Received: 31 March 2017; Accepted: 15 June 2017; Published: 18 June 2017

Abstract: Background: The aim of our study was to investigate the safety and efficacy of the LDV Z8 femtosecond laser in cataract surgery compared to the conventional procedure. Methods: This prospective study was performed at the Swiss Eye Research Foundation, Eye Clinic ORASIS, Reinach, Switzerland. The study included 130 eyes from 130 patients: 68 treated with femtosecond laser-assisted cataract surgery (FLACS) using the FEMTO LDV Z8 and 62 treated with conventional phacoemulsification. Capsulotomy and lens fragmentation in the laser group were performed with the FEMTO LDV Z8 femtosecond laser system, which employs a new, low-energy, high repetition rate laser process for cataract surgery. In the conventional group, the capsulotomy was performed by a cystotome, and lens fragmentation was achieved by the stop-and-chop. Results: Ease of phacoemulsification (on a 4-point scale), the completeness of capsulotomy (on a 10-point scale), effective phacoemulsification time (seconds), uncorrected distance visual acuity (UCVA), best spectacle-corrected distance visual acuity (BSCVA), spherical equivalent (SE), and safety of the procedure were evaluated. The total follow-up time was three months. Conclusions: FLACS with the FEMTO LDV Z8 system was characterized by complete and reproducible capsulotomy and highly effective lens fragmentation. Postoperative visual outcomes were excellent, and the safety of the procedure was optimal.

Keywords: femtosecond laser; physical properties; cataract surgery; clinical outcomes; complications

1. Introduction

Femtosecond laser technology was first introduced in corneal refractive surgery for performing LASIK flaps. Compared to the microkeratome, an increase in precision and safety was observed [1,2]. Femtosecond technology was soon expanded to cataract surgery where its application introduced a higher predictability, safety, and potentially improved refractive outcome. Femtosecond laser systems are designed to perform anterior capsulotomy, lens fragmentation using different patterns, clear corneal incisions, and arcuate incisions. In the past few years, a significant amount of research investigating the advantages of femtosecond laser-assisted cataract surgery compared to conventional ultrasound phacoemulsification cataract surgery has been conducted. These studies have demonstrated that femtosecond laser-assisted capsulotomies have a higher precision regarding circularity and placement versus achieved diameter than those created by manual continuous curvilinear capsulorhexis. The femtosecond laser lens fragmentation results in a significant decrease in phacoemulsification energy exposure to the eye [3–8]. In the literature, it has been shown that the cut quality of clear corneal incisions done by femtosecond laser improves the tunnel morphology with less tissue damage compared with the conventional procedure. Due to its high precision and excellent surgical planning, femtosecond use in cataract surgery has also reduced the occurrence of high-order aberrations [9–11]. Femtosecond laser technology is, at the moment, more expensive compared to conventional cataract surgery but offers several advantages. A slightly greater amount of time is necessary for the femtosecond laser procedure compared with conventional phacoemulsification.

Femtosecond Laser

The Femto LDV Z8 (Ziemer Ophthalmic Systems AG, Port, Switzerland) is a high frequency femtosecond laser system for corneal surgery, corneal-refractive surgery, and cataract surgery. Unique among cataract laser systems, the Z8 applies the concept of overlapping low-energy near-infrared (1030 nm) femtosecond laser pulses in the nano-Joule range. This concept was originally developed by Ziemer Ophthalmic Systems for corneal surgery but was later adapted for cataract surgery applications such as lens fragmentation, capsulotomy, clear corneal incisions, and arcuate incisions. In order to shorten surgery time because small spots with large numerical aperture are used (Figure 1a), the laser system runs in the MHz range applying up to 1 billion pulses per surgery. Conventional femtosecond lasers with small numerical apertures (Figure 1b) that run in the kHz range, leads to a larger spot with a higher pulse energy and more gas creation.

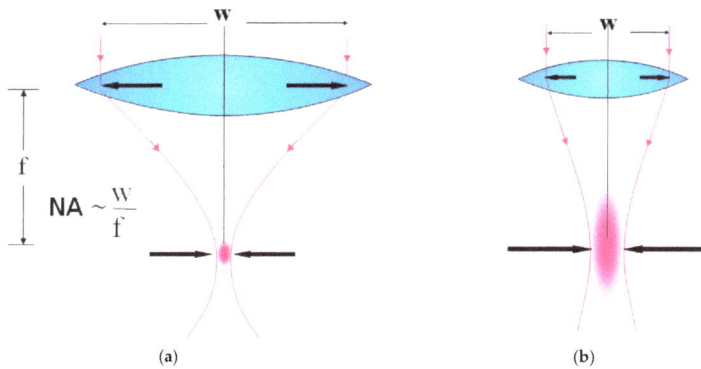

(a)   (b)

Figure 1. (**a**) The large numerical aperture is the key for minimizing the focal volume which leads to low pulse energy and less bubbles (LDV Z8 femtosecond laser). (**b**) The small numerical aperture leads to higher pulse energy and more bubbles (conventional laser systems).

Each pulse creates a cavitation bubble approximately a few microns wide, which gently separates tissue. The handpiece (Figure 2) is the size of a compact camera and integrates all required electronics, optics, and actuators to perform visualization and resection in the anterior chamber of the eye. Visual esolution is possible down to 5 microns and is performed with a combination of a color camera and spectral-domain optical coherence tomography (OCT) operated at 840 nm (Figure 3).

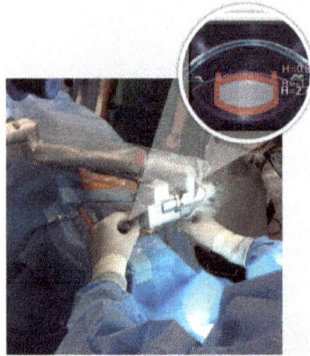

Figure 2. Femtosecond laser handpiece of the LDV Z8.

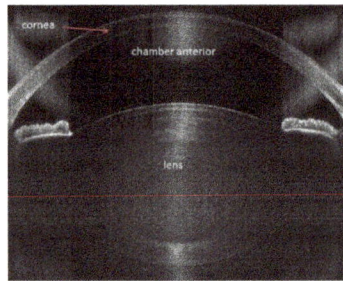

Figure 3. High-resolution OCT at a wavelength of 840 nm is mandatory for receiving a precise cut in the right position.

The FEMTO LDV Z8 uses a high focusing power microscope lens integrated in the handpiece to achieve focusing to a small spot size (<2 µm), which enables cuts to be made with nJ pulse energy. Low pulse energy with high-frequency applications is very precise and allows a spot diameter of less than 2 µm (Figure 4a). Conventional femtosecond lasers with a small numerical aperture and pulse energies in the µJ range has spot diameters greater than 5 µm and spot separation greater than the spot diameter (typically 10–20 µm), which can lead to tissue bridges (Figure 4b).

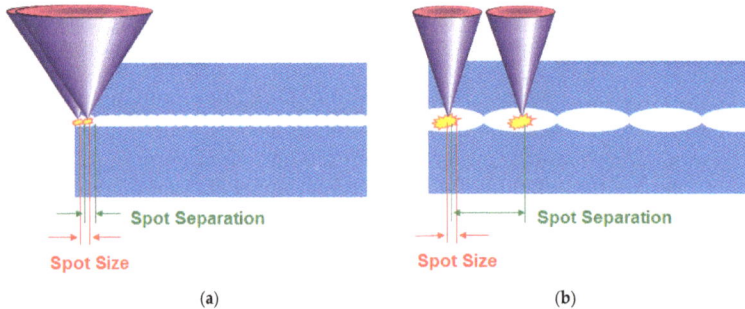

Figure 4. (**a**) The cutting process is limited to the focal spot size. Many pulses are needed to cut the tissue, so a high frequency repetition rate is needed. (**b**) The cutting process is mainly performed by mechanical forces of the expanding gas bubbles). Fewer pluses are needed but stress is generated in the tissue.

Given this unique combination of technical parameters, FLACS is able to create a more precise and circular capsulorhexis that could improve phacoemulsification and IOL centration, so a more precise refractive outcome after surgery could be expected [4,11–15].

2. Materials and Methods

This prospective randomized operative-interventional case–control study compares the performance and safety of femtosecond laser-assisted cataract procedures with those of conventional phacoemulsification cataract surgery.

The inclusion criteria required eligibility to undergo lens extraction by phacoemulsification followed by IOL implantation, an ability to complete patient interface docking with the femtosecond laser, an age of 50 years of older, willingness and ability to return for scheduled follow-up examination, and no current infections. Exclusion criteria consisted of minimal and maximal K-values of the central 3 mm zone that differ by more than 5D on topographic map of the cornea, a maximum K-value that exceeds 50D, a minimum K-value of less than 37D, corneal disease or pathology, such as corneal scaring or opacity, that precludes the transmission of laser wavelength or that distorts laser light, poorly dilating pupils of less than 6 mm or any other defect of the pupil that prevents the iris from adequate refraction peripherally, manifest glaucoma and ocular hypertension, and pseudoexfoliation. Additionally, any systemic or ocular pathology or previous ocular surgery was also excluded. All surgery procedures were performed by an experienced surgeon (BP) at the Eye Clinic ORASIS between January 2015 and September 2016.

The Z8 is a mobile femtosecond laser system that can be used in a sterile environment of the operating theatre. The hand-held patient interface allows for surgery to be performed without making significant alterations to the operation room layout in terms of space and equipment, thus preserving existing workflows. In the current study, all femtosecond laser cataract surgeries and conventional cataract surgeries were performed under the surgeon's microscope, and no patients were moved into or out of the operating room during the procedure. All surgeries were performed under topical anesthesia rapidocain intracameral. Preoperative the pupil dilation was achieved by application of Mydriasert (combination of phenylephrine hydrochlorid (5.4 mg) and Tropicamide (0.28 mg)).

2.1. Femtosecond Laser-Assisted Cataract Surgery Technique

The suction ring of a disposable liquid–patient interface was applied to the eye with centration over the limbus. The system contains a liquid interface (no applanation), which prevents posterior corneal descemet folds, ensuring an unhindered laser beam transmission. As soon as the suction vacuum reached 400 mbar, the suction ring was filled with a balanced salt solution (BSS). The handpiece, which is attached to an articulating arm of the laser system, was docked over the corneal apex. In the handpiece, there is a color camera and an integrated ocular coherence tomography (OCT) system that images the ocular structures. Treatment parameters were customized to accommodate each individual patient. Custom surgical planning is performed by the precise placement of surgical incisions based on OCT images that identify ocular structures and automatically determine and display safety margins and suggested cut locations. Via a touchscreen, the surgeon has the ability to reposition treatment patterns. Laser treatment begins with lens fragmentation (an eight-piece pie-cut pattern) followed by anterior capsulotomy (5.0 mm in diameter). Unlike other FLACS systems, lens fragmentation before anterior capsulotomy is possible with the Z8, as the low energy results in minimal gas production, which significantly reduces the risk of intra-operative complications. As shown in Figure 5, the capsular button in the OCT image can be seen free-floating, while the fragmented lens shows no accumulation of gas.

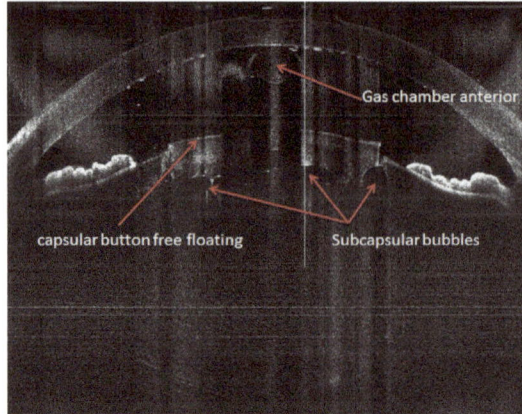

Figure 5. A complete capsulotomy is seen with the capsular button free floating in the anterior chamber, while there is nearly no accumulation of gas in the fragmented lens. There are minimal subcapsular bubbles in the anterior chamber.

2.2. Conventional Cataract Surgery Technique

Two paracentesis 0.8 mm in diameter were performed. Intracameral anesthesia was administered (Lidocaine hydrochlorid and Epinephrine, 0.005 mg). A capsulorhexis 5 mm in diameter was attempted. For phacoemulsification, the stop-and-chop technique was applied. The remainder of the surgical steps required to complete the operation were identical between FLACS and conventional groups.

Minimal gas accumulation was visible at the posterior surface of the cornea, which was observed in the OCT through the creation of shadows seen on the lower part of the image. For all patients, the phacoemulsification device Catharex 3 system (Oertli Instrumente AG, Berneck, Switzerland) was used. By using the bimanual irrigation/aspiration system, residual cortex was removed. In all cases, an IOL was implanted in the capsular bag. Patients were scheduled for postoperative examination at Day 1, Day 12, and 4, 8, and 12 weeks after surgery. The main outcome measures evaluated in this study were best corrected visual acuity (BCVA), effective phacoemulsification time (EPT, seconds), and complications. Cataract severity was graded according to nuclear opalescence on the Lens Opacities Classification System III [16] with Grades 1–4.

Statistical analysis was computed with IBM SPSS Statistics version 20.0 (IBM Corp., Armonk, NY, USA). Normal distribution of data was determined by the Shapiro–Wilk test (data was considered normal if $p > 0.05$). Normal values were shown as mean $\pm$ standard deviation, whereas the median value was shown as non-parametric data. The level of significance was set at $p < 0.05$. BCVA was measured with Snellen projector charts, and data were converted to logarithm of the minimum angle of resolution (logMAR) units for statistical analysis. Related-samples Wilcoxon signed rank test was used to compare preoperative and postoperative BCVA and intended versus measured capsulotomy diameters.

3. Results

There were 33 males (48.5%) and 35 females (51.5%) in the FLACS group and 25 (40.3%) males and 37 females (59.7%) in the conventional cataract surgery group enrolled in the study.

The ethics committee of Northwest and Central Switzerland (EKNZ) approved the study. A total of 130 eyes from 130 patients were recruited for cataract treatment, with 68 patients recruited to the FLACS group (Group 1) and 62 patients recruited to the conventional cataract surgery group (Group 2). The mean age of patients in the FLACS group was 70.4 $\pm$ 8.4 years (range: 50–83 years) and 69.6 $\pm$ 8.2 years (range: 50–85 years) for the conventional cataract surgery group. There was no statistically significant difference in age ($p = 0.25$) between the two groups. Regarding the preoperative BCVA, there were no significant differences between the groups ($p = 0.49$). According to the Lens Opacities Classification System III, the preoperative cataract grade density in the femtosecond laser cataract surgery group was 2.57 ± 0.58 and the conventional cataract surgery group was 2.23 ± 0.42, which is highly significant ($p < 0.001$).

All patients in both groups underwent a successful operation. The intended capsulotomy diameter was set at 5.0 mm in all cases. The achieved capsulotomy diameter in the FLACS group was 5.0 ± 0.12 mm (range: 4.6–5.4 mm), median 5.0 mm, and in the conventional cataract surgery group 4.7 ± 0.36 mm (range: 4.0–5.6 mm), median 4.7 mm, which is highly significant ($p < 0.001$). The mean phacoemulsification time in Group 1 was 1.9 ± 2.25 s (range: 0–11 s), median 1.0 s, and in Group 2, 2.3 ± 2.41 s (range: 0.3–14 s), median 1.7 s, which is significant ($p = 0.042$). The effective phacoemulsification time (EPT) in Group 1 was found to be 1.48 ± 1.80 s (range: 0–8.8 s), median 0.8 s, and in Group 2 1.81 ± 1.93 s (range: 0.24–11.2 s), median 1.36 s, which is significant ($p = 0.044$) (Table 1).

Table 1. Mean phacoemulsification time/effective phacoemulsification time for Groups 1 and 2.

	Group 1	Group 2	*p*-Value
mean phacoemulsification time (s)	1.9 ± 2.25	2.3 ± 2.41	0.042
effective phacoemulsification time (EPT)	1.48 ± 1.80	1.81 ± 1.93	0.044

Overall surgery time in Group 1 was 7.5 ± 1.22 min (range: 5–12 min) and 6.6 ± 1.76 min (range: 4.6–12 min) in Group 2, that is slightly significant ($p = 0.048$).

The mean preoperative BCVA was 0.29 logMAR (range 1.30–0.01 logMAR) in Group 1 and 0.30 logMAR (range 1.30–0.01 logMAR) in Group 2 ($p = 0.50$). There is no difference between the groups. The mean BCVA, 1 day post-operation, was 0.16 logMAR (range 1.30–0 logMAR) in Group 1 and 0.22 logMAR (range 1.30–0 logMAR) ($p = 0.038$) in Group 2; 12 days post-operation, 0.06 logMAR (range 0.49–0 logMAR) in Group 1 and 0.06 logMAR (range 0.60–(−0.10) logMAR) in Group 2 ($p = 0.48$); 4 weeks post-operation, 0.03 logMAR (range 0.49–(−0.10) logMAR) in Group 1 and 0.06 logMAR (range 0.30–(−0.10) logMAR) in Group 2 ($p = 0.31$); 8 weeks post-operation, 0.03 logMAR (range 0.40–(−0.10) logMAR) in Group 1 and 0.06 logMAR (range 0.49–(−0.10) logMAR) in Group 2 ($p = 0.41$); 12 weeks post-operation, 0.01 logMAR (range 0.30–(−0.10) logMAR) in Group 1 and 0.02 logMAR (range 0.49–(−0.10) logMAR) in Group 2 ($p = 0.37$). Only the value at 1 day is significant, whereas at any later follow-up there are no significant differences between the groups (Table 2).

Table 2. Mean BCA for Group 1 and Group 2 in the follow-up.

Mean BCVA	Group 1	Group 2	
preoperative	0.29 logMAR (range 1.30–0.01)	0.30 logMAR (range 1.30–0.01)	$p = 0.50$
1 day post-operation	0.16 logMAR (range 1.30–0)	0.22 logMAR (range 1.30–0)	$p = 0.038$
12 days post-operation	0.06 logMAR (range 0.49–0)	0.06 logMAR (range 0.60–(−0.10))	$p = 0.48$
4 weeks post-operation	0.03 logMAR (range 0.49–(−0.10))	0.06 logMAR (range 0.30–(−0.10))	$p = 0.31$
8 weeks post-operation	0.03 logMAR (range 0.40–(−0.10))	0.06 logMAR (range 0.49–(−0.10))	$p = 0.41$
12 weeks post-operation	0.01 logMAR (range 0.30–(−0.10))	0.02 logMAR (range 0.49–(−0.10))	$p = 0.37$

The vacuum time for FLACS patients 139 ± 26 s.

Follow-up was 3 months for all patients. No intraoperative complications were recorded.

4. Discussion

Numerous studies have reported advantages of femtosecond laser over conventional phacoemulsification cataract surgery [3,4,6,8,13,14,17–23]. Our study shows that a targeted 5 mm capsulotomy could be achieved very precisely with the femtosecond laser treatment, demonstrating only small variance in reproducibility, whereas the manual capsulorhexis differed significantly. Other studies have demonstrated very similar results, where the capsulotomies created using the femtosecond laser were more accurate in size than those created by manual continuous curvilinear capsulorhexis [4,8,13,14,22]. The accuracy of the capsulotomy is very important because it provides the surgeon access to the capsular bag for fragmentation and removal of natural lens and placement of the IOL. The diameter of the capsulotomy should allow overlap between the capsul rim and the IOL optic and haptic for correct IOL positioning. In special IOL, like toric IOL, the alignment is particularly important. Thus, the diameter, shape, and centration of the capsulorhexis can influence IOL position and may have an impact on refractive outcomes.

According of Lens Opacities Classification System III, the preoperative cataract grade density in the femtosecond laser-assisted cataract surgery group (Group 1) was significantly higher ($p < 0.001$) than in the conventional cataract surgery group (Group 2) in our study. Despite this potential disadvantage, we needed significantly less phacoemulsification time and effective phacoemulsification time in the femtosecond laser group (Group 1) compared with the conventional phacoemulsification surgery group (Group 2). Other studies have shown that the reduction of ultrasound energy from phacoemulsification can reduce the risk of capsule complication. Phacoemulsification time and effective phacoemulsification time are known to increase with nuclear density, but other groups have reported similar findings regarding FLACS and EPT [4] as we have observed. In our study, it was seen that, even with a low-energy laser application, the lens fragmentation was perfectly cut. Low energy creates smaller gas bubbles, which reduces the tension on the capsular bag during the procedure. Thus, the Femto LDV Z8 femtosecond laser is able to perform the optimal procedure algorithm, where the cut procedure begins with the lens fragmentation followed by capsulotomy and clear corneal incisions. We did not observe any bubbles during any of the stages of the laser procedure, which could disturb the optimal cut quality.

In our study, we detected an improvement in visual acuity one day post-operation, an improvement that was significantly greater with the femtosecond laser compared with the conventional procedure. This may reveal that the rehabilitation time in the first postoperative day is faster. In all other follow-up times after 12 days, no significant differences regarding the visual acuity were observed.

FLACS with the LDV Z8, a low-energy high frequency femtosecond laser, shows very high precision, with a significant decrease in effective phacoemulsification time (EPT) compared to the conventional procedure, even when the lens density was higher. Our results indicate that the healing time involved in visual acuity is faster in the first postoperative days, demonstrating the clinical advantages of a gentle technique with the femtosecond laser. However, regarding the overall surgery time, we report that slightly more time is needed to perform femtosecond laser treatment, but the potential to optimize workflow further and eliminate this difference is a future aim.

5. Conclusions

One of the main goals is providing repeatable and precise outcomes, with an aim to offer customized medical solutions for patients. The low-energy LDV Z8 with its advanced OCT visualization allows the best placement of the capsulotomy and optimizes surgical planning. All of this influences the strength of capsulotomy and significantly improves refractive outcomes due to reduced IOL tilt [14,24]. A high-frequency device with low pulse energy enables minimal gas creation during lens fragmentation. This sets it apart from other cataract laser devices with higher energy and low frequency, where larger bubbles and tissue bridges are created.

Acknowledgments: A special thanks goes to Holger Lubatschowski, Hannover, Germany, for distributing the images (Figures 1 and 4).

Author Contributions: Bojan Pajic and Brigitte Pajic-Eggspuehler conceived and designed the experiments; Bojan Pajic performed the experiments; Zeljka Cvejic contributed analysis tools; all authors wrote the paper.

Conflicts of Interest: The authors declare no conflict of interest.

References

1. Ratkay-Traub, I.; Juhasz, T.; Horvath, C.; Suarez, C.; Kiss, K.; Ferincz, I.; Kurtz, R. Ultra-short puls (femtosecond) laser surgery: Initial use in LASIK flap creation. *Ophthalmol. Clin. N. Am.* **2001**, *14*, 347–355.
2. Kim, P.; Sutton, G.L.; Rootman, D.S. Applications of femtosecond laser in corneal refractive surgery. *Curr. Opin.* **2011**, *22*, 238–244. [CrossRef] [PubMed]
3. Conrad-Hengerer, I.; Al Juburi, M.; Schultz, T.; Hengerer, F.H.; Dick, H.B. Corneal endothelial cell loss and corneal thickness in conventional compared with femtosecond laser-assisted cataract surgery: Three-month follow-up. *J. Cataract Refract. Surg.* **2013**, *39*, 1307–1313. [CrossRef] [PubMed]
4. Conrad-Hengerer, I.; Hengerer, F.H.; Schultz, T.; Dick, H.B. Effect of femtosecond laser fragmentation on effective phacoemulsification time in cataract surgery. *J. Refract. Surg.* **2012**, *28*, 879–883. [CrossRef] [PubMed]
5. Abell, R.G.; Kerr, N.M.; Vote, B.J. Toward zero effective phacoemulsification time using femtosecond laser pretreatment. *Ophthalmology* **2013**, *120*, 942–948. [CrossRef] [PubMed]
6. Abell, R.G.; Kerr, N.M.; Vote, B.J. Femtosecond laser-assisted cataract surgery compared with conventional cataract surgery. *Clin. Exp. Ophthalmol.* **2013**, *41*, 455–462. [CrossRef] [PubMed]
7. Reddy, K.P.; Kandulla, J.; Auffarth, G.U. Effectiveness and safety of femtosecond laser-assisted lens fragmentation and anterior capsulotomy versus the manual technique in cataract surgery. *J. Cataract Refract. Surg.* **2013**, *39*, 1297–1306. [CrossRef] [PubMed]
8. Nagy, Z.Z.; Kranitz, K.; Takacs, A.I.; Mihaltz, K.; Kovacs, I.; Knorz, M.C. Comparison of intraocular lens decentration parameters after femtosecond and manual capsulotomies. *J. Refract. Surg.* **2011**, *27*, 564–569. [CrossRef] [PubMed]
9. Grewal, D.S.; Basti, S. Comparison of morphologic features of clear corneal incisions created with a femtosecond laser or a keratome. *J. Cataract Refract. Surg.* **2014**, *40*, 521–530. [CrossRef] [PubMed]
10. Alió, J.L.; Abdou, A.A.; Soria, F.; Javaloy, J.; Fernández-Buenaga, R.; Nagy, Z.Z.; Filkorn, T. Femtosecond laser cataract incision morphology and corneal higher-order aberration analysis. *J. Refract. Surg.* **2013**, *29*, 590–595. [CrossRef] [PubMed]
11. Mastropasqua, L.; Toto, L.; Mastropasqua, A.; Vecchiarino, L.; Mastropasqua, R.; Pedrotti, E.; Di Nicola, M. Femtosecond laser versus manual clear corneal incision in cataract surgery. *J. Refract. Surg.* **2014**, *30*, 27–33. [CrossRef] [PubMed]
12. Moshirfar, M.; Churgin, D.S.; Hsu, M. Femtosecond laser-assisted cataract surgery: A current review. *Middle East Afr. J. Ophthalmol.* **2011**, *18*, 285–291. [CrossRef] [PubMed]
13. Friedman, N.J.; Palanker, D.V.; Schuele, G.; Andersen, D.; Marcellino, G.; Seibel, B.S.; Batlle, J.; Feliz, R.; Talamo, J.H.; Blumenkranz, M.S.; et al. Femtosecond laser capsulotomy. *J. Cataract Refract. Surg.* **2011**, *37*, 1189–1198. [CrossRef] [PubMed]
14. Kranitz, K.; Takacs, A.; Mihaltz, K.; Kovacs, I.; Knorz, M.C.; Nagy, Z.Z. Femtosecond laser capsulotomy and manual continuous curvilinear capsulorrhexis parameters and their effects on intraocular lens centration. *J. Refract. Surg.* **2011**, *27*, 558–563. [CrossRef] [PubMed]
15. Assia, E.I.; Apple, D.J.; Tsai, J.C.; Morgan, R.C. Mechanism of radial tear formation and extension after anterior capsulectomy. *Ophthalmology* **1991**, *98*, 432–437. [CrossRef]
16. Chylack, L.T., Jr.; Wolfe, J.K.; Singer, D.M.; Leske, M.C.; Bullimore, M.A.; Bailey, I.L.; Friend, J.; McCarthy, D.; Wu, S.Y. The Longitudinal Study of Cataract Study Group The Lens Opacities Classification System III. *Arch. Ophthalmol.* **1993**, *111*, 831–836. [CrossRef] [PubMed]
17. Takács, A.I.; Kovács, I.; Miháltz, K.; Filkorn, T.; Knorz, M.C.; Nagy, Z.Z. Central corneal volume and endothelial cell count following femtosecond laser-assisted refractive cataract surgery compared to conventional phacoemulsification. *J. Refract. Surg.* **2012**, *28*, 387–391. [CrossRef] [PubMed]
18. Filkorn, T.; Kovács, I.; Takács, A.; Horváth, E.; Knorz, M.C.; Nagy, Z.Z. Comparison of IOL power calculation and refractive outcome after laser refractive cataract surgery with a femtosecond laser versus conventional phacoemulsification. *J. Refract. Surg.* **2012**, *28*, 540–544. [CrossRef] [PubMed]
19. Nagy, Z.; Takacs, A.; Filkorn, T.; Sarayba, M. Initial clinical evaluation of an intraocular femtosecond laser in cataract surgery. *J. Refract. Surg.* **2009**, *25*, 1053–1060. [CrossRef] [PubMed]
20. Conrad-Hengerer, I.; Hengerer, F.H.; Joachim, S.C.; Schultz, T.; Dick, H.B. Femtosecond laser-assisted cataract surgery in intumescent white cataracts. *J. Cataract Refract. Surg.* **2014**, *40*, 44–50. [CrossRef] [PubMed]

21. Conrad-Hengerer, I.; Dick, H.B.; Schultz, T.; Hengerer, F.H. Femtosecond laser-assisted capsulotomy after penetrating injury of the cornea and lens capsule. *J. Cataract Refract. Surg.* **2014**, *40*, 153–156. [CrossRef] [PubMed]
22. Palanker, D.V.; Blumenkranz, M.S.; Andersen, D.; Wiltberger, M.; Marcellino, G.; Gooding, P.; Angeley, D.; Schuele, G.; Woodley, B.; Simoneau, M.; et al. Femtosecond laser-assisted cataract surgery with integrated optical coherence tomography. *Sci. Trans. Med.* **2010**, *2*, 58ra85. [CrossRef] [PubMed]
23. Naranjo-Tackman, R. How a femtosecond laser increases safety and precision in cataract surgery? *Curr. Opin. Ophthalmol.* **2011**, *22*, 53–57. [CrossRef] [PubMed]
24. Packer, M.; Teuma, E.V.; Glasser, A.; Bott, S. Defining the ideal femtosecond laser capsulotomy. *Br. J. Ophthalmol.* **2015**, *99*, 1137–1142. [CrossRef] [PubMed]

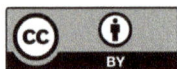

sensors

MDPI

Article

Image-Guided Laparoscopic Surgical Tool (IGLaST) Based on the Optical Frequency Domain Imaging (OFDI) to Prevent Bleeding

Byung Jun Park [1,†], Seung Rag Lee [1,†], Hyun Jin Bang [1], Byung Yeon Kim [1], Jeong Hun Park [1], Dong Guk Kim [1], Sung Soo Park [2,*] and Young Jae Won [1,*]

[1] Medical Device Development Center, Osong Medical Innovation Foundation, Cheongju, Chungbuk 361-951, Korea; yachon.park@gmail.com (B.J.P.); naviman78@gmail.com (S.R.L.); crisenc@kbiohealth.kr (H.J.B.); nick.kimby@gmail.com (B.Y.K.); pjh8311@kbiohealth.kr (J.H.P.); dgkim@kbiohealth.kr (D.G.K.)
[2] Department of Surgery, Korea University College of Medicine, Seoul 02841, Korea
* Correspondence: sungsoo.park.md@gmail.com (S.S.P.); yjwon000@gmail.com (Y.J.W.); Tel.: +82-2-920-6772 (S.S.P.); +82-43-200-9714 (Y.J.W.)
† These authors contributed equally to this work.

Academic Editors: Dragan Indjin, Željka Cvejić and Małgorzata Jędrzejewska-Szczerska
Received: 21 February 2017; Accepted: 19 April 2017; Published: 21 April 2017

Abstract: We present an image-guided laparoscopic surgical tool (IGLaST) to prevent bleeding. By applying optical frequency domain imaging (OFDI) to a specially designed laparoscopic surgical tool, the inside of fatty tissue can be observed before a resection, and the presence and size of blood vessels can be recognized. The optical sensing module on the IGLaST head has a diameter of less than 390 μm and is moved back and forth by a linear servo actuator in the IGLaST body. We proved the feasibility of IGLaST by in vivo imaging inside the fatty tissue of a porcine model. A blood vessel with a diameter of about 2.2 mm was clearly observed. Our proposed scheme can contribute to safe surgery without bleeding by monitoring vessels inside the tissue and can be further expanded to detect invisible nerves of the laparoscopic thyroid during prostate gland surgery.

Keywords: laser and laser optics; optical frequency domain imaging; optical coherence tomography; laparoscopic surgical tool; medical optics instrumentation

1. Introduction

Laparoscopic surgery, which is also called minimally invasive surgery (MIS) with laparoscopy, has become widely accepted as a part of general, gynecological, urological, and thoracic surgeries. Because laparoscopic surgery is performed with a laparoscope and thin rod-shaped surgical instruments through trocars settled on the body wall (the hole size is usually 0.5–1.5 cm), it provides many advantages to the patient compared with open surgery in terms of pain, incision size, and postoperative recovery [1].

While laparoscopic surgery is clearly advantageous in terms of patient outcomes, there are some drawbacks on the surgeon's side, such as a loss of dexterity, poor depth perception, the fulcrum effect, and a decreased sense of touch [2,3]. In particular, the loss of tactile sensation by depending on tools makes it difficult to avoid invisible blood vessels surrounded by the fatty tissues of the dissection area before resection. In open surgery, surgeons are not only able to feel pulsating blood vessels with their own hands but also use their comprehensive knowledge of gross human anatomy to trace specific local areas that need to be dissected. However, MIS takes away the surgeon's tactile senses of the tissue and applications of a wide anatomical map due to the magnified local camera view of the laparoscopic system. These inevitable drawbacks of MIS force surgeons to dissect tissues very meticulously to find vessels and expose them until they are nearly naked because they need to confirm them on the monitor and have no tactile sense. Even minor bleeding can make the laparoscopic surgical field very dirty and confusing. This situation sometimes lengthens the duration of MIS. To ensure perfect bleeding control from vessels, surgeons use more hemoclips than they actually need. Moreover, if a blood vessel is not fully captured within the sealing area of the advanced energy device, bleeding cannot be avoided.

The optical frequency domain imaging (OFDI) technique, which is also known as swept source optical coherence tomography (SS-OCT), is a high-sensitivity and high-resolution optical cross-sectional imaging technique based on optical frequency-domain interferometry with a wavelength sweeping laser [4]. Because the optical cross-sectional imaging technique is fast and minimally invasive compared to non-optical techniques such as MRI, CT, and X-rays, it has been extensively studied in a number of medical fields. Clinically, OFDI is used in ocular and cardiovascular applications and has been demonstrated to accurately image the normal eye and coronary artery in vivo as well as diseased states [5–9]. Typically, the penetration depth is about 1–3 mm in tissue, and the depth resolution is about 10–15 μm [10]. OFDI has also been applied to studying the structural features of skin, gynecological tissues, and gastrointestinal tract [11–14]. Most previous studies on medical devices using OFDI focused on discriminating between normal and diseased or cancerous tissues based on microstructural features. When the OFDI technique is applied in a laparoscopic surgical device such as a tissue dissector, safe surgery without unwanted bleeding can be realized by monitoring blood vessels inside a tissue before resection.

We developed an image-guided laparoscopic surgical tool (IGLaST) to observe blood vessels inside a tissue that uses a clinically qualified OFDI technique and the specially designed laparoscopic surgical tool. We demonstrated our proposed scheme in vivo by observing the blood vessels surrounded by the fatty tissues of a porcine model.

2. Materials and Methods

2.1. Design of IGLaST

Compared to previous medical devices using OFDI, IGLaST is for laparoscopic surgical devices that grasp a tissue or blood vessel for dissection or sealing. The proposed IGLaST comprises an optical imaging part based on the OFDI technique and a specially designed laparoscopic surgical part, as shown in Figure 1. We designed the laparoscopic surgical part to scan an optical sensing module with a linear actuator and operate the head with a handle. The optical imaging part consists of the OFDI system and an optical sensing module.

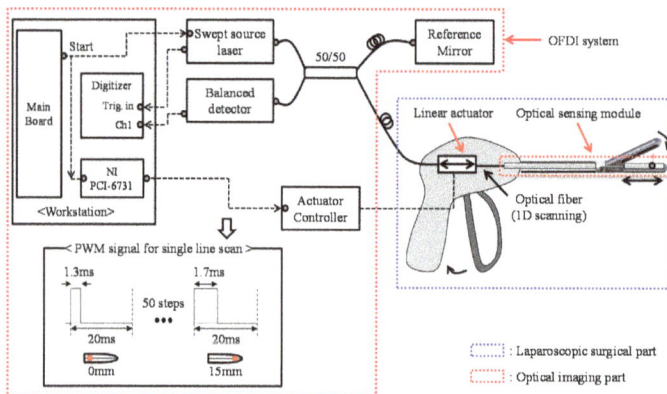

Figure 1. Schematic diagram of an image-guided laparoscopic surgical tool (IGLaST) based on the optical frequency domain imaging (OFDI) technique.

Because laparoscopic surgery is minimally invasive, the head size for the surgical instruments is restricted to a diameter of 5–10 mm. The optical sensing module can be simply realized by an optical fiber with a diameter of less than 0.35 mm. Such an optical fiber is inexpensive and easily separated and combined by an optical connector. Thus, OFDI can be an effective technique for realizing an image-guided disposable laparoscopic surgical tool.

2.2. OFDI for IGLaST

A swept sourced laser with a center wavelength λ_0 of 1300 nm and a spectral bandwidth λ_{full} of 100 nm at a cutoff point of -20 dB (SL1310V1-10048, Thorlabs, Sterling, VA, USA) was used as the light source. The swept source is separated by a 3 dB fiber coupler. One of two beams after the 3 dB fiber coupler goes to a reference mirror, and the other goes to the sample. The two reflected beams from the reference mirror and sample pass through the same root in opposite directions and are interfered with. The interference optical signal is detected by a balanced detector and acquired by a digitizer with a sampling rate of up to 500 MS/s at a 12 bit resolution.

In an experiment, the mechanical movement of the optical sensing module was performed by using a linear servo actuator (PLS-5030, POTENIT, Seoul, Korea) for 15 mm transverse line scanning within 1 s. Generally, OFDI imaging requires a high-speed line scanning system (HSLS) for biomedical applications [5–9]. However, HSLS-based OFDI is not required for laparoscopic surgical applications because the sample is tightly fixed by the IGLaST head. Our proposed line scanning scheme with a linear servo actuator provides a low-cost and miniaturized device for practical use in laparoscopic surgical applications. To control the linear servo actuator, an NI PCI-6731 board (National Instruments, Austin, TX, USA) was equipped with a workstation, and pulse-width modulation (PWM) signals were generated as described in Figure 1.

To facilitate clear imaging, the swept source laser, digitizer, and linear servo actuator were synchronized, as represented in Figure 1.

The repetition rate of the light source was 100 kHz, and 100,000 interference signals were generated in a single scan. For a higher signal-to-noise ratio (SNR), the 20 adjacent interference signals were averaged after fast Fourier transform (FFT). Finally, a 5000 × 701 pixel OFDI image was acquired.

2.3. Realization of IGLaST

To apply the proposed method to a laparoscopic tissue dissector, we developed the IGLaST head with an optical sensing module and tissue cutter. The IGLaST head with biocompatible material (SUS304) contains two routes for the optical sensing module and tissue cutter, as shown in Figure 2. The size of the area for grasping the tissue is about 5.3 mm × 20 mm. Each route for the optical sensing module and tissue cutter has the same width of 0.5 mm, and the route for the optical sensing module has a length of 17 mm.

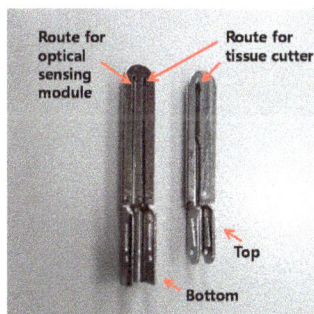

Figure 2. IGLaST head with the route for the optical sensing module.

In order to transmit the laser beam into a sample, a ball-lens fiber functioning as a reflective mirror at the end of a fiber was manufactured, as shown in Figure 3a. This was predetermined by using a simulation tool (Light Tools, Synopsys, Mountain View, CA, USA) to satisfy a spot size (Full width at half maximum) of 27 μm at a working distance of 1.6 mm, as shown in Figure 3b. A coreless fiber (FG125LA, Thorlabs, Sterling, VA, USA) was fusion-spliced to the SMF (SMF-28, Corning, Corning, NY, USA) and cleaved to a predetermined length. Then, the distal end of the coreless fiber was heated, while being translated in a tungsten filament furnace to form a ball lens. The translation length and speed, the temperature of the filament, and the duration of heating were empirically adjusted to form the optimal ball-lens fiber. The entire ball lens fabrication process was performed at a computer-controlled fusion splicing workstation (GPX-3000, Vytran, Morganville, NJ, USA). To perpendicularly reflect the beam into the tissue, the distal tip of the ball lens was polished with a fiber polishing machine (Ultrapol, Ultra Tech., Santa Ana, CA, USA). The angle between the fiber axis and polished surface was about 39°. We confirmed the spot size (FWHM) of the beam was about 22.8 μm at a working distance of 1.6 mm by using a beam profiler (SP620U, Spiricon, Jerusalem, Israel), as shown in Figure 3c. The distance between the SMF/coreless fiber interface and front of the ball lens was 302 μm, and the coronal diameter of the ball lens was 323 μm.

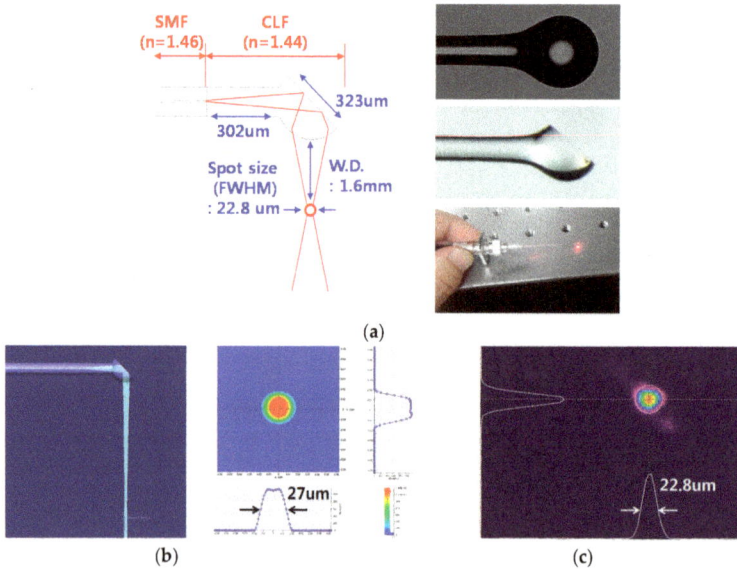

Figure 3. (**a**) Design and manufacture of the ball-lens fiber. (**b**) Simulation results for the ball-lens fiber. (**c**) Experimentally measured beam profile of the ball-lens fiber at a working distance of 1.6 mm.

Figure 4 shows the structure of proposed optical sensing module. To protect the ball-lens fiber, a polyimide with an inner diameter of 350 μm and outer diameter of 390 μm was used. The polyimide was inserted into the groove on the bottom of the IGLaST head and secured with epoxy, as shown at the bottom of Figure 4. The rest of the ball-lens fiber was guided by Shrinkable Tube 1. Between the polyimide and Tube 1, Shrinkable Tube 2 was used as a spacer and had a smaller inner diameter than Tube 1. The length of Tube 1 was about 500 mm, which is similar to the length of a laparoscopic surgical tool. After the end of Tube 1, a linear servomotor was used for one-dimensional scanning of the ball-lens fiber. To minimize twisting or bending of the ball-lens fiber, the linear servomotor was placed close to the end of Tube 1.

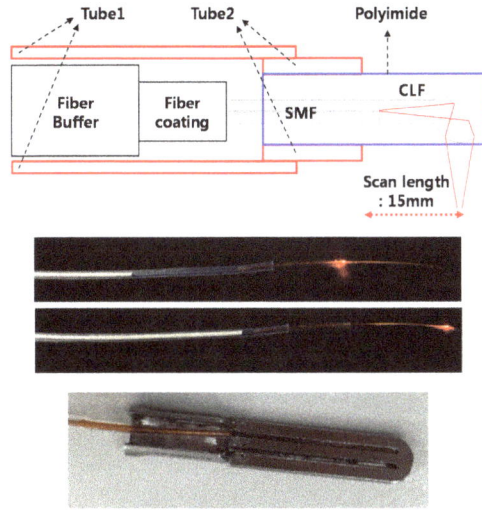

Figure 4. Optical sensing module for IGLaST.

One-dimensional scanning of the ball-lens fiber inside the optical sensing module was tested by using a laser diode with a central wavelength of 633 nm, as shown at the middle of Figure 4. After the optical sensing module was assembled, the head was attached to the IGLaST body.

3. Results

3.1. Optical Properties

Figure 5 plots the experimentally measured beam diameter (FWHM) of the optical sensing module of IGLaST. The beam shape was measured by using a microscope equipped with an IR camera [15]. The beam diameter plot started at 400 µm considering the air gap between the optical sensing module and IGLaST head surface. The beam profile was elliptically shaped after passing through the polyimide. The ratio of the x-axis/y-axis crossed at the focal plane. The measured x- and y-axis beam diameters were 29.3 and 31.8 µm, respectively. The lateral resolution expected by the FWHM beam width ranged from 20 to 65 µm in the first 2 mm after the IGLaST head.

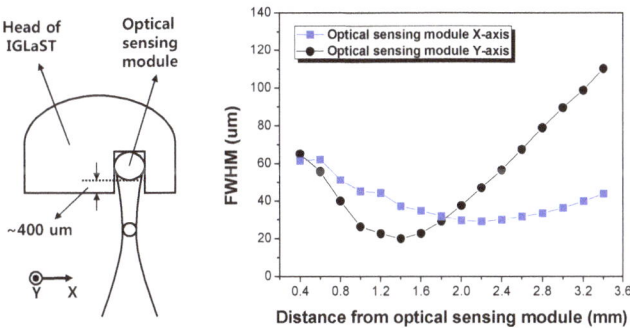

Figure 5. Beam diameter (FWHM) of the optical sensing module.

3.2. Imaging of a Vessel Inside the Fatty Tissues of a Porcine Model with IGLaST

As a demonstration, IGLaST was used to observe blood vessel inside fatty tissue during laparoscopic surgery. We prepared a 40 kg porcine model that was 3 months old. The pig underwent surgical procedures under general anesthesia. Three incisions with a length of 0.5–1 cm were made on the abdomen of the pig, and trocars were placed in the incisions. A laparoscope, laparoscopic dissection tool, and laparoscopic clamp were inserted inside the body through the trocars, and an operation was performed to find the region of interest. The animal experiment protocol was approved by the Institutional Animal Care and Use Committee (IACUC) of Korea University.

Figure 6 shows the in vivo imaging inside the fatty tissue of the pig with IGLaST. In laparoscopic surgery, tissues to be dissected should consist of adipose, lymphatics, and collagen, and blood vessels must be surrounded by the tissue complex. Therefore, the tissue complex that may cover major blood vessels of an artery or vein usually needs to be dissected to find them. In most cases, blood vessels inside the tissue are invisible, as shown in Figure 6a. We inserted our developed IGLaST inside the pig body through a trocar and grasped the tissue with the head of IGLaST to observe invisible blood vessels inside the tissue, as shown in Figure 6b. The red light is a guide source to inform the position of the head of the ball-lens fiber. The blood vessel inside the fatty tissue of the pig appeared with OFDI, as shown in Figure 6c. The yellow bar in Figure 6c represents a length of 0.5 mm. The size of the image was about 15×1.75 mm^2. After the tissue was grasped, the tissue was compressed, and the thickness of the tissue was reduced to about 0.5–0.6 mm. In this experiment, a blood vessel with a length of about 2.2 mm was clearly observed.

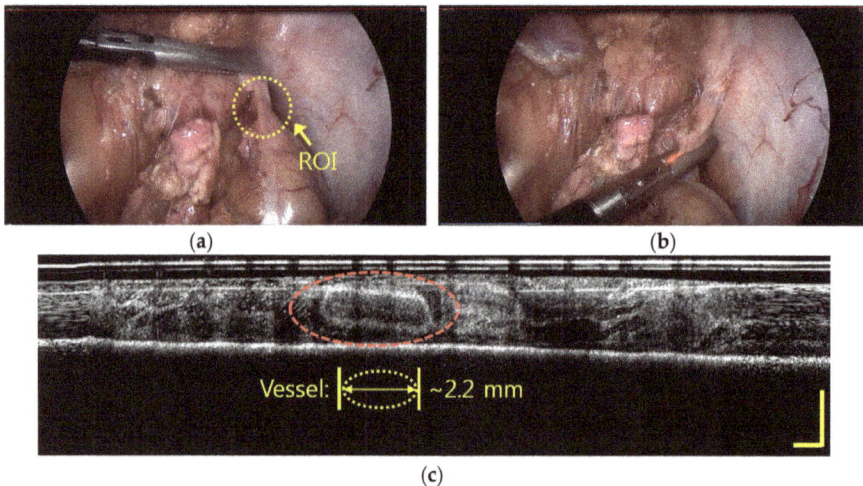

Figure 6. In vivo imaging inside the fatty tissue of a porcine model with IGLaST; the blood vessel inside the tissue is visible. (**a**) Laparoscopic image of the porcine model. (**b**) Laparoscopic image of the porcine model after the tissue is grasped with IGLaST. (**c**) OFDI image inside the fatty tissue.

When the IGLaST head grasping the tissue was slightly released, image blurring occurred at the vessel position because of blood flow, as shown in Figure 7a. If the morphological image processing technique to extract blurring pixels is applied, the contrast can be increased to improve awareness of the blood vessels inside the tissue, as shown in Figure 7b. This technique provides the functions of erosion, smooth filtering, simple threshold, and area sort to isolate the blurred part [16]. IGLaST can be further improved to discriminate arteries and veins by the application of Doppler and angiographic techniques [17–19].

(a)

(b)

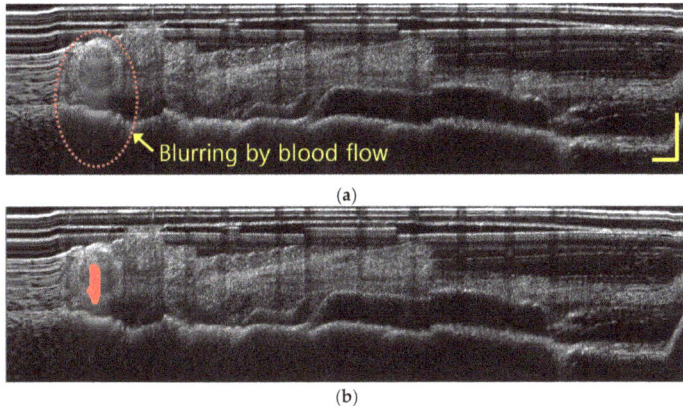

Figure 7. (a) In vivo imaging of the blood flow inside the fatty tissue of a porcine model with IGLaST. (b) Identification of blood flow with the morphological image processing technique.

4. Discussion and Conclusions

We proposed and developed IGLaST based on the OFDI technique to prevent bleeding. To observe within tissue that may cover invisible blood vessels of a vein or artery, we specially designed a laparoscopic surgical tool and applied the OFDI technique. We successfully demonstrated that our proposed scheme can be used to prevent unwanted bleeding by observing a blood vessel with a diameter of about 2.2 mm inside the fatty tissues of a porcine model during laparoscopic surgery. The experimental results suggest that IGLaST can be a useful tool for investigating blood vessels inside the tissue before resection. The utility of IGLaST may extend to other surgical devices such as laparoscopic surgical staplers, laparoscopic vessel sealing devices, and surgical scissors.

The use of a low-speed linear servo actuator may be unfamiliar for researchers interested in high-speed OFDI-based medical devices for cardiovascular imaging and ocular imaging. However, it is sufficient to prove the feasibility and usability of IGLaST because the sample was tightly fixed by the IGLaST head. The proposed line scanning scheme with a linear servo actuator provides a low-cost and miniaturized device for the practical use of laparoscopic surgical applications. In future IGLaST designs, we will apply the high-speed OFDI technique to the laparoscopic surgical tool to identify the blood flow of blood vessels inside the tissue so that arteries and veins can be discriminated based on Doppler and angiographic techniques.

For the optical sensing module, a beam diameter (FWHM) of less than 65 µm was obtained in the first 2 mm after the IGLaST head. In this study, the size of the observed blood vessel inside the tissue was a few millimeters, so the achieved lateral resolution was acceptable. However, the lateral resolution of IGLaST needs to be further improved to observe small blood vessels or nerves inside the tissue.

We believe that techniques using IGLaST can also be applied to identify invisible nerves or lymphatic vessels inside the tissue to avoid injuring them during minimally invasive surgery (MIS). Moreover, our proposed scheme has tremendous potential as a smart image-guided laparoscopic surgical tool for robot-assisted surgery.

Acknowledgments: This work was supported by the Industrial Strategic Technology Development Program (10051331) funded by the Ministry of Trade, Industry and Energy (MOTIE) of Korea.

Author Contributions: Young Jae Won and Sung Soo Park made the idea and designed the system; Byung Jun Park, Seung Rag Lee, and Byung Yeon Kim built the system; Hyun Jin Bang contributed to make optical head for IGLaST; Jung Hun Park and Dong Guk Kim contributed to make mechanical head for IGLaST; all authors performed the experiments; Byung Jun Park and Seung Rag Lee analyzed the data; Young Jae Won and Sung Soo Park wrote the paper.

Conflicts of Interest: The authors declare no conflict of interest.

References

1. Swanstrom, L.L.; Soper, N.J. *Mastery of Endoscopic and Laparoscopic Surgery*; Lippincott Williams & Wilkins: Philadelphia, PA, USA, 2013.
2. Der Putten, E.P.W.; Goossens, R.H.M.; Jakimowicz, J.J.; Dankelman, J. Haptics in minimally invasive surgery—A review. *Minim. Invasive Ther. Alied Technol.* **2008**, *17*, 3–16. [CrossRef] [PubMed]
3. Gallagher, A.G.; McClure, N.; McGuigan, J.; Ritchie, K.; Sheehy, N.P. An ergonomic analysis of the fulcrum effect in the acquisition of endoscopic skills. *Endoscopy* **1998**, *30*, 617–620. [CrossRef] [PubMed]
4. Fercher, A.F.; Drexler, W.; Hitzenberger, C.K.; Lasser, T. Optical coherence tomography—Principles and applications. *Rep. Prog. Phys.* **2003**, *66*, 239–303. [CrossRef]
5. Zysk, A.M.; Nguyen, F.T.; Oldenburg, A.L.; Marks, D.L.; Boppart, S.A. Optical coherence tomography: A review of clinical development from bench to bedside. *J. Biomed. Opt.* **2007**, *12*, 051403. [CrossRef] [PubMed]
6. Costa, R.A.; Skaf, M.; Melo, L.A.S.; Calucci, D.; Cardillo, J.A.; Castro, J.C.; Huang, D.; Wojtkowski, M. Retinal assessment using optical coherence tomography. *Prog. Retin. Eye Res.* **2006**, *25*, 325–353. [CrossRef] [PubMed]
7. Dogra, M.R.; Gupta, A.; Gupta, V. *Atlas of Optical Coherence Tomography of Macular Diseases*; Taylor & Francis: Boca Raton, FL, USA, 2004.
8. Brezinski, M.E.; Tearney, G.J.; Bouma, B.E.; Izatt, J.A.; Hee, M.R.; Swanson, E.A.; Southern, J.F.; Fujimoto, J.G. Optical coherence tomography for optical biopsy: Properties and demonstration of vascular pathology. *Circulation* **1996**, *93*, 1206–1213. [CrossRef] [PubMed]
9. Cho, H.S.; Jang, S.-J.; Kim, K.; Dan-Chin-Yu, A.V.; Shishkov, M.; Bouma, B.E.; Oh, W.-Y. High-frame-rate intravascular optical frequency-domain imaging in vivo. *Biomed. Opt. Exp.* **2014**, *5*, 223–232. [CrossRef] [PubMed]
10. Fujimoto, J.G.; Pitris, C.; Boppart, S.A.; Brezinski, M.E. Optical coherence tomography: An emerging technology for biomedical imaging and optical biopsy. *Neoplasia* **2000**, *2*, 9–25. [CrossRef] [PubMed]
11. Cogliati, A.; Canavesi, C.; Hayes, A.; Tankam, P.; Duma, V.-F.; Santhanam, A.; Thompson, K.P.; Rolland, J.P. MEMS—Based handheld scanning probe with pre-shaped input signals for distortion-free images in Gabor-domain optical coherence microscopy. *Opt. Express* **2016**, *24*, 13365–13374. [CrossRef] [PubMed]
12. Testoni, P.A.; Mangiavillano, B. Optical coherence tomography in detection of dysplasia and cancer of the gastrointestinal tract and bilio-pancreatic ductal system. *World J. Gastroenterol.* **2008**, *14*, 6444–6452. [CrossRef] [PubMed]
13. Suter, M.J.; Vakoc, B.J.; Yachimski, P.S.; Shishkov, M.; Lauwers, G.Y.; Mino-Kenudson, M.; Bouma, B.E.; Nishioka, N.S.; Tearney, G.J. Comprehensive microscopy of the esophagus in human patients with optical frequency domain imaging. *Gastrointest. Endosc.* **2008**, *68*, 745–753. [CrossRef] [PubMed]
14. Boppart, S.A.; Goodman, A.; Libus, J.; Pitris, C.; Jesser, C.A.; Brezinski, M.E.; Fusimoto, J.G. High resolution imaging of endometriosis and ovarian carcinoma with optical coherence tomography: Feasibility for laparoscopic-based imaging. *Br. J. Obstet. Gynaecol.* **1999**, *106*, 1071–1077. [CrossRef] [PubMed]
15. Lee, J.B.; Chae, Y.G.; Ahn, Y.C.; Moon, S.B. Ultra-thin and flexible endoscopy probe for optical coherence tomography based on stepwise transitional core fiber. *Biomed. Opt. Express* **2015**, *6*, 1782–1796. [CrossRef] [PubMed]
16. Dougherty, E.R.; Lotufo, R.A. *Hands-on Morphological Image Processing*; SPIE: Bellingham, WA, USA, 2003.
17. Rollins, A.M.; Yazdanfar, S.; Barton, J.K.; Izatt, J.A. Real-time in vivo color Doppler optical coherence tomography. *J. Biomed. Opt.* **2002**, *7*, 123–129. [CrossRef] [PubMed]

18. De Carlo, T.E.; Romano, A.; Waheed, N.K.; Duker, J.S. A review of optical coherence tomography angiography (OCTA). *Int. J. Retin. Vitr.* **2015**, *1*. [CrossRef] [PubMed]

19. Choi, W.J.; Li, Y.D.; Qin, W.; Wang, R.K. Cerebral capillary velocimetry based on temporal OCT speckle contrast. *Biomed. Opt. Express* **2016**, *7*, 4859–4873. [CrossRef] [PubMed]

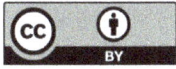

sensors

MDPI

Article

Body Weight Estimation for Dose-Finding and Health Monitoring of Lying, Standing and Walking Patients Based on RGB-D Data

Christian Pfitzner [1,2,*], Stefan May [1] and Andreas Nüchter [2,*]

1 Department of Electrical Engineering, Precision Engineering, Information Technology at the Techniche Hochschule Nürnberg Georg Simon Ohm; Keßlerplatz 12, 90489 Nuremberg, Germany; stefan.may@th-nuernberg.de

2 Department of Informatics VII: Robotics and Telematics at the Julius-Maximilians University Würzburg, Am Hubland, 97074 Wuerzburg, Germany

* Correspondence: christian.pfitzner@th-nuernberg.de (C.P.); andreas.nuechter@uni-wuerzburg.de (A.N.)

Received: 28 January 2018; Accepted: 20 April 2018; Published: 24 April 2018

Abstract: This paper describes the estimation of the body weight of a person in front of an RGB-D camera. A survey of different methods for body weight estimation based on depth sensors is given. First, an estimation of people standing in front of a camera is presented. Second, an approach based on a stream of depth images is used to obtain the body weight of a person walking towards a sensor. The algorithm first extracts features from a point cloud and forwards them to an artificial neural network (ANN) to obtain an estimation of body weight. Besides the algorithm for the estimation, this paper further presents an open-access dataset based on measurements from a trauma room in a hospital as well as data from visitors of a public event. In total, the dataset contains 439 measurements. The article illustrates the efficiency of the approach with experiments with persons lying down in a hospital, standing persons, and walking persons. Applicable scenarios for the presented algorithm are body weight-related dosing of emergency patients.

Keywords: image processing; machine learning; perception; sensor fusion; segmentation; RGB-D; thermal camera; kinect; human body weight; stroke

---

1. Introduction

When it comes to the treatment of ischemic stroke patients, it is crucial to solve the blood clot in the brain vessel as fast as possible. For the treatment of ischemic strokes, the medicament rtPA was approved in 1996 by the U.S. Food and Drug Administration [1]. The medicine has to be given with a dosage of 0.9 mg per kilogram of the patient's body weight. Furthermore, a maximum dose of 90 mg is specified for patients weighing more than 100 kilograms. It is best used within the first hour after the appearance of stroke symptoms. After three hours, side effects can prevail over the solving of the blood clot. Because of this narrow time window, physicians are in a hurry for treatment. Weighing a patient on a common standing scale is often not possible because the patient is in pain or is not able to stand due to other symptoms of stroke, e.g., paralysis. The obvious way to determine the body weight of someone quickly is to ask the person. However, if it comes to stroke, only half of the patients are knowledgeable and are not handicapped by stroke symptoms [2]. Additionally, elderly patients might suffer from dementia and cannot provide a reliable value for their body weight. Furthermore, relatives who could be asked might not be available in the trauma room or do not know the body weight of the patient. In addition, anthropometric methods exist, where lengths and circumferences of body parts are measured with a measuring tape. Based on an empirical equation, e.g., the equation for stroke patients presented by Lorenz et al. [3], gives an estimation of body weight.

The disadvantage of those anthropometric methods is that the patient has to be moved and the measuring is time-consuming.

Therefore, visual estimation of the patient's body weight by the attending physician in the emergency room has become routine worldwide. In a registry with 27,910 stroke patients, only 14.6 percent were weighed [4]. However, several studies [5–7] illustrate that such a weight estimation by a visual guess from a physician is often not sufficient for dosing: Every third patient receives a dosage out of the ±10 percent bound. This result can be improved if the average estimation of several persons from medical staff is taken. Furthermore, the estimations from nursing staff are more reliable than the visual guesses by physicians [2].

The observation of body weight is also essential in elder care: People with a healthy weight can recover better from sickness than people who are underweight or obese. However, older people often have a reduced appetite, coupled with a decline in biological and physiological functions [8]. In elder care, people are weighed on common standing scales to observe changes in body weight. Multiple approaches with 3D sensors are being tested in the field of elder care, especially since the release of the low-cost Microsoft Kinect camera [9]. Some applications of these approaches are fall detection or the monitoring of breathing [10,11]. The contact-less body weight approach can be combined in context with these other approaches to monitor changes in body weight to improve elder care.

In contrast to the scenario of patients being measured on a stretcher, the weighing of standing people can be easily done on a spring scale. However, the automatic weighing of several people in a short time can bring a benefit in some applications: Since 2017, the Finnish airline Finnair weighs passengers to determine the total weight of an airplane for take-off. While the weight of baggage is measured with a scale, the weight of the passengers is only roughly rated with standardized weights [12]. The precise knowledge about the weight gives possibilities to optimize fuel requirements and therefore operating costs [13]. In 1985, a McDonnell Douglas DC-8 jetliner crashed with 256 people on board. One reason for the crash might have been the underestimated onboard weight, which was mentioned in the occurrence report [14]. Furthermore, the motivation for a visual weight system is gained as objects that the subject is wearing or carrying, e.g., a backpack, can be filtered out for weight estimation.

The presented approach is an extension of Pfitzner et al. [15]: While this previous work had the clear focus on clinical use, the work presented here extends the approach towards standing and walking people. First, this article contributes a summary about the visual body weight estimation for various situations. The settings for the different approaches are compared, as well as the results of the experiments. Second, the article shows that the feature set from previous work is also suitable for body weight estimation of standing or walking subjects. To obtain the body weight of walking subjects, a clustering method is presented, combining the estimations from each frame, to a single and also a more robust estimation. Finally, the article provides the 3D data used for experiments so that other research groups can contribute to this topic.

The paper is structured as follows: First, the related work concerning the body weight estimation based on a camera system is presented, focusing on lying, standing, and walking people. Second, the here applied and published dataset for body weight estimation based on RGB-D-T (color, depth and thermal) data is explained. In the following section, the approach for body weight estimation is presented and separated for standing and walking persons. Experiments with the here applied dataset and a dataset from related work demonstrate the efficiency of the developed algorithm. The results are examined in comparison to other approaches for visual weight estimation from related work. Finally, the paper concludes with a discussion and plans for future work.

2. Related Work

The related work is subdivided for lying, standing and walking people and further provides a summary of weighing and estimation devices for clinical usage.

2.1. Common Weighing and Medical Estimation Devices

Scales come in a wide range. The most common type is standing scales. Analog scales use a reference weight or a spring to obtain the body weight, while modern digital scales use strain gauges and a change in resistance to get a value for body weight. In the clinical scenario, chair scales exist, so a patient does not need to stand for the process of weighing. Different types of bed scales are available to weigh patients who are lying down. First, scales can be designed as a single plate integrated into the floor where the bed is placed. Second, bed scales are available with multiple weighing devices, which are attached to each wheel. The sum of all weight is the total weight of the bed, including the patient. In both scenarios, the tare weight of the empty bed has to be known. Consequently, either the bed is weighed in advance without the patient or the tare weight of the bed has to be identified. Choosing the wrong type of bed can result in a high degree of error concerning the patient's weight. Furthermore, different attachments, such as medical devices or handrails, can cause a change in tare weight. In addition, it is possible to integrate multiple strain gauges directly into the mattress. This solves the issue of determining the tare weight of the bed. It is also possible to integrate weighing directly into the computer tomography to speed up the process of weight acquisition [16].

Furthermore, rulers exist to approximate body weight for medical usage: Approximation rulers are common to estimate the body weight of young children; the Broselow tape was developed in 1985 by James Broselow and Robert Luten. It provides nine different weight groups for children younger than 12. A colored scale on the measuring tape relegates to different medical sets, prepared for emergency treatment of the different weight groups in case of an emergency. Several studies illustrate that the Broselow tape is reliable for first aid personnel [17]. However, for children, the estimation of the parents can be even more reliable, if available [18].

2.2. Estimation from Lying People

The body weight estimation of lying people is important mainly in the scenario of clinical usage. Most patients are already lying on a stretcher or a bed. Furthermore, the here presented approaches are suitable for bedridden patients.

Pirker et al. [19] employed 16 stereo cameras around a stretcher. Additional projectors are needed for complete illumination. A parametric human model complements the back side of the body. Composed images are filtered for noise reduction and, finally, the volume is calculated with the help of cross-sections along the body. Because of the high amount of cameras around the patient's bed, physicians would be constricted during treatment.

The here presented algorithm for the estimation of lying, walking and standing people is the continuation of preceding work: In 2015, Pfitzner et al. [20] showed an approach for body weight estimation with a depth camera. The algorithm extracts only the volume of a subject lying on a medical stretcher, multiplying it with a fixed value for the density. Color and depth gradient achieve the segmentation. The focus of this application was set on the body weight estimation of stroke patients within the treatment process in the trauma room. Although the approach is straightforward, the system was more reliable than the visual guess performed by the medical staff: 79 percent of all patients received a sufficient body weight estimation, while the visual guess from a physician could only provide a sufficient estimation in 68 percent of patients.

Figure 1 shows the scene in the trauma room with a patient on the stretcher and the complete system, as presented in Pfitzner et al. [20]. The setup with the patient lying on a medical stretcher and the sensors integrated into the ceiling is the same as in the following previous work.

The approach was extended in 2016 by the work of Pfitzner et al. [15]. An additional thermal camera improves the segmentation, and the patient in the fused field of view can be clearly segmented from the mattress that the subject is lying on. Furthermore, this paper introduced an extended feature extraction, as well as a machine learning approach—here an ANN—to improve the outcome in body weight estimation, by minimizing outliers and improving the standard deviation for the relative error.

In total, 89.9 percent of all subjects received an estimate of ±10 percent. For this approach, a patent exists [21].

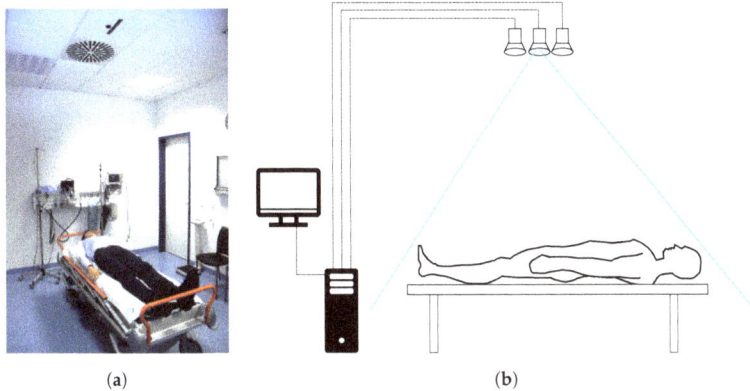

Figure 1. Clinical integration of sensors into the trauma room, as shown in [15]. Within the scenario of trauma room in which physicians mostly treat emergency patients, the sensor system is integrated into the ceiling (**a**); The system does not hinder the physician while treating the patient, who is often lying on a medical stretcher. Besides the sensors in the ceiling, the system consists of a computer system—including a keyboard and a mouse for interaction, a monitor for visualization and a barcode scanner to identify patients with their ID (**b**). The connection between the sensors and the computer is achieved by USB cables. (**a**) Trauma room with sensors integrated into the ceiling; (**b**) Schematic of the sensor system and its connections to a computer.

Pfitzner et al. [22] presented a comparison of different depth sensors for the scenario of body weight estimation. In conclusion, the Kinect One can provide better results in body weight estimation—95.3 percent for the ±10 percent range—compared to the estimation based on the data of the Kinect with 94.8 percent. Additionally, this work also presents a correlation analysis of the extracted features, and how a different configuration of the available features can provide a reliable result.

2.3. Estimation from Standing People

In contrast to the estimation of lying people, the scenario for standing or walking people is more complex: The person is not aligned to a fixed surface on the back. Furthermore, the posture and the position of the subject changes in a sequence of frames.

Robinson and Parkinson [23] developed an approach for the body weight estimation of standing people. Here, anthropometric features are extracted from a scene's point cloud and the raw sensor data from an RGB-D sensor with a person standing in front of it can be seen. This approach also demonstrated that these raw features from the point cloud could lead to a bias because of un-calibrated sensor or noise. Furthermore, even thin clothes can confuse the extraction of the features, like the circumference of a body part, e.g., waist or hip circumference.

Cook et al. [24] presented a framework based on a structured light sensor for radiation dose estimation in CT examinations. In preliminary experiments, they showed results for five persons standing in front of a structured light sensor. The measured volume of the patient differs due to different positions of their arms.

With the help of skeleton tracking, Velardo and Dugelay showed a computer vision system to prove the health of a person with the help of a structured light sensor [25]. Apart from sensing the age of the subject, the sensor measures anthropometric features from arms, legs, and the body. The authors provide a trained statistical model from a medical database, containing anthropometric measurements from more than 28,000 subjects, as well as the ground truth body weight. This approach has the benefit of a large sample size for training. However, the estimation of the anthropometric features based on the RGB-D data is hard due to the sensor's noise. Additionally, the system provides information about obesity and nutrition to the user.

Based on a side-view feature, Nguyen et al. [26] developed a method to estimate the human body weight of standing people captured with an RGB-D camera. A model is trained based on regression. Together with handling the gender data, the algorithm can reach the mean average error of 5.20 kg over 300 subjects. In an additional experiment, the authors proved that the body weight estimation based on RGB-D data is more reliable compared with the human estimation. Furthermore, the utilized dataset with 300 subjects is published as an open-access source, containing the RGB-D data, the ground truth gender, and the ground truth body weight. This dataset is also applied to the following experiments.

2.4. Estimation from Walking People

Beside the body weight estimation from a single frame, it is also possible to estimate it by a sequence of sensor data. Labati et al. [27] developed a body weight estimation suitable for walking persons. The focus was set on a contact-less and low-cost method. The method is based on frame sequences from two cameras, which are placed to get a frontal and a side-view of the walking person. The feature vector consists of the height of a person, an approximation of the body volume, an approximation for the body shape and the walking direction. The extracted features are forwarded to an ANN to obtain body weight. Experiments are performed with 20 subjects, walking in eight different directions. A maximum absolute mean error was recorded with less than 2.4 kg.

Arigbabu et al. [28] demonstrated the extraction of soft biometrics, e.g., body height and weight, based on video frames from a single monocular camera. Due to a homogeneous background, the people's silhouette can be extracted easily with state of the art image processing techniques like background subtraction. The silhouette is converted into a binary mask, where 13 features are extracted depending on the pixel density in segmented regions. The feature vector is finally forwarded to an ANN to estimate the body weight. In experiments with 80 subjects, they reached a mean average error of 4.66 kg the estimation of body weight. The update rate of the extraction of all described soft biometrics was about 1 Hz. The approach was compared with the previously presented approach by Labati et al. [27] and Velardo and Dugelay [25].

Most of the approaches presented here use neural networks as a machine learning approach to generate a model for body weight estimation. The difference in the approaches can be found in the types of features forwarded to a neural network. In contrast to related work, the approach in this paper is not limited to a particular application. The selected features for machine learning are suitable for the scenarios of subjects who are lying, standing or walking. They can be used in general for the estimation of body weight. Furthermore, Table 1 compares the results of related work as a summary. The approaches presented by Nguyen et al. [26], Velardo and Dugelay [25], Labati et al. [27] and Arigbabu et al. [28] are compared in the experiment section.

Table 1. Results for contact-less human body weight estimation from related work in alphabetic order. The results are not directly comparable due to different evaluation metrics.

Method	Sensor	Approach	Constrains	Results
Cook et al. [24]	RGB-D structured light	image processing to reconstruct the volume	sample size 6 subjects	only volume estimation
Pirker et al. [19]	8 stereo cameras	image processing to reconstruct the volume	scene has to be known	only volume estimation
Nguyen et al. [26]	RGB-D structured light	machine learning with l2-regularization and support vector regression		5.2 kg MAE
Velardo and Dugelay [25]	RGB-D structured light	machine learning with multiple regression analysis	sample size 15 subjects	2.7 kg for a single subject
Pfitzner et al. [20]	RGB-D structured light	image processing to reconstruct the volume	person is lying on a flat surface	79.1 % within relative error of 10 %

Table 1. *Cont.*

Method	Sensor	Approach	Constrains	Results
Pfitzner et al. [15]	RGB-D structured light	machine learning with ANN	person is lying on a flat surface	89.6 % within relative error of 10 %
Pfitzner et al. [22]	RGB-D structured light and ToF	machine learning with ANN	person is lying on a flat surface	95.3 % within relative error of 10 %
Labati et al. [27]	2 RGB cameras	machine learning with ANN	sample size 20 subjects	2.3 kg std error
Arigbabu et al. [28]	RGB cameras	machine learning with ANN		4.66 kg MAE

3. Approach for Visual Body Weight Estimation

The algorithm is subdivided into sections for sensor fusion, segmentation, and feature extraction. It leads to a learning approach based on an ANN to obtain the body weight of a single person. Figure 2 illustrates the procedure in body weight estimation based on the previously segmented point cloud.

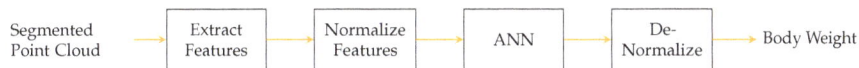

Figure 2. Process of body weight estimation.

3.1. System Description

The system uses different sensors, depending on the recorded dataset. It was developed for previous work [15,20] to be integrated into the clinical environment. There the system includes a Microsoft Kinect, a Microsoft Kinect One and an Optris PI400 thermal camera. A single depth sensor is sufficient for body weight extraction. However, the developed algorithm should not depend on the applied sensor. Therefore, experiments are performed with different sensors. Table 2 compares the sensors to each other.

Table 2. Property table of used sensors: The three sensors are selected for the body weight estimation because of their similar FOV, which provides a total view of the patient on the stretcher. For the 3D sensors, the measurement range is sufficient. The frame rate of at least 30 Hz is acceptable, while the thermal camera provides a frame rate of 80 Hz.

Model	Kinect	Kinect One	Optris PI400
Principle	Structured Light	Time-of-Flight	Thermal Camera
Resolution	320×240	512×424	382×288
Field of View	$57° \times 43°$	$70° \times 60°$	$62° \times 49°$
Frame rate	30 fps	30 fps	80 fps
Dimensions	$73 \times 283 \times 73$ mm^3	$249 \times 66 \times 67$ mm^3	$46 \times 56 \times 90$ mm^3
Weight	564 g	1400 g	320 g
Power consumption	12 W	32 W	<2.5 W via USB
Interface	USB 2.0	USB 3.0	USB 2.0
Price	$100	$200	$3500

Both the Kinect and the Kinect One are RGB-D cameras providing a color stream RGB, and a depth per pixel D. The first Kinect camera was released in 2011 bringing a low-cost consumer product into robotics. The sensor brought multiple applications and made an impact well beyond the gaming industry [29]. The Kinect holds a sensor for infrared (IR) and a sensor for color. Both sensors are calibrated to each other. The structured light principle obtains depth: A projector emits a known pattern in the environment. This pattern is seen by the IR sensor from a different pose to calculate the depth for an arbitrary pixel. Khoshelham and Elberink [30] illustrate the sensor's characteristics in image quality and noise.

In contrast to that, the Kinect One works by the Time-of-Flight (ToF) principle [31]: Having a highly precise measurement device for the time, it would be possible to calculate the distance between a light source and an object by measuring the time. The range of a given point can be calculated by the time *t* the light travels with the help of the speed of light *c* with $d = 0.5 \cdot t \cdot c$. Due to the fast traveling light, the distance measurement is obtained by modulated light: A source emits a light pulse towards an object. The frequency for modulation is known, and a phase shift can be measured from the reflected signal.

The here applied depth sensors differ not only in their resolution, but also the different principle provides a diverse characteristic of depth. Both sensors are compared to each other by Sarbolandi et al. [32]. Today, there exist various types of RGB-D sensors, which are suitable for the body weight estimation approach, e.g., Asus Xtion cameras from the Intel RealSense series [33]. The thermal camera is state of the art and is added to the sensor set to ease segmentation based on a simple thermal threshold. In this presented sensor configuration, the thermal camera is the most expensive part. It was used because it was already available from an earlier project. However, a cheaper thermal camera with a lower resolution and frame rate can be used for the segmentation. Pfitzner et al. [20] illustrated that the visual body weight estimation is possible without a thermal camera, but outliers due to insufficient segmentation can occur.

The algorithm—including the sensor fusion, the feature extraction and the forwarding to an artificial neural network—is implemented on a conventional desktop computer, which is installed in the trauma room. The computer in the trauma room, which is equipped with an Intel i7 of the 4th generation, can provide the result in body weight estimation within 300 ms, including the saving of the sensor data. The software does not rely on specialized hardware, like a high-end graphics card, although the processing speed could benefit from parallelization. For offline processing, a mobile computer (Dell M4800) is used, having a maximum power consumption of less than 80 Watt [34]. Therefore, the complete hardware could be designed with less than 100 W, including the mobile computer, the thermal camera (<2.5 Watt) and the Microsoft Kinect (12 Watt). Table 3 illustrates that the processing time for the desktop computer and the mobile computer is similar. A small experiment in our laboratory showed that the approach is also suitable for small size embedded computers, e.g., a Raspberry PI. With a reduced visualization, and without the saving of the sensor's data to the database, this configuration provided the estimation of body weight in around 5 s, see Table 3. The system is then limited in real-time visualization, as well as process time, and the estimation of the body weight is available with a higher delay. However, the embedded computer can have the benefit of lower power consumption and a smaller footprint, which provides easier integration in the clinical environment.

Table 3. Tested hardware including time measurements for the estimation: The biggest part of processing time is used to segment the patient from the environment. In contrast to that, the extraction of the features and the processing via an artificial neural network is small. The total time includes visualization and logging during the processing.

	Desktop Computer	Dell M4800 Mobile Computer	Raspberry PI 3	Asus Tinkerboard
Processor	Intel i7-4820K	Intel i7-4900MQ	ARM Cortex-A53	Rockchip RK3288
Nr. of Threads	8	8	4	4
max. Clock	3.90 GHz	3.80 GHz	1.2 GHz	1.8 GHz
TDP	130 W	47 W	<3.7 W	5 W
Time for Segmentation	239 ms	245 ms	5321 ms	2661 ms
Time for Estimation	22 ms	23 ms	267 ms	212 ms
Total Processing Time	263 ms	270 ms	5604 ms	2885 ms

3.2. Sensor Fusion

All applied projective depth, color, and thermal sensors are calibrated intrinsically based on the method presented by Zhang [35]. Therefore, a single calibration pattern is used, which is visible in depth, color, and thermal frame. Gonzalez-Jorge et al. [36] present different types of suitable calibration targets. The here applied calibration target consists of a metal plate on the back which is colored white and a black wooden plate on top. The wooden plate has holes in a circular pattern. The metal plate can be heated. Because of a space between the metal and the wood plate, a thermal gradient is visible, and the wholes appear to be warmer than the top surface. The circle pattern is therefore visible in the spectrum of the thermal camera [15].

The results of sensor fusion can be displayed in different settings. Besides the typical representation on the screen as a color image of the scene, the depth can be visualized by a color mapping. Furthermore, it is also possible to illustrate the scene as a false-color representation for temperature or fused with the color stream, similar to that presented by Vidas et al. [37]. This is achieved by comparing the color channel of every point in the cloud. Figure 3 illustrates the sensor fusion and its visualizations: In Figure 3c, the data from the color sensor of the Kinect camera is fused with its depth stream. In the fused image, the color stream provides the intensity of each pixel as a grayscale, while the color of a pixel arranges the depth in the scene, as shown in Figure 3b. In addition, the color data and the thermal data are aligned to be visible at the same time, see Figure 3d. From the given data, further data can be calculated to enhance the point cloud or the depth image, e.g., with normals.

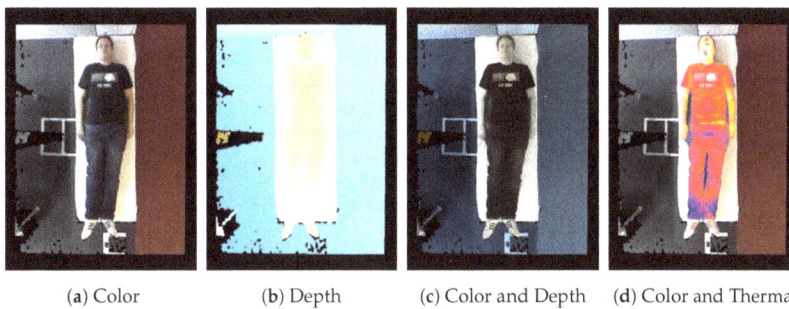

    (a) Color   (b) Depth   (c) Color and Depth   (d) Color and Therma

Figure 3. Visualization of sensor fusion: Figure (**a**) shows the raw color stream from an RGB-D camera. The depth stream can be visualized using a colormap, here drawing blue values for far objects and drawing white and orange for nearer objects (**b**). The stream from the thermal camera can be visualized in several ways: either it is drawn with false-color representation (**c**) or can be combined with other streams—here a combination of the color stream, highlighted with temperature (**d**). The here presented image-based sensor fusion is achieved by intrinsic and extrinsic camera calibration, which is presented in Figure 4.

Figure 4 presents the process of calibration for sensor fusion: The frames from the sensor are differentiated by indices, K for the Kinect, $K2$ for the Kinect One and T for the thermal camera. All three sensors are calibrated intrinsically. First, the raw streams from the sensors $\mathbf{I}$ are forwarded to rectification based on the determined intrinsic parameters $\mathbf{P}$ and $\mathbf{d}$ [35]. Second, the rectified images $\mathbf{I}$ are then calibrated extrinsically based on the previously estimated transformations $\mathbf{T}$. Third, the aligned data $\mathbf{I}$ is synchronized in time by the method presented by Lussier and Thrun [38] with $\Delta t_T, \Delta t_K, \Delta t_{K2}$. Finally, a point cloud $\mathcal{P} = (\mathbf{p}_1\ \mathbf{p}_2\ \dots\ \mathbf{p}_n)$ containing n points, can be generated with the help of the pinhole camera model.

The intrinsic calibration aims to remove the aberrations from the lens, bringing the image in the form of the pinhole camera model. For the intrinsic calibration, the projection matrix $\mathbf{P}$ has to be determined. The matrix contains the focal length , as well as the offset to the sensor's center. Therefore, based on the pinhole camera model, a point $\mathbf{p} = (x\ y\ z)^T \in \mathbb{R}^3$ can be projected onto the sensor as a pixel $\mathbf{q} = (u\ v)^T$. For the extrinsic calibration, the world frame's origin is set the same as the origin of the infrared sensor of the Kinect. The extrinsic factory calibration of both Kinect cameras is left as it is. The transformations between the two Kinect cameras and the thermal camera is estimated with the help of the same calibration pattern.

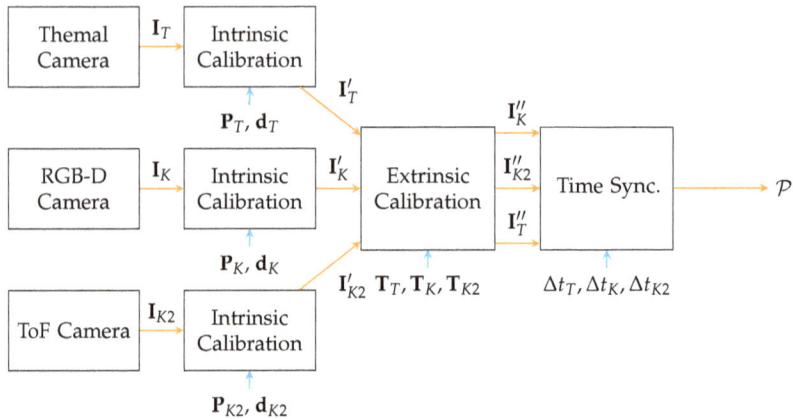

Figure 4. Process of sensor calibration: First, all projective sensors are calibrated intrinsically to remove distortions from the image and to obtain the projection matrix for each sensor $\mathbf{P}_T$, $\mathbf{P}_K$ and $\mathbf{P}_{K2}$. Furthermore, the coefficients for distortions $\mathbf{d} = (k_1\ k_2\ k_3\ p_1\ p_2)$ are necessary for rectification. The vector contains the parameters for radial distortion (k_1, k_2, k_3), as well as the parameters for tangential distortion (p_1, p_2) [35]. Second, the sensors are calibrated extrinsically, estimating the transformations between the sensors $\mathbf{T}$. The calibrated images are noted by $\mathbf{I}'_T$, $\mathbf{I}'_K$, and $\mathbf{I}'_{K2}$. Finally, the data from the sensors are synchronized in time based on $\Delta t_T, \Delta t_K, \Delta t_{K2}$. The synchronized images are noted by $\mathbf{I}''_K$, $\mathbf{I}''_{K2}$, and $\mathbf{I}''_T$. After this process of calibration, sensor fusion can be applied and data is converted towards a Cartesian point cloud $\mathcal{P} \in \mathbb{R}^3$.

Figure 5 illustrates the transformation between the sensors. The extrinsic parameters—the rotation $\mathbf{R}$ and the translation $\mathbf{t}$—are combined to a pose $^A\xi_B$ describing the relative pose of $\{B\}$ with respect to $\{A\}$. After sensor fusion, every point can contain the Cartesian coordinates (x, y, z), color (rgb) and thermal data (t) with $\mathbf{p} = (x\ y\ z\ rgb\ t)^T$. For calibration and sensor fusion, OpenCV was applied [39].

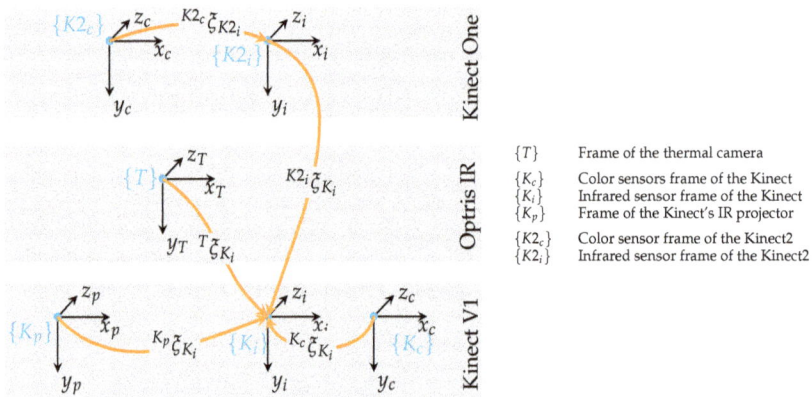

$\{T\}$	Frame of the thermal camera
$\{K_c\}$	Color sensors frame of the Kinect
$\{K_i\}$	Infrared sensor frame of the Kinect
$\{K_p\}$	Frame of the Kinect's IR projector
$\{K2_c\}$	Color sensor frame of the Kinect2
$\{K2_i\}$	Infrared sensor frame of the Kinect2

Figure 5. Transformation tree for the system's sensors: The infrared frame of the Kinect is used as reference for the world coordinate origin $\{0\}$. The manufacturer already calibrates the 3D sensor's own sensor frames. To obtain the transformation between the Kinect V1 and Kinect One, the IR sensors from both cameras are taken as a reference.

3.3. Segmentation

The process of segmentation differs with the scene: A patient lying on a medical stretcher with physicians on his side is harder to segment than someone standing in an empty room with a clear distance to the wall behind him. The point cloud $\mathcal{P}$ is segmented in a set belonging to the person $\mathcal{P}^p$ and a set for the environment $\mathcal{P}^E$ with $\mathcal{P} = \mathcal{P}^E + \mathcal{P}^p$. Therefore, a point can only belong to the person's point cloud, or the environment. The segmentation for clinical applications is described by Pfitzner et al. [15]. For the reader's convenience, it is also presented as follows: The patient is placed in a set range within the field of view (FOV) of the sensors mounted on the ceiling. This range is visible with markers on the floor. In an initial step, the amount of data in the point cloud is reduced. Therefore, the floor and all data outside the range of the markers on the floor is removed from the point cloud. After this step, the point cloud should contain mostly the patient and the stretcher he or she is lying on. Based on the available thermal data from the thermal camera, the segmentation can be done with a threshold in temperature. Points having a higher temperature than a fixed limit are included in the patient's point set $\mathcal{P}^p$. Physicians or family members close to the patient can be removed by finding the most significant contour easily under the assumption that the most significant part of the remaining scene is the patient and the stretcher. Based on the Random Sample Consensus (RANSAC) algorithm [40], the surface of the stretcher is obtained with a model for a plane. On one side, this is necessary to improve the outcome of segmentation. On the other side, the surface of the stretcher is necessary for the upcoming feature extraction. Morphological operations like erosion and dilation improve the outcome of segmentation [41]. Finally, the scene's point cloud $\mathcal{P}$ is segmented, and the patient's point cloud $\mathcal{P}^p$ is available. To check if a patient is within the FOV of the camera, state of the art algorithms like the histogram of oriented gradients can be used [42]. Further, the measurement can be started by the medical staff by pressing a button attached to the wall in the trauma room. The segmentation in this medical scenario is reliable and robust. The data from the thermal camera provides good results in segmentation, sufficient for feature extraction. However, also without a thermal camera, the segmentation can be achieved, but outliers can occur, as illustrated in previous work [20].

The segmentation of a standing or walking person is less complex: To segment the person from the background, a reference frame $\mathcal{P}_{ref}$ without the person is recorded in advance. The current frame containing the person is subtracted from the reference frame $\mathcal{P}^P = \mathcal{P} - \mathcal{P}_{ref}$. Due to the sensor's noise, a threshold in distance should be applied to get a good outcome of background subtraction. Furthermore, to improve the outcome of the segmentation on the floor, the RANSAC algorithm can be applied to detect points on the floor and remove them from the scene's point cloud. Therefore, the segmentation of the feet gets more accurate and robust. Outliers and jumping edge errors can be removed by morphological filters or statistical outlier filters. Figure 6 illustrates the segmentation based on background subtraction with a person walking towards the camera. This procedure is similar as presented in related work by Labati et al. [27] and Nguyen et al. [26].

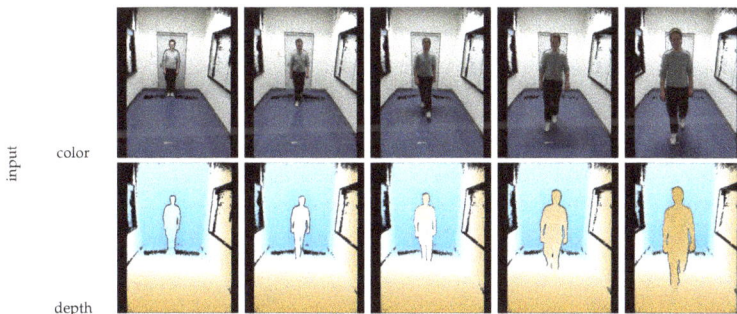

Figure 6. *Cont.*

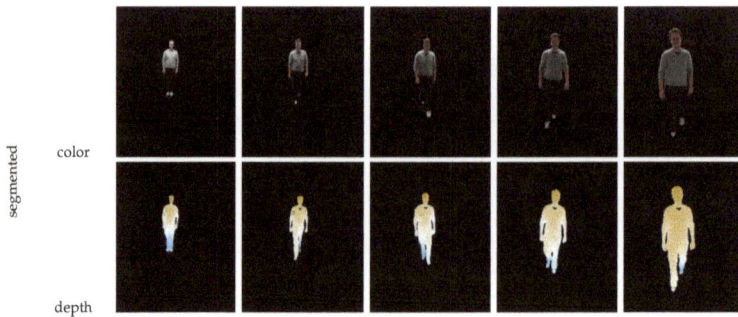

Figure 6. Sequence of someone walking towards the camera: The first two rows in the table illustrate the raw scene in color and depth representation, while the lower part of the table shows the segmented person. The sequence was recorded over four to five seconds. The scene is recorded with the Kinect One.

3.4. Feature Extraction

Based on the segmentation, features are obtained from the person's point cloud $\mathcal{P}^P$. The position of a patient does not vary much in the clinical scenario with the patient on a medical stretcher in a previously defined position of the bed and in a fixed distance from the sensors. In contrast to that, the pose of multiple persons standing in front of a camera can vary more; while walking the pose of the person changes from frame to frame. Therefore, it is necessary that the extracted features are robust against changes in scale, translation, and perspective. The difference in posture is small for most people standing in front of the camera or lying on a stretcher: most of them have their arms aside their body and a few have their arms crossed over their stomach.

The extracted features are presented in Table 4. The correlation of those features to the ground truth body weight is shown in Pfitzner et al. [22]. A good feature is invariant against scale (s), rotation (r), translation (t), perspective (pe) and posture of the person (po) in front of the camera. However, while most of the here presented features are invariant for scale, due to the applied 3D data, no feature is invariant against changes in posture. Therefore, the data applied for training the model should cover many different common postures for standing and walking people.

The features can be grouped: The features f_1 to f_4 are simple geometric features. The estimation of the volume is only possible due to the stretcher the patient is lying on. The volume is calculated based on a triangle mesh of the person's frontal surface s. The not visible surface on the back of the person is modeled by a single plane. The calculation of the volume is presented in detail in Pfitzner et al. [20]. Further, the triangle mesh is taken to calculate the frontal surface of a person. Although both features, the volume, and the surface, are only estimations and can be far from ground truth values, they can be a hint for an estimator: A person having a higher value for volume tends to be heavier compared to someone having a lower volume value. In addition, this first feature group contains the number of points belonging to the person's point cloud $|\mathcal{P}^P|$ and the calculated density of the scene, setting the number of points from the person in relation to the number of points of the whole scene $|\mathcal{P}|$.

The second group of features (f_5 to f_{10}) is based on eigenvalues and the eigenvalues itself: The normalized eigenvalues have the benefit that they are invariant against coordinate transformations like scale, rotation, and translation. Therefore, the features based on these eigenvalues — sphericity, flatness, and linearity — are also invariant against transformations.

The third group consists of features from statistics: Compactness and kurtosis are normalized and therefore invariant against scale, rotation, and translation.

Features from the silhouette of a person are grouped in the fourth section: The area and length of the contour and the convex hull are invariant against rotation, and translation, but not against scale. However, a small change in posture can change the outcome from the calculation of contour and convex hull.

Table 4. List of features for body weight estimation $\forall \, \mathbf{p}_j \in \mathcal{P}^P$. The table further lists the invariance of each feature by scale (s), rotation (r), translation (t), perspective (pe) and posture of the person (po) with + (invariant), 0 (invariant with limitations) and - (not invariant). The equations in the table are taken from the previous work [22].

	Feature	\multicolumn{5}{c}{Invariance}	Equation
		s	r	t	pe	po	
f_1	volume	+	+	+	0	-	v
f_2	surface	+	+	+	0	-	s
f_3	number of patient's points	-	+	+	0	-	$|\mathcal{P}^P|$
f_4	density	-	+	+	0	-	$|\mathcal{P}^P|/|\mathcal{P}|$
f_5	1. eigenvalue	+	+	+	0	-	λ_1
f_6	2. eigenvalue	+	+	+	0	-	λ_2
f_7	3. eigenvalue	+	+	+	0	-	λ_3
f_8	sphericity	+	+	+	0	-	$\lambda_3/\sum_i \lambda_i$
f_9	flatness	+	+	+	0	-	$2\cdot(\lambda_2-\lambda_3)/\sum_i \lambda_i$
f_{10}	linearity	+	+	+	0	-	$(\lambda_1-\lambda_2)/\sum_i \lambda_i$
f_{11}	compactness	+	+	+	0	-	$\sqrt{1/n \sum_i (\mathbf{p}_j - \bar{\mathbf{p}})^2}$
f_{12}	kurtosis	+	+	+	0	-	$1/n \sum_j ||\mathbf{p}_j - \bar{\mathbf{p}}||$
f_{13}	alt. compactness	+	+	+	0	-	$\sum_j (\mathbf{p}_j - \bar{\mathbf{p}})^4/f_9$
f_{14}	distance to person	+	+	+	+	0	d
f_{15}	contour length	-	+	+	-	-	l_c
f_{16}	contour area	-	+	+	-	-	a_c
f_{17}	convex hull length	-	+	+	-	-	l_h
f_{18}	convex hull area	-	+	+	-	-	a_h
f_{19}	gender	+	+	+	+	+	g

Related work showed that the body weight estimation could be improved if the gender is known [26]. The gender was here taken from ground truth, but could also be estimated by algorithm [26,43]. Apparently, the gender does not change in any way with applied transformation. Further, the cited algorithms are robust in detecting gender [43].

Table 5 demonstrates the changes in the feature values with different postures: The first scene shows a subject standing straight with the arms aside. The features are listed and calculated by the previously presented equations. In the second scene, the subject raises both hands a bit. The values for surface and density do not change much. In addition, the first eigenvalue nearly stays the same. However, the value for the third eigenvalue changes, due to the arms raised in front of the person. Flatness and sphericity—which correlate with the third eigenvalue—also change significantly. Compared to the third scene, where the subject stands with legs apart, the second eigenvalue changes most. Therefore, flatness and also linearity change. Comparing the first and the fourth scene, the subject crosses the arms: The surface lowers, as well as all features from contour and convex hull. The second eigenvalue lowers while the third eigenvalue increases. In the last scene, the subject is wearing a backpack. Comparing the features from this scene with the first scene, most of the features are within the same range. However, there are differences due to slight differences in posture. Apparently, the body weight estimation can ignore such objects as backpacks, if not visible to the sensor.

Concerning all the poses presented here, the features from contour and convex hull are able to vary the most: A subject having the arms aside can cause a much higher length in contour when there is a small gap between the body and the arm. However, as shown in [22], the length and area of the contour correlate with the body weight and therefore it can be useful to enclose such features for body weight estimation.

Table 5. Changes in features with different poses: Five different scenes illustrate the change in feature values depending on the posture.

Features	Scene 1	Scene 2	Scene 3	Scene 4	Scene 5
Surface	9.5×10^{-1}	9.7×10^{-1}	9.6×10^{-1}	8.6×10^{-1}	9.7×10^{-1}
Density	1.1×10^{-1}	1.1×10^{-1}	1.2×10^{-1}	1.0×10^{-1}	1.3×10^{-1}
1st eigenvalue	4.7×10^{3}	4.7×10^{3}	5.1×10^{3}	4.5×10^{3}	5.4×10^{3}
2nd eigenvalue	3.9×10^{2}	4.6×10^{2}	6.9×10^{2}	2.5×10^{2}	5.2×10^{2}
3rd eigenvalue	7.1×10^{1}	3.2×10^{2}	7.9×10^{1}	9.4×10^{1}	7.7×10^{1}
Sphericity	4.1×10^{-2}	1.8×10^{-1}	4.0×10^{-2}	5.8×10^{-2}	3.8×10^{-2}
Flatness	1.2×10^{-1}	5×10^{-2}	2.0×10^{-1}	6×10^{-2}	1.4×10^{-1}
Linearity	8.3×10^{-1}	7.7×10^{-1}	7.5×10^{-1}	8.8×10^{-1}	8.1×10^{-1}
Compactness	4.6×10^{-1}	4.6×10^{-1}	4.6×10^{-1}	4.7×10^{-1}	4.5×10^{-1}
Kurtosis	5.4×10^{3}	5.5×10^{3}	6.2×10^{3}	5.0×10^{3}	6.0×10^{3}
AltCompactness	8.6×10^{-1}	8.7×10^{-1}	8.6×10^{-1}	8.6×10^{-1}	8.7×10^{-1}
Contour length	1.0×10^{3}	1.4×10^{3}	1.4×10^{3}	1.1×10^{3}	1.4×10^{3}
Contour area	2.5×10^{4}	2.5×10^{4}	2.8×10^{4}	2.1×10^{4}	1.4×10^{3}
Convex hull length	8.2×10^{2}	8.3×10^{2}	9.3×10^{2}	8.0×10^{2}	8.8×10^{2}
Convex hull area	3.0×10^{4}	3.5×10^{4}	4.3×10^{4}	2.6×10^{4}	3.7×10^{4}
Distance	1.8	1.8	1.7	1.8	1.6
color					
segmented depth					

Machine learning minimizes the invariances in selected features. However, a suitable set for training and testing should cover most of the various poses, especially when the subject is moving during body weight estimation.

3.5. Weight Estimation Based on a Single Frame

The previously extracted features are forwarded to an ANN. The network is designed as a three-layer feedforward network, having one layer as input, one hidden layer, and a single output layer. The output layer consists of a single neuron representing the body weight in kilograms. The number of input units is set by the number of features forwarded to the network. For every element of the feature vector, an input unit exists.

The network is trained with a subset of the available data. For the upcoming experiments, 70 percent of a dataset is forwarded to the neural network for training. The remaining 30 percent of each dataset is used to evaluate the network. Those data are never used for training so the network cannot overfit for the training data. Learning is achieved by resilient propagation [44]. Regularization is applied with weight decay to improve the outcome. First, the error of training and testing decreases. After a while the error in testing dataset increases while the training error is still decreasing. This is the moment to abort the training to prevent an over-fitting. Due to randomized starting points, the learning via the neural network approach can come to different solutions for every trial.

3.6. Estimation of a Sensor Stream

The FOV, the person's height, and the maximum distance for 3D data acquisition mark the starting and end markers on the floor, see Figure 7b. Figure 7a illustrates the poses of all people walking towards the camera. Due to different settings for the experiments, the path people tend to walk differs. Further, the camera did not always have the same orientation towards the floor and was not always mounted at the same height.

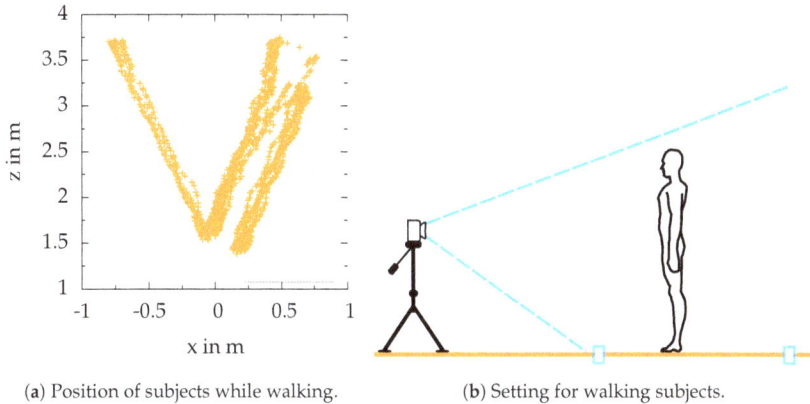

(a) Position of subjects while walking.   (b) Setting for walking subjects.

Figure 7. Poses of people walking towards the camera (**a**): The complete datasets consist of several independent experiments. Therefore, the poses of the people walking differ, depending on the orientation of the camera. The people stand at the first marker (**b**). While walking towards the second marker close to the camera, every frame from the sensor is saved for offline processing. The recording is stopped when the second marker is reached.

First, the person is segmented from the background by the methods described in the previous section. Second, for every frame of the dataset, the body weight estimation is applied. In a scatter plot together with the ground truth body weight, a line becomes visible for every single person. Some of the estimations are close to the ground truth body weight. Even outliers of more than 30 percent occur. Therefore, taking an arbitrary frame from a person's dataset will likely lead to a close to random result. Third, a clustering method is applied, so not only an arbitrary frame from a person's dataset provides an estimation of the body weight. A Euclidean clustering method is applied to improve the outcome. The clustering is applied as follows: A dataset of a person $\mathcal{D}$ consists out of N frames from the sensor $D_0, D_1, \ldots, D_N$. Every frame consists of a point cloud $\mathcal{P}$.

1. For every frame in the dataset $D_i \in \mathcal{D}$ estimate the body weight based on the calculated features $w_i(D_i \to \mathbf{f})$.
2. Calculate the mean distance $\bar{d}$ for every estimation of a dataset $\mathcal{D}$ to all other estimations by

$$\bar{d}_i(D_i) = \frac{1}{N} \sum_{j=1}^{N} |w_i - w_j| \quad \text{where } i \neq j \tag{1}$$

and store the calculated average distances in a vector $\bar{\mathbf{d}}$.
3. Sort the calculated distances in an ascending order $\bar{d}_0 \leq \bar{d}_1 \leq \ldots \leq \bar{d}_N$.
4. Remove values with the highest distances. Keep a fixed amount of distances, e.g., 20 percent.

5.   Calculate the centroid of the remaining estimations containing $n_{0.2} = 0.2 \cdot N$ estimations

$$\bar{w} = \frac{1}{n_{0.2}} \sum_{i=1}^{n_{0.2}} w_i \qquad (2)$$

which is the result of the body weight estimation based on a stream of data.

The principle in clustering is demonstrated in the upcoming section with experiments.

4. A Dataset for Body Weight Estimation

In addition to the here presented algorithm, a dataset is published to boost research in this field. Public datasets, as provided by Nguyen et al. [26] help to improve models for body weight estimation. Furthermore, developed algorithms and models can be applied to the dataset to generate comparable results. Depending on the recorded dataset, different sensors are used for recording. First, the Microsoft Kinect camera from the first generation of the XBox is used to obtain 3D data from the environment. Another sensor used for data acquisition is the second generation Kinect camera, the Kinect One. Additionally, a thermal camera is added and fused to the 3D data. This should ensure an easy segmentation approach based on a thermal threshold.

Table 6 illustrates the characteristics of the subjects in the dataset. The datasets are the following:

- **HospitalNoThermo**: From May 2014 to September 2014 a dataset was recorded from the Universitätsklinikum Erlangen, Germany, for preliminary testing. In this early dataset only RGB-D data is available without thermal data. The thermal camera was added after this experiment. The dataset contains 192 measurements.
- **Hospital**: This dataset includes feature values from trauma room patients from the Universitätsklinkum Erlangen, Germany. The dataset contains 127 measurements from people lying on a medical stretcher, recorded with a Microsoft Kinect. For this dataset a proper distribution is achieved consisting of people of different ages, body weights and shapes, see Table 4. Additionally, this dataset contains the patients' self-estimation, age, sex, as well as anthropometric features like body height, abdominal girth, and waist circumference. The distance between the sensors and the subjects was around 2 m.
- **Event**: The features from this dataset were recorded at a public event, called Long Night of Science in 2015 in Nuremberg, Germany. People in this dataset were visitors of the public event. This dataset contains 106 people. For this public event, it was not convenient to take anthropometric measurements. Ground truth was validated with a standard digital scale. The dataset consists of sensor values from Kinect and thermal camera. Additionally, this dataset includes point clouds from Microsoft Kinect One.
- **Walking**: Based on the results of the previous three datasets, experiments with people standing and walking in front of the camera are complemented. The dataset consists of 14 people, mostly employees, and students from the laboratory.

For the first three datasets, the camera is mounted over a stretcher. The stretcher at the event and the hospital datasets are different. Furthermore, the installation of the sensors did not pay attention to the same height or distance to the stretcher. Therefore, the distance to the stretcher differs between the datasets.

Table 6. Datasets applied for this article: The first two datasets are recorded in a trauma room of the University Hospital Erlangen, Germany. The third dataset is based on a public event in a laboratory, containing visitors of this event. The fourth set is recorded with employees and students of the laboratory. For comparison, the average body weight of the German population in 2009 is 73.9 kg [45]. This average value is close to the first three datasets. The last dataset W8-300 is recorded by [26], showing people standing in the front of a Kinect camera.

Dataset	Sensors	Scenario	Real Weight in kg				Gender		Total
			min	max	Mean	σ	Female	Male	
HospitalNoThermo	K	lying	48.8	165	78.3	17.3	93	99	192
Hospital	K, T	lying	48.6	129	77.8	17.1	72	55	127
Event	K, K2,T	lying	48.8	114	78.6	12.0	24	82	106
Walking	K2	walking	68	134	84.2	16.4	0	14	14
W8-300 [26]	K1	standing	40	104	67.2	14.7	97	207	299

Due to privacy issues, the datasets only contain the depth and the thermal information. The datasets are available via https://osf.io/rhq3m/ [46]. Each frame from the sensors is stored as a point cloud within the common PCD file format, used by the point cloud library [47]. An arbitrary point in the cloud contains the Cartesian coordinates **p** and three values for color—red, green and blue channel. The data can be enhanced with temperature values t.

The name of each frame contains the metadata of each person in front of the camera. The data name is structured as follows GENDER_GROUNDTRUTH_PERSONID_FRAME_ID.pcd. Besides the raw data from the sensors, an already segmented version of each frame exists within the repository. Furthermore, the parameters from intrinsic and extrinsic calibration are available. The authors gratefully acknowledge collaboration and joint work to improve the outcome of body weight estimation based on RGB-D data, especially for the clinical application.

5. Experiments and Results

For the upcoming section, the presented algorithm is evaluated for standing and walking people. Experiments for lying people are presented and discussed in the previous work [15,20].

The validate the experiments, different metrics are used for comparison: For each measurement the absolute error e can be calculated, having the ground truth value $\hat{x}$ as well as the estimated value $\tilde{x}$ by $e_i = \hat{x} - \tilde{x}$. The absolute error would be good to compare a group of people having the same body weight and differ only in their visual appearance. The here presented group of people for testing has a high variety of body weight and visual appearance. Therefore, the absolute error is not sufficient for comparison. Better for comparison of variant datasets is the relative error which is defined for an arbitrary dataset with

$$\epsilon = \frac{\hat{x}_i - \tilde{x}_i}{\hat{x}_i} = \frac{e_i}{\hat{x}_i} \tag{3}$$

Another way to prove and benchmark the body weight estimation approach is the mean absolute error (MAE). The absolute error of each dataset e_i is summed up and divided by the total number of datasets for benchmarking. It is defined by

$$e_{mae} = \frac{1}{N} \sum_{i=1}^{N} |e_i|. \tag{4}$$

Further, the mean square error (MSE) can be used for validation. Here the absolute error is squared before summation. It is defined by

$$e_{mse} = \frac{1}{N} \sum_{i=1}^{N} e_i^2. \tag{5}$$

Compared to the mean absolute error, outliers were weighted stronger.

5.1. Standing

In contrast to experiments for people who were lying down, the most correlating feature—the volume—cannot be used because no reference surface for the back of a person exists. Therefore, the body weight estimation has to rely on the remaining features. A previous experiment with the two datasets from a hospital and the event dataset illustrated that the body weight estimation gets worse if the volume is missing. Nevertheless, the decrease in accuracy can be sufficient for other applications.

For the experiment, the dataset W8-300 generated by Nguyen et al. [26] is applied. It contains 299 people standing in front of a Microsoft Kinect camera. The color and the depth frame are saved separately with a resolution for each channel of 8 bit. The segmentation has been done in advance based on ground detection with RANSAC model [40]: The images in the dataset are already segmented, only containing the person's data as a depth and color image; the background is not visible. The file name of each dataset contains first the gender, second the ground truth body weight, and lastly the surname of the person. The ground truth body weight varies within a range starting from 40 kg up to 104 kg. In the experiments, 202 males and 97 females participated.

Figure 8 illustrates the result from the dataset: First, the ground truth ordered datasets are shuffled. For training of the ANN, 70 percent of the dataset were used; the other 30 percent were applied for testing.

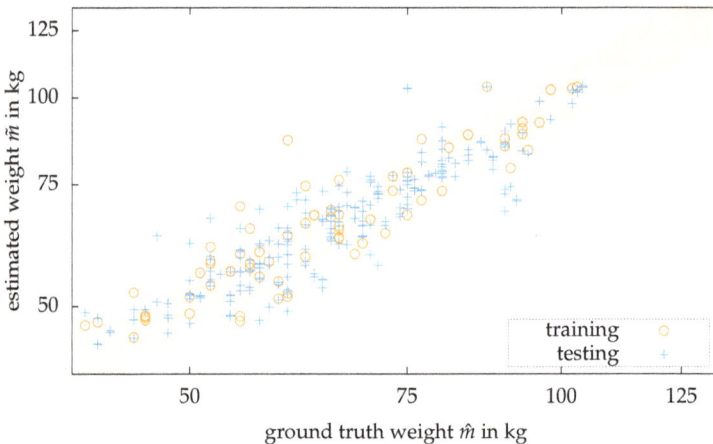

Figure 8. Results of the experiment with people standing in front of the camera based on the here proposed algorithm and the W-300 dataset contributed by Nguyen et al. [26]. The orange area marks the range for the relative error of ±10 percent.

All people were not told to hold a fixed posture but most of them were standing normally with their arms aside.

Nguyen et al. [26] compared the MAE in their publication: They reached a MAE of 4.62 kg for female and 5.59 kg for male persons. Without the discrimination in gender, the algorithm performs with a MAE of 5.20 kg. This experiment also includes the ground truth of the gender for the applied model. Compared to their results, the here performed experiment reaches an MAE of 4.3 kg. The approach presented by [25] can outperform the here presented results with a MAE of 2.7 kg. However, the sample size in the published article contains only six subjects.

5.2. Walking

In addition to the previous experiments, walking people should also be estimated for their body weight. Therefore, a dataset was recorded with students and employees of the Technische Hochschule Nürnberg, Georg Simon Ohm, walking in front of a Microsoft Kinect One. The person is walking towards the sensor, starting at a fixed distance. A marker on the floor shows the limitation of the recorded scene, due to the FOV of the sensor. The sensor is mounted on a tripod in a height of around 1.5 m.

The setting for this experiment is described in detail in the previous section. Figure 9 illustrates the results of this experiment as a scatter plot:

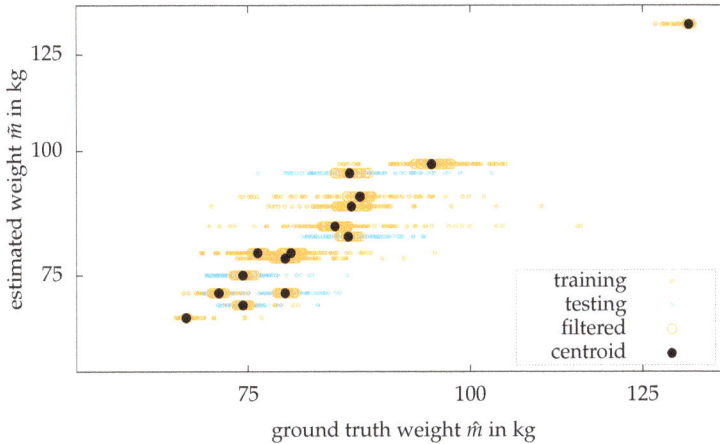

Figure 9. Results of the experiment with people walking towards the camera: The estimations for every frame for an arbitrary person generate a set of estimations, formed as a line together with the ground truth value in the scatter plot. Based on Euclidean clustering, 80 percent of the estimations are removed from the dataset. The final estimation is given based on the centroid of the remaining estimations. The orange area marks the range for the relative error of ± 10 percent.

The estimations for an arbitrary person lead in the scatter plot points, aligning on a horizontal line. Often, most of the estimations are outside of the ± 10 percent bound. However, some estimations appear to be more dense to other estimations than some outliers. The previously presented approach for clustering now minimizes the set of estimations of an arbitrary person (here marked in bigger points) and calculates the centroid of these sets. For this small sample size of 14 subjects, all of the final estimations were within a range of ± 10 percent.

The results provided by Labati et al. [27] outperform the here presented approach when comparing the standard deviation. In contrast to that, the proposed approach outperforms the estimation for walking people presented by Arigbabu et al. [28].

6. Discussion

All presented experiments rely on the same set of features. Table 7 compares the result from walking and standing people for body weight estimation: The estimation works best if the subject is lying on a medical stretcher, comparing the results for the relative error and the percentage of in range estimations. This result occurs because in this configuration the volume of the subject can be extracted easily. Further, the variety of posture and position of the subject is low in the overall datasets [22]. The algorithm works with different types of sensors, e.g., a structured light sensor (Kinect) as well as a time of flight sensor (Kinect One). Figure 10 illustrates the relative error in a cumulative plot for lying, standing and walking subjects.

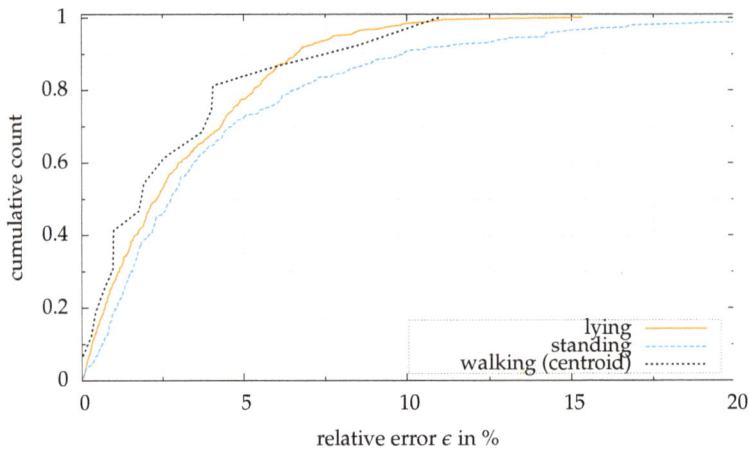

Figure 10. Comparison between the different settings for body weight estimation: Although the results for the estimation with standing people from the W8-300 dataset is the worst in this cumulative plot, the results can be sufficient for a certain applications. Due to the clustering approach, the estimation of walking subjects outperforms the other settings within the range of ±5 percent. The results for the lying patients are taken from Pfitzner et al. [22].

Table 7. Results from experiments for standing and walking people. Additionally, the results from Pfitzner et al. [22] are added for comparison. The lower part of the table illustrates the results from related work, when available in detail. The best result is marked in bold for each category.

	Dataset	Size	Relative Error in %				In Range in %			Error in kg / kg^2	
			min	max	Mean	σ	5	10	20	MAE	MSE
Lying [22]	Event	106	−8.7	14.3	0.90	4.80	75.6	95.3	**100**	2.86	13.8
Standing	W8-300	299	−28.8	16.76	−0.1	5.80	70.5	91.3	99.3	4.31	33.5
Walking	Walking	14	**−6.7**	**9.38**	0.32	**3.88**	**78.5**	**100**	**100**	3.30	20.5
Nguyen et al. [26]	W8-300	299								5.2	
Velardo and Dugelay [25]		6			3.6					**2.7**	
Labati et al. [27]		20				**2.3**					
Arigbabu et al. [28]		13								4.66	

The results for subjects standing in front of a camera are less accurate in nearly every category. However, over 90 percent of the body weight estimation is within a range of ±10 percent. Comparing the here presented approach with the algorithm presented by Nguyen et al. [26], the experiment performs better for the dataset W8-300 with a MAE of 4.31 kg, facing 5.20 kg. In contrast to that, the estimation of subjects walking towards the camera is outstanding. However, the results rely on a small set of subjects. Therefore, the experiment is far from being statistically significant, but it proves the concept.

Although the system with its features is suitable for body weight estimation of lying, standing and walking subjects, there are some limitations. The previously trained ANN can only provide a sufficient result for the body weight estimation when a similar subject has been seen in advance, which is common for machine learning approaches. At a public laboratory event, children were estimated with relative errors in body weight of up to 50 percent—due to not being seen before. The used model was trained with patients from the hospital, where subjects younger than 18 years were excluded in the dataset. While the pose of the subjects lying in the clinical scenario is similar, the pose for walking subjects can vary strongly from frame to frame. For the here presented small experiment, all subjects are facing the camera and walking towards it. In a scenario with the people walking differently, e.g., walking sideways, the algorithms would not provide sufficient estimation results.

7. Conclusions and Future Work

This paper presented a novel approach for the estimation of body weight. In contrast to related work, the approach with its feature vector was tested for lying, standing and walking subjects. Experiments proved that the estimation is possible within a given range. The algorithm and the extracted features previously presented in [15] are also able to provide an estimation of standing and walking people. The missing volume—which correlates with the body weight the most [22]—is the reason the estimation for a single frame of a walking subject is worse than for a lying person. However, the estimation on a sequence of frames combined with the presented clustering provides a sufficient body weight estimation. In direct comparison with the approach for body weight estimation approach from Nguyen et al. [26], the approach presented here can outperform the results, while being applied to the same dataset.

For future work, it is the aim of the here presented project to obtain a bigger dataset: The estimation of standing people should be expanded to an approach where people do not need to face in the direction of the sensors. Further, the path for the estimation of walking people should be made more variable so people can move freely in front of the camera. This approach needs a higher demand for varying data. The authors gratefully acknowledge future joint work to improve the outcome of the algorithm and to develop a bigger dataset for experiments and modeling.

Author Contributions: Christian Pfitzner designed the algorithm and the experiments for the here presented multimodal sensor system; Stefan May and Andreas Nüchter contributed to the methology with conception and ideas for the experiment for the approach and experiments for visual body weight estimation. Furthermore, they improved the content of the article with their annotations.

Acknowledgments: Christian Pfitzner was supported by the BayWISS research training group "Digitization". This publication was funded by the German Research Foundation (DFG) and the University of Würzburg in the funding programme Open Access Publishing.

Conflicts of Interest: The authors declare no conflict of interest.

Abbreviations

The following abbreviations are used in this manuscript:

ANN	artificial neural network
FPV	field of view
IR	infrared
MAE	mean average error
MSE	mean square error
RANSAC	random sample consensus
RGB	red green blue
RGB-D	red green blue depth
RGB-D-T	red green blue depth thermal
PCD	point cloud data
rtPA	recombinant tissue plasminogen activator
TDP	thermal design power
ToF	time of flight

References

1. Zivin, J.A. Acute stroke therapy with tissue plasminogen activator (tPA) since it was approved by the U.S. Food and Drug Administration (FDA). *Annal. Neurol.* **2009**, *66*, 6–10. [CrossRef] [PubMed]
2. Breuer, L.; Nowe, T.; Huttner, H.B.; Blinzler, C.; Kollmar, R.; Schellinger, P.D.; Schwab, S.; Köhrmann, M. Weight Approximation in Stroke Before Thrombolysis The WAIST-Study: A Prospective Observational "Dose-Finding" Study. *Stroke* **2010**, *41*, 2867–2871. [CrossRef] [PubMed]

3. Lorenz, M.W.; Graf, M.; Henke, C.; Hermans, M.; Ziemann, U.; Sitzer, M.; Foerch, C. Anthropometric approximation of body weight in unresponsive stroke patients. *J. Neurol. Neurosurg. Psychiatry* **2007**, *78*, 1331–1336. [CrossRef] [PubMed]
4. Diedler, J.; Ahmed, N.; Glahn, J.; Grond, M.; Lorenzano, S.; Brozman, M.; Sykora, M.; Ringleb, P. Is the Maximum Dose of 90 mg Alteplase Sufficient for Patients With Ischemic Stroke Weighing >100 kg? *Stroke* **2011**, *42*, 1615–1620. [CrossRef] [PubMed]
5. Coe, T.; Halkes, M.; Houghton, K.; Jefferson, D. The accuracy of visual estimation of weight and height in pre-operative supine patients. *Anaesthesia* **1999**, *54*, 582–586. [CrossRef] [PubMed]
6. Cubison, T.; Gilbert, P. So much for percentage, but what about the weight? *Emerg. Med. J.* **2005**, *22*, 643–645. [CrossRef] [PubMed]
7. Menon, S.; Kelly, A.M. How accurate is weight estimation in the emergency department? *Emerg. Med. Australas.* **2005**, *17*, 113–116. [CrossRef] [PubMed]
8. Ahmed, N.N.; Pearce, S.E. Acute care for the elderly: A literature review. *Popul. Health Manag.* **2010**, *13*, 219–225. [CrossRef] [PubMed]
9. Webster, D.; Celik, O. Systematic review of Kinect applications in elderly care and stroke rehabilitation. *J. Neuroeng. Rehabil.* **2014**, *11*, 108. [CrossRef] [PubMed]
10. Gasparrini, S.; Cippitelli, E.; Spinsante, S.; Gambi, E. A Depth-Based Fall Detection System Using a Kinect® Sensor. *Sensors* **2014**, *14*, 2756–2775. [CrossRef] [PubMed]
11. Procházka, A.; Schätz, M.; Vyšata, O.; Vališ, M. Microsoft Kinect Visual and Depth Sensors for Breathing and Heart Rate Analysis. *Sensors* **2016**, *16*, 996. [CrossRef] [PubMed]
12. Publication, C.A.A. *Civil Aviation Safety Authority—Standard Passenger and Baggage Weights*; Civil Aviation Safety Authority: Woden Valley, Australia, 1990. Available online: https://www.casa.gov.au/file/104861/download?token=E70-zaqD (accessed on 19 April 2018)
13. Elliott, A.F. Why a Finnish Airline Is Weighing Passengers Before They Board, 2017. Available online: https://www.telegraph.co.uk/travel/news/why-a-finnish-airline-is-weighing-every-passenger-before-they-board/ (accessed on 2 April 2018).
14. Board, C.A.S. *Aviation Occurrence Report*; Arrow Air Inc. Douglas DC-8-63 N950JW; Gander International Airport: Gander, NL, Canada, 1988.
15. Pfitzner, C.; May, S.; Nüchter, A. Neural network-based visual body weight estimation for drug dosage finding. *Proceedings of the SPIE Medical Imaging 2016*; SPIE: San Diego, CA, USA, 2016.
16. Ragoschke-Schumm, A.; Razouk, A.; Lesmeister, M.; Helwig, S.; Grunwald, I.Q.; Fassbender, K. Dosage Calculation for Intravenous Thrombolysis of Ischemic Stroke: To Weigh or to Estimate? *Cerebrovas. Dis. Extra* **2017**, *7*, 103–110. [CrossRef] [PubMed]
17. Argall, J.A.W.; Wright, N.; Mackway-Jones, K.; Jackson, R. A comparison of two commonly used methods of weight estimation. *Arch. Dis. Child.* **2003**, *88*, 789–790. [CrossRef] [PubMed]
18. Krieser, D.; Nguyen, K.; Kerr, D.; Jolley, D.; Clooney, M.; Kelly, A.M. Parental weight estimation of their child's weight is more accurate than other weight estimation methods for determining childrens weight in an emergency department? *Emerg. Med. J.* **2007**, *24*, 756–759. [CrossRef] [PubMed]
19. Pirker, K.; Rüther, M.; Bischof, H.; Skrabal, F. Human Body Volume Estimation in a Clinical Environment, 2010. Available online: http://citeseerx.ist.psu.edu/viewdoc/download?doi=10.1.1.173.3803&rep=rep1&type=pdf (accessed on 2 January 2018).
20. Pfitzner, C.; May, S.; Merkl, C.; Breuer, L.; Braun, J.; Dirauf, F. Libra3D: Body Weight Estimation for Emergency Patients in Clinical Environments with a 3D Structured Light Sensor. In Proceedings of the IEEE International Conference on Robotics and Automation, Seattle, WA, USA, 26–30 May 2015.
21. Pfitzner, C.; May, S.; Merkl, C. Vorrichtung und verfahren zur optischen erfassung eines gewichtes einer person. Available online: https://patents.google.com/patent/DE102016103543A1/de (accessed on 5 January 2018).
22. Pfitzner, C.; May, S.; Nüchter, A. Evaluation of Features from RGB-D Data for Human Body Weight Estimation. In Proceedings of the 20th World Congress of the International Federation of Automatic Control (WC '17), Toulouse, France, 9–14 July 2017.
23. Robinson, M.; Parkinson, M.B. Estimating Anthropometry with Microsoft Kinect. In Proceedings of the 2nd International Digital Human Modeling Symposium, Ann Arbor, MI, USA, 11–14 June 2013.

24. Cook, T.S.; Couch, G.; Couch, T.J.; Kim, W.; Boonn, W.W. Using the Microsoft Kinect for Patient Size Estimation and Radiation Dose Normalization: Proof of Concept and Initial Validation. *J. Dig. Imaging* **2013**, *26*, 657–662. [CrossRef] [PubMed]

25. Velardo, C.; Dugelay, J.L. What can computer vision tell you about your weight? In Proceedings of the 20th European Signal Processing Conference EUSIPCO, Bucharest, Romania, 27–31August 2012.

26. Nguyen, T.V.; Feng, J.; Yan, S. Seeing Human Weight from a Single RGB-D Image. *J. Comput. Sci. Technol.* **2014**, *29*, 777–784. [CrossRef]

27. Labati, R.; Genovese, A.; Piuri, V.; Scotti, F. Weight Estimation from Frame Sequences Using Computational Intelligence Techniques. In Proceedings of the IEEE International Conference on Computational Intelligence for Measurement Systems and Applications (CIMSA), Tianjin, China, 2–4 July 2012; pp. 29–34.

28. Arigbabu, O.A.; Ahmad, S.M.S.; Adnan, W.A.W.; Yussof, S.; Iranmanesh, V.; Malallah, F.L. Estimating body related soft biometric traits in video frames. *Sci. World J.* **2014**, *2014*, doi:10.1155/2014/460973. [CrossRef] [PubMed]

29. Zhang, Z. Microsoft Kinect Sensor and Its Effect. *IEEE MultiMedia* **2012**, *19*, 4–10. [CrossRef]

30. Khoshelham, K.; Elberink, S.O. Accuracy and resolution of kinect depth data for indoor mapping applications. *Sensors* **2012**, *12*, 1437–1454. [CrossRef] [PubMed]

31. May, S. *3D Time-of-Flight Ranging for Robotic Perception in Dynamic Environments*; VDI-Verlag: Dusseldorf, Germany, 2009.

32. Sarbolandi, H.; Lefloch, D.; Kolb, A. Kinect range sensing: Structured-light versus Time-of-Flight Kinect. *Comput. Vis. Image Underst.* **2015**, *139*, 1–20. [CrossRef]

33. Draelos, M.; Qiu, Q.; Bronstein, A.; Sapiro, G. Intel realsense; Real low cost gaze. In Proceedings of the 2015 IEEE International Conference on Image Processing (ICIP), Quebec City, QC, Canada, 27–30 September 2015; pp. 2520–2524.

34. Winkler, T. Review Dell Precision M4800 Notebook. Available online: https://www.notebookcheck.net/Review-Dell-Precision-M4800-Notebook.104416.0.html (accessed on 3 April 2018).

35. Zhang, Z. A Flexible New Technique for Camera Calibration. *IEEE Trans. Pattern Anal. Mach. Intell.* **2000**, *22*, 1330–1334. [CrossRef]

36. Gonzalez-Jorge, H.; Rodríguez-Gonzálvez, P.; Martínez-Sánchez, J.; González-Aguilera, D.; Arias, P.; Gesto, M.; Díaz-Vilariño, L. Metrological comparison between Kinect I and Kinect II sensors. *Measurement* **2015**, *70*, 21–26. [CrossRef]

37. Vidas, S.; Moghadam, P.; Bosse, M. 3D thermal mapping of building interiors using an RGB-D and thermal camera. In Proceedings of the 2013 IEEE International Conference on Robotics and Automation, Karlsruhe, Germany, 6–10 May 2013; pp. 2311–2318.

38. Lussier, J.T.; Thrun, S. Automatic calibration of RGBD and thermal cameras. In Proceedings of the 2014 IEEE/RSJ International Conference on Intelligent Robots and Systems (IROS 2014), Chicago, IL, USA, 14–18 September 2014; pp. 451–458.

39. Bradski, G.; Kaehler, A. *Learning OpenCV*, 1st ed.; O'Reilly Media: Sebastopol, CA, USA, 2008.

40. Fischler, M.A.; Bolles, R.C. Random Sample Consensus: A Paradigm for Model Fitting with Applications to Image Analysis and Automated Cartography. *Commun. ACM* **1981**, *24*, 381–395. [CrossRef]

41. Szeliski, R. *Computer Vision: Algorithms and Applications*, 1st ed.; Springer: New York, NY, USA, 2010.

42. Dalal, N.; Triggs, B. Histograms of oriented gradients for human detection. In Proceedings of the IEEE Computer Society Conference on Computer Vision and Pattern Recognition, CVPR, San Diego, CA, USA, 20–25 June 2005; Volume I, pp. 886–893.

43. Linder, T.; Wehner, S.; Arras, K.O. Real-time full-body human gender recognition in (RGB)-D data. In Proceedings of the IEEE International Conference on Robotics and Automation, ICRA 2015, Seattle, WA, USA, 26–30 May 2015; pp. 3039–3045.

44. Riedmiller, M.; Braun, H. A Direct Adaptive Method for Faster Backpropagation Learning: The RPROP Algorithm. In Proceedings of the IEEE International Conference on Neural Networks, San Francisco, CA, USA, 28 March–1 April 1993; pp. 586–591.

45. Deutschland, S.B. Mikrozensus - Fragen zur Gesundheit 2009. Available online: https://www.destatis.de/DE/ZahlenFakten/GesellschaftStaat/Gesundheit/GesundheitszustandRelevantesVerhalten/Tabellen/GesundheitszustandBehandlungsanlaesse.pdf?__blob=publicationFile (accessed on 3 April 2018).

46. Pfitzner, C. RGB-D(-T) Datasets for Body Weight Estimation of Stroke Patients from the Libra3D Project, 2018. Available online: https://osf.io/h93ry/ (accessed on 30 March 2018).
47. Rusu, R.B.; Marton, Z.C.; Blodow, N.; Dolha, M.; Beetz, M. Towards 3D Point cloud based object maps for household environments. *Robot. Auton. Syst.* **2008**, *56*, 927–941. [CrossRef]

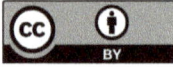

![sensors logo] *sensors*

MDPI

Article

Vibration and Noise in Magnetic Resonance Imaging of the Vocal Tract: Differences between Whole-Body and Open-Air Devices

Jiří Přibil [1,*], Anna Přibilová [2] and Ivan Frollo [1]

[1] Institute of Measurement Science, Slovak Academy of Sciences, 841 04 Bratislava, Slovak Republic; ivan.frollo@savba.sk
[2] Faculty of Electrical Engineering and Information Technology, Slovak University of Technology in Bratislava, 812 19 Bratislava, Slovak Republic; anna.pribilova@stuba.sk
* Correspondence: umerprib@savba.sk; Tel.: +421-2-59104543

Received: 12 March 2018; Accepted: 4 April 2018; Published: 5 April 2018

Abstract: This article compares open-air and whole-body magnetic resonance imaging (MRI) equipment working with a weak magnetic field as regards the methods of its generation, spectral properties of mechanical vibration and acoustic noise produced by gradient coils during the scanning process, and the measured noise intensity. These devices are used for non-invasive MRI reconstruction of the human vocal tract during phonation with simultaneous speech recording. In this case, the vibration and noise have negative influence on quality of speech signal. Two basic measurement experiments were performed within the paper: mapping sound pressure levels in the MRI device vicinity and picking up vibration and noise signals in the MRI scanning area. Spectral characteristics of these signals are then analyzed statistically and compared visually and numerically.

Keywords: magnetic resonance imaging; acoustic noise; mechanical vibration

1. Introduction

The magnetic resonance imaging (MRI) tomograph is basically a huge intelligent sensor used for biomedical purposes. Two different types of MRI equipment were analyzed and compared in the framework of this paper. They both work with a weak stationary magnetic field B_0 up to 0.2 T but with totally different mechanical construction and different physical principle of this magnetic field creation. A pair of permanent magnets is usually incorporated in the open-air MRI device being normally used in clinical diagnostic practice for scanning smaller parts of human body such as a hand, a neck, a coxa, a knee, etc., or various biological tissues [1]. On the other hand, a resistive magnet containing a water-cooled multi-section coil is used for generation of a basic magnetic field in larger whole-body device enabling MR scans of more complex parts of the human body. Every MRI device consists of a gradient system to select x, y, and z slices of a tested subject. In the open-air MRI system, planar gradient coils [2] are mostly used to minimize space requirements. For the whole-body devices, there is typical use of cylindrical gradient coils distributed around the tube in which an examined person/object lies. There are also many differences in construction and practical realization of open-air and whole-body types of these devices. In spite of all the differences, both devices have in common undesirable production of significant mechanical pulses during execution of a scan sequence. Although magnetic translational forces and torques on diamagnetic and paramagnetic tissues are not of safety concern, this does not apply to acoustic noise as a result of rapid switching of large currents accompanied with rapid direction reversal of Lorenz forces [3]. The radiated acoustic noise can be measured by a microphone and its sound pressure level (SPL) can be mapped in the MRI neighborhood. The component frequencies of this acoustic noise fall into the standard audio frequency range, so it can be processed in the spectral domain and analyzed using methods similar to those of audio and speech signal analysis.

These MRI devices can also be successfully used for analysis of the human vocal tract structure and its dynamic shaping during speech production [4]. For this purpose, the speech signal must be recorded simultaneously in real time while the MR scan sequence is being executed [5]. The speech signal should be recorded with high signal-to-noise ratio (SNR), but an acoustic noise produced by the MRI gradient system degrades its quality [6]. Thus, noise reduction techniques must be applied to improve the SNR of the speech signal [7,8]. One group of enhancement methods is based on spectral subtraction of the estimated background noise [9]. However, noise estimation techniques based on statistical approaches are not able to track real noise variations; thereby they result in an artificial residual musical noise and a distorted speech [10]. Therefore, spectral properties of both vibration and noise generated by the gradient system of the MRI device must be analyzed with high precision so that the noise could be efficiently suppressed while preserving maximum quality of the processed speech signal [11].

The main motivation of this study was to measure and compare intensity, distribution, and spectral properties of mechanical vibration and acoustic noise produced by the low magnetic field MR imagers. As both types of investigated tomographs use the same physical principles for modulation of the basic magnetic field, we suppose comparable results of measured vibration and noise signals. These results can be generalized for next use, e.g., when direct measurement is difficult or practically impossible or undistorted values cannot be obtained. Hence, it is helpful that we can use results from the alternative type of MRI with the final aim to suppress negative influence of noise in the recorded speech signal while using a similar device. The original contribution of our paper lies in investigation and comparison of two low-field MRI devices with similar magnetic flux density differing in construction.

The study also describes measurement experiments performed in the scanning area and in the neighborhood of the MRI equipment. First, for both types of investigated MRI devices, mapping of the SPL was performed in their vicinity. The main experiment consisted of real-time recording of the vibration and noise signals which were subsequently off-line processed—the determined spectral features were statistically analyzed, and the obtained results were visually and numerically compared. Attenuation and reflection of the acoustic wave caused by the enclosing metal shielding cage, and influence of the mass of a tested person/object in the scanning area during execution of an MR scan sequence on the properties of vibration and noise signals were also discussed. Finally, the time delay between the vibration signal and the excitation impulse in the gradient coil from simultaneously recorded electrical excitation, vibration, and noise signals was analyzed and evaluated.

2. Subject and Methods

2.1. Differences in Construction of the Gradient System in the Open-Air and the Whole-Body MRI Equipment

Basic vibration and noise analysis was performed on the open-air MRI device [12] normally used in clinical diagnostic practice. This type of equipment has a stationary magnetic field with magnetic induction of 0.178 T produced by a pair of permanent magnets. The gradient system consists of 2×3 planar coils situated between the magnets and an RF receiving/transmitting coil with a tested object/subject. Different RF coils with cylindrical diameter not exceeding 18 cm are used for MR scans of a human knee, an arm, a leg, thin layers of botanical and zoological samples, or testing phantoms. Due to electromagnetic compatibility and reduction of possible RF signal interference, the whole MRI scanning equipment is located inside a metal cage. It is made of 2-mm thick steel plate with symmetrically placed holes of 2.5-mm diameter in 5-mm grid to eliminate electromagnetic field propagation to the surrounding space (control room with operator console, etc.). Such a perforated surface successfully attenuates low-frequency sound if its wavelength is much larger than perforation thickness and diameter [13,14]. The orifice together with the backing air cavity forms a Helmholtz resonator whose frequency of sound absorption depends on size of these acoustic elements [15]. Since volume of air behind the apertures (surrounding air in a room with a cage inside) is rather great, the Helmholtz resonance frequency is rather low, and this effect can be neglected. However, each flat part of the metal surface (between perforations) may reflect sound energy towards inside if the wavelength of the sound is much lower than the size of this flat part.

The situation is totally different when the whole-body MRI device is investigated. In this case, the gradient system is made up of six cylindrical coils. Size of the gradient coils is also greater, since the tube diameter must enable insertion of the patient's bed with an examined person. In the case of an experimental whole-body MR imager TMR96 used in measurements for this study, the device works with a magnetic field $B_0 = 0.1$ T created by a resistive water-cooled magnet with a diameter of 1414 mm and a length of 2240 mm. The active part of the equipment is enclosed in a shielding metal cage with the size of a small room (550 × 340 × 230 cm) made of 2-mm thin copper sheet with a smooth surface that is fully sealed except for four ventilation holes. For this reason, it is supposed to be a good acoustic reflector. On the other hand, although the pick-up sensors are arranged outside the scanning area to eliminate interaction with the working magnetic field, they are very close to the examined person lying inside the scan tube, so the effect of reflected acoustic wave superposition can be neglected in the recorded sound signal. More robust construction and greater mass of this device would inhibit its vibration. However, higher energy of the impulse current must be applied to select 3D coordinates of a tested subject, so stronger Lorentz forces [16] act in the gradient coil system. In the final effect, vibration and noise levels inside the scanning area are usually higher than those in the open-air MRI with planar gradient coils.

Preliminary performed experiments have shown that the produced vibration and acoustic noise are principally influenced by a mechanical load of a person lying in the scanning area of the open-air MRI machine [17] where the examined person lies directly on the plastic cover of the bottom gradient coil. The whole-body MRI contains a movable bed which is not directly connected with the gradient coils, but for larger volume of the sample inserted in larger gradient coils, higher electric current must flow through the gradient coils to perform equivalent change in the magnetic field to choose each of the x, y, z coordinates in the selected field of view (FOV) [18]. Higher energy used for generation of the vibration signal also has an effect on its spectral properties. From the acoustic point of view, the test person/sample/phantom placed on the patient's bed changes the overall mass and stiffness of the whole scanning system including the gradient coil structure. These changed mechanical properties result in different vibration than in the case of the plate weighted by the mass of a tested person. It means that, first of all, the spectral properties of the picked-up vibration signal are changed depending on the applied mechanical weight.

2.2. Sensors for Measurement in a Weak Magnetic Field Environment

In general, the interaction with a stationary magnetic field B_0 in the scanning area must be eliminated during measurement experiments to obtain MR images of sufficient quality without any artifacts. The same applies for measurement of noise SPL, excitation signal of the gradient coil system, and vibration and noise signals. In the case of MRI equipment working with a weak magnetic field (up to 0.2 T), the interaction problem can be solved by a proper choice of the arrangement where the measuring device (SPL meter and/or pick-up microphone) is located in an adequate distance from the noise signal source outside the magnetic field area. The choice of a suitable recording microphone was led by its good sensitivity and proper directional pickup pattern. Since the noise depends on the position of the measuring microphone, the directional pattern of the noise distribution in the MRI equipment neighborhood had to be mapped using optimal selection of the recording microphone position and parameters (distance from the central point of the MRI scanning area, direction angle, working height, type of the microphone pickup pattern). The sensors measuring vibration and electrical excitation signals must be placed inside the MRI scanning area where they are affected by a stationary magnetic field—see the documentary photo of measurement in and around the TMR96 device in Figure 1. In the scanning area, there is a high voltage generated by the excitation RF coil of the MRI device during execution of the MR sequence. This would result in large disturbance of a signal from the sensor or in damage of electronics integrated with the sensor. The vibration sensor with a piezoelectric transducer can be successfully used in these circumstances [11,12,17]. It is important that the sensor has good sensitivity and maximally flat frequency response. Its frequency range should cover harmonic frequencies of vibration and noise signals. These are concentrated in the low band due to frequency-limited gradient pulses [19], which is similar to the frequency range used for basic processing of speech signals. The above-mentioned requirements can be fulfilled by the sensor constructed for acoustic musical instrument pick up [20]. Finally, the sensing coil measuring the excitation signal must be designed with appropriate physical parameters (impedance, number of turns, mechanical construction, etc.) together with the input circuits for signal processing.

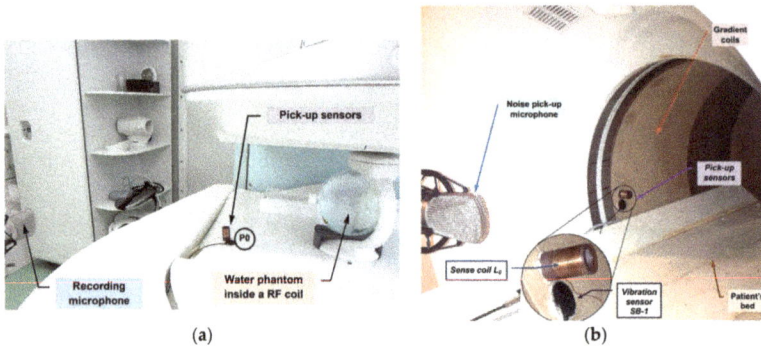

(a) (b)

Figure 1. Photo of sensors placement for recording of vibration, noise, and electrical excitation signals in open-air and whole-body devices; (**a**) E-scan Esaote Opera with the spherical water phantom inside the knee RF coil; (**b**) MR imager TMR-96.

2.3. Features for Description of Vibration and Noise Signal Properties

For basic visual comparison of spectral properties of the recorded vibration or noise signals, a periodogram representing an estimate of a power spectral density (PSD) can be successfully used. Another useful graphical rendering is a spectrogram showing all PSD values in a time window moving through the whole analyzed signal.

Basic spectral properties of the vibration/noise are determined from the spectral envelope and subsequently histograms of spectral values are calculated and compared. MRI parameters of repetition time (TR) and echo time (TE) affect the dominant resonance F_{V0} (reciprocal of TR) and the secondary resonances $F_{V1,2}$ (first two local maxima of the spectral envelope where its gradient changes from positive to negative or poles of the linear predictive coding transfer function). Spectral decrease ($S_{decrease}$) is a parameter representing a degree of fall of the power spectrum. It can be calculated by a linear regression using the mean square method. A similar parameter is spectral tilt (S_{tilt}) as an angle between a line connecting spectral envelope values at low and high frequencies and a horizontal line. Supplementary spectral features describe a shape of the power spectrum of the analyzed signal. Spectral centroid (S_{centr}) determines a centre of gravity of the spectrum—the average frequency weighted by the values of the normalized energy of each frequency component in the spectrum. Spectral flatness (S_{flat}) determining a degree of periodicity in the signal is calculated as a ratio of geometric and arithmetic means of the power spectrum. Shannon spectral entropy (S_{entrop}) is a measure of randomness of the spectral probability density represented by normalized spectral components. Spectral spread (S_{spread}) represents the dispersion of the power spectrum around its mean value.

In the last step, relationship between the primary electrical excitation of the gradient coils and the secondary generated acoustic noise is described. For this purpose, the time delay between these two signals must be analyzed. Indirect determination is based on statistical analysis of mutual positions of signal peaks of excitation and noise signals recorded in parallel. From the obtained distances, the histograms of percentage occurrence are calculated in dependence on the signal polarity and the maximum values of time delays Td_{pos}, Td_{neg} are determined [12]. These two maxima are not equal for a non-planar surface of the lower cover of the gradient coil system. This means that vibration travels in two different paths between the point of its generation and the target position of the pick-up microphone. Then the final result is given by a median value of both maxima. The second method of time delay determination is based on direct calculation using formulae

$$c = \sqrt{\frac{\gamma \cdot R \cdot T}{M}}, \qquad \Delta t = \frac{D_{X0}}{c} = \frac{\Delta n}{f_s}, \tag{1}$$

where c is velocity of sound propagation in the air at a given temperature, $\gamma = 1.4$ is air adiabatic constant, $R = 8.31446$ J K^{-1} mol^{-1} is universal gas constant, T [K] $= t$ [°C] $+ 273.15$ is thermodynamic temperature, $M = 28.9647 \times 10^{-3}$ kg mol^{-1} is air molar mass, D_{X0} is real distance between the noise microphone location and the excitation signal measuring point Δn is corresponding number of samples, and f_s is sampling frequency. These two approaches (direct and indirect) of time delay determination can be used to compare theoretical and real distances between the vibrating gradient coils and the noise sensor. However, this time delay involves superposition of a delay between the electrical excitation signal and the consequent vibration signal. Being a small delay, it is difficult to be determined in practice, but it causes an increase of the resulting theoretical distance D_X.

3. Experiments and Results

This study encompasses three basic parts dealing with different comparisons in the area of MRI. The first part describes experiments for analysis of vibration and noise conditions in the scanning area and in the neighborhood of the open-air MRI equipment E-scan Opera by Esaote company Esaote S.p.A., Genoa, Italy [21], and the experimental whole-body experimental MR imager TMR96 device built at the Institute of Measurement Science (IMS) in Bratislava, using the Apollo (Tecmag Inc., Houston, TX, USA) console for control by the NTNMR ver. 1.4 software package [22]. Both investigated MRI devices are located at the IMS, in the laboratories of the department of imaging methods.

At first, different recording microphone positions and parameters (distance between the central point of the MRI scanning area and the microphone membrane, direction angle, working height, and microphone pickup pattern) are tested, and their effect on spectral properties of the recorded noise signal is analyzed. Next, the recorded electrical excitation, vibration, and noise signals are processed for visual comparison of spectrograms and periodograms. Then, basic and supplementary spectral features are statistically analyzed. Time delays between the electrical excitation impulses in the gradient coils and the subsequently generated mechanical vibration/acoustic noise are determined from the simultaneously picked-up signals. These delay times are visualized by histograms and occurrence density plots.

Two basic types of MR scan sequences called Spin Echo (SE) and Gradient Echo (GE) arising from physical principles of MRI [18] are used in the performed experiments. For real-time recording of the vibration signal, the piezoelectric SB-1 bass pickup was used. The acoustic noise was recorded by the 1'' dual diaphragm condenser microphone B-2 PRO (by Behringer GmbH, Kirchardt, Germany) with final choice of a cardioid pickup pattern. For sensing the excitation signal, a special coil with an inductance L_0 was designed and used—see documentary photos of measurement arrangement for both investigated MRI devices in Figure 1. The whole recording was performed by the Behringer Podcast Studio equipment used for connection to an external computer by the USB interface. A typical duration of the recorded signal was 30 s and for further signal processing the stationary parts lasting 15 s were selected using the sound editor program Sound Forge 8.0 by Sony Media Software, WI, USA.

Subsequently, spectral properties of the recorded noise signals were analyzed. The temperature was always kept by air conditioning at 23 °C, giving the sound velocity of 345 m/s.

3.1. Mapping of Vibration and Noise Conditions in the Scanning Area of the Open-Air MRI Device

Basic mapping of vibration and noise conditions in the scanning area and in the neighborhood of the open-air MRI E-Scan Opera was performed within our previous research [12]. In the framework of the present study, two additional experiments were performed:

1. Measurement of the acoustic noise SPL in the MRI neighborhood in directions of 30°, 90°, and 150°—see the overview photo together with the principal angle diagram of the MRI scanning area in Figure 2a. Discrete MRI noise SPL values measured at distances of 45, 60, and 75 cm from the central point of the scanning area are shown in Figure 3a. The detailed measurement of the directional pattern of the acoustic noise SPL distribution was practically executed in the range of <0°~165°> in 15° steps (excluding the last one because of a patient bed at the position of 180°), at the distance of $D_L = 60$ cm from the MRI device central point—see the resulting diagram in Figure 3b. In both cases, the measurement was realized with the help of the sound level meter of the multi-function environment meter Lafayette DT 8820.

2. Parallel real-time recording of the signals from the electrical excitation, the vibration sensor, the microphone and/or the sound level meter. Comparison of both MRI devices in the form of histograms and occurrence density plots of basic and supplementary spectral properties together with the calculated time delays between the electrical excitation of the gradient coils and the subsequently generated noise can be found in Section 3.3.

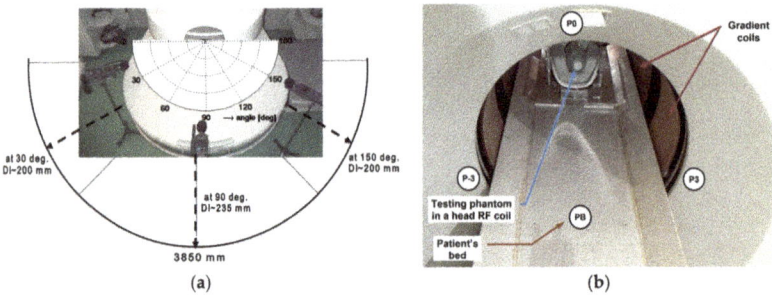

Figure 2. Arrangement of the noise and vibration measurements: in the open-air magnetic resonance imaging (MRI) device Opera together with principal angle diagram of the MRI scanning area; (a) sound pressure level (SPL) meter situated at 30°, 90°, and 150°; (b) in the whole-body imager TMR-96.

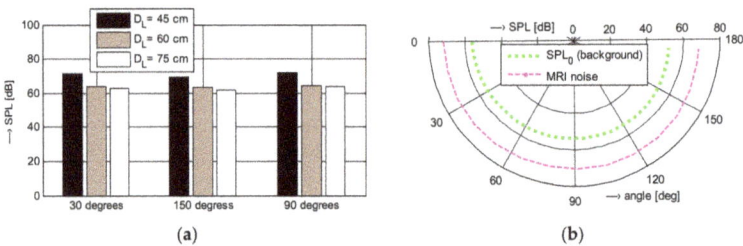

Figure 3. Visual comparison of obtained noise SPL values; (a) measured in the directions of 30°, 90°, and 150° at the distances of $D_L = \{45, 60, 75\}$ cm; (b) measured directional patterns of the noise source and the background noise SPL_0, $D_L = 60$ cm.

The baseline measurement in the open-air device Opera was carried out during the execution of 3-D and Hi-Resolution (Hi-Res) sequences that are used for scanning of a human vocal tract [11,12,17]. In order to obtain results comparable with those for the whole-body MRI device, the parameters of used Hi-Res SE HF scan sequence were set to TE = 26 ms and TR = 500 ms. The auxiliary parameters were adjusted to 10 slices of 4-mm thickness and sagittal orientation, the spherical test phantom filled with doped water was inserted in the scanning RF knee coil. The sensors of electrical excitation and vibration signals were mounted directly on the lower plastic holder of the gradient coils in the direction of 45° at the point P0—see the arrangement photo in Figure 1a.

3.2. Analysis of Vibration and Noise Conditions of the Whole-Body MRI Equipment

The second collection of experiments was aimed at mapping noise conditions in the scanning area and in the vicinity of the experimental whole-body MR imager TMR-96 [23]. These experiments consist of

1. Measurement of the acoustic noise SPL in MRI neighborhood in the direction of 0° at three heights (2, 25, and 55 cm) above the patient's bed level. Then, the SPL meter was located in ±120° (points P3 and P-3) at the height of 85 cm above the floor—see the arrangement photo in Figure 2b. The SPL meter was always placed at the distance of D_L = 60 cm from the front plastic panel to minimize interaction with the magnetic field. The measurement itself was carried out during the SE scan sequence with TE = 18 ms, TR = 400 ms under three noise conditions (obtained discrete noise *SPL* values are presented in Table 1).

   - SPL_{00}—the background noise when all devices are stopped,
   - SPL_{01}—the ventilators inside the copper cage are running,
   - SPL_X—the scanning MR sequence is being executed with ventilation fans running.

2. The detailed measurement of the directional pattern of the acoustic noise SPL distribution in the MRI tube vicinity in the range of 0°~180° with 15° steps, at the distance of D_L = 45 cm from the MRI center (point PC) of the scanning area, in the high h = 120 cm above the floor level (25 cm above the patient's bed)—see the arrangement photo in Figure 4a and the resulting diagram for GE/SE sequence (TE = 18 ms, TR = 400 ms) together with SPL_{01} curve in Figure 4b. In both cases, the measurement was realized with the help of the sound level meter of the multi-function environment meter Lafayette DT 8820.

3. Real-time recoding of the voltage signal from a piezoelectric transducer of the SB-1 sensor during execution of a chosen scan MR sequence (SE/GE type with different TE and TR parameter settings) and parallel recording of the electrical excitation signal (impulses from the MRI device gradient coil system) and/or the signals from the vibration sensor/pick-up microphone for time delay calculation and spectral properties comparison.

The succession of sampling, resampling to 16 kHz, off-line signal processing, and analysis of spectral properties was similar to that in the open-air device. Here, the test phantom consists of a 1-liter plastic bottle filled with doped water [24] inside the head RF coil located on the patient's bed in the middle of the MRI device scanning area. The second comparison experiment was focused on testing the influence of different locations of the vibration sensor and different scan sequences on spectral properties of the vibration signal. The succeeding analysis and comparison were aimed at:

- Mapping of vibration in different parts of the MRI device—the sensor mounted directly on the surface of the front plastic cover at the points P0, P3, P-3, and on the surface of the patient's bed (PB). The numerical results of the basic spectral features can be seen in Table 2 and the box-plot statistics of the supplementary spectral properties in Figure 6.
- Determination of differences between two mostly used MR scan sequences of SE and GE types; the pick-up sensor at the P3 point—see the visualization of differences of the selected signal features in Figure 5.

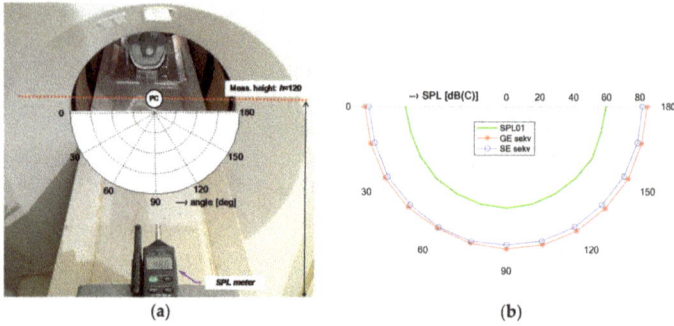

(a)   (b)

Figure 4. Arrangement of measurement of the acoustic noise SPL distribution in the vicinity of the TMR96 scanning tube; (**a**) SPL meter situated at the distance $D_L = 45$ cm from the scanning area center (point PC), in the height $h = 120$ cm above the floor level; (**b**) directional pattern for SE/GE sequences together with SPL_{01} values.

Table 1. Measured SPL [dB(C)] at different positions.

Noise Condition/Measuring Position	at 0°		at 120°	at 120°	
	$h_0{}^1 = 55$ cm	$h_0{}^1 = 25$ cm	$h_0{}^1 = 2$ cm	$h_1{}^2 = 85$ cm	$h_1{}^2 = 85$ cm
SPL_{00} silent	47.9	47.7	47.5	47.4	47.5
SPL_{01} + ventilators	54.1	56.8	56.9	61.8	59.6
SPL_X scan sequence	77	79.1	80.1	79.5	78.7

[1] Height above the patient's bed level. [2] Height above the floor.

Table 2. Mean values of basic spectral features of the recorded vibration signals [1].

Sensor Position/Feature	Signal$_{RMS}$ (-)	En$_{c0}$ (-)	S_{tilt} (°)	F_{V1} (Hz)	F_{V2} (Hz)
0° (TR = 400)	4.3	0.47	−22	429	1380
120° (TR = 400/500)	2.7/2.4	0.38/0.31	−1/−14	352/260	1105/1048
−120° (TR = 400)	2.5	0.27	−13	368	930
Patient's bed (TR = 400)	7.9	0.95	3	398	1662

[1] Used SpinEcho sequence with TE = 18 ms in all cases.

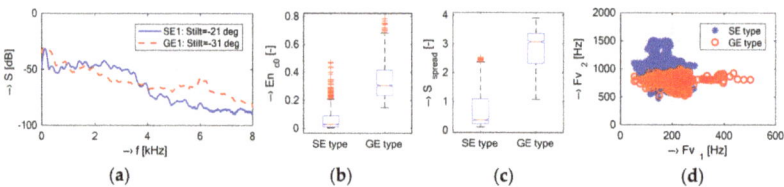

(a)   (b)   (c)   (d)

Figure 5. Visualization of differences of selected features of the recorded vibration signals; (**a**) spectral envelopes and calculated spectral tilts; (**b**) boxplot of basic statistical properties for En_{c0}; (**c**) S_{spread}; (**d**) mutual positions of F_{v1} and F_{v2} for SE/GE scan sequences with TE = 18 ms and TR = 500 ms.

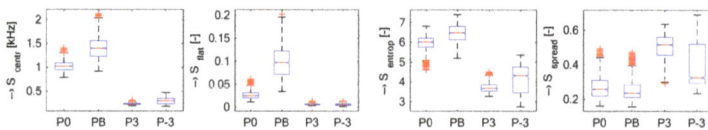

Figure 6. Box-plot of basic statistical parameters of supplementary spectral properties (centroid, flatness, entropy, spread) determined from the vibration signal picked up at different measuring positions {P0, PB, P3, P-3} during the SE sequence (TE = 18 ms, TR = 400 ms).

3.3. Comparison of Spectral Properties of Vibration and Noise Signals Recorded in Open and Closed MRI Devices

The vibration and/or noise signals recorded in the open-air Opera and the whole-body TMR96 MRI devices using the test phantom placed in the RF coil were compared graphically and grouped for both types of devices. If not stated otherwise, the signals were taken at the position P0 during execution of the MR sequence Hi-Res SE 26 HF (TR = 400 ms) for the Opera MRI device and the position P3 using the SE1-18 (TR = 400 ms) for the TMR96 device. The processed signals were used to compare

- Basic spectral properties of vibration signals including spectral density, its envelope, spectral tilt, and spectrograms presented in the set of graphs in Figure 7;
- Histograms of supplementary spectral properties of vibration signals shown in Figure 8;
- Time delays between an electrical excitation signal and a generated acoustic noise (calculated from positive and negative pulses using the statistical method described in [12])—see the set of graphs in Figure 9.

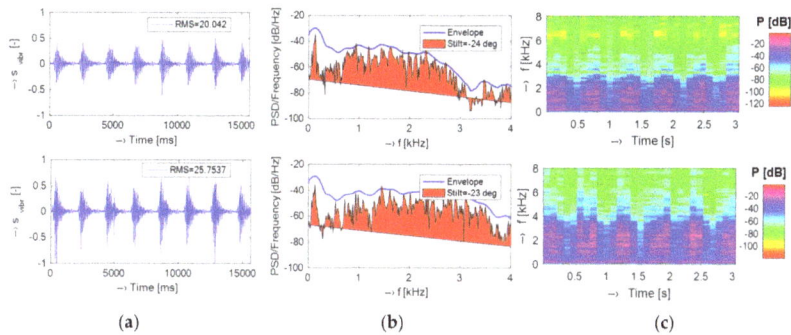

(a)   (b)   (c)

Figure 7. Visualization of basic spectral properties of recorded vibration signals; (**a**) stationary part of a normalized signal with its RMS value; (**b**) spectral density together with its envelope and calculated spectral tilt; (**c**) corresponding spectrograms for MRI Opera (upper set) and TMR96 (lower set).

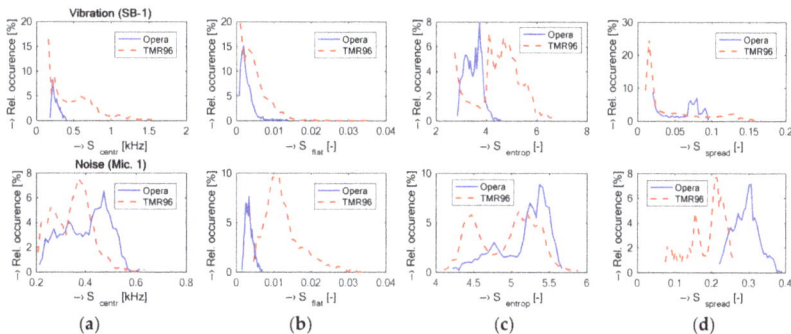

(a)   (b)   (c)   (d)

Figure 8. Histograms of supplementary spectral properties; (**a**) S_{centr}; (**b**) S_{flat}; (**c**) S_{entrop}; (**d**) S_{spread}, determined from picked-up vibration signals inside the Opera and TMR96 MRI devices.

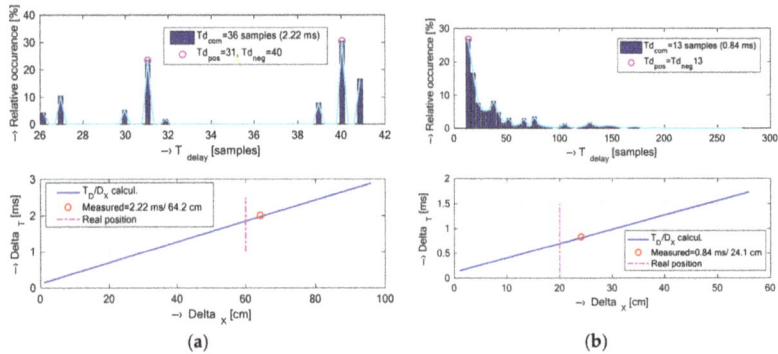

Figure 9. Histograms of evaluated time delays [samples] between electrical excitation and acoustic noise signals recorded in the MRI device (upper set), comparison of calculated and estimated mean values of time delays [ms] together with theoretical and real microphone distances (lower set); (**a**) for MRI Opera microphone Mic. 1 at a distance 60 cm and a direction 30°, sensing coil L_0 at 45°; (**b**) for TMR96 Mic. 1 at a distance 16 cm from the patient's bed position, L_0 at P3, sequence SE1-18 (TR = 400 ms); t = 23 °C, c = 346 m/s.

4. Discussion and Conclusions

The measurements in the vicinity of the open-air MRI equipment E-scan Esaote Opera have shown that the maximum sound pressure level of about 72 dB(C) was achieved for the SPL meter located in the direction of 30°, the height of 85 cm (in the middle between the upper and the lower gradient coils), and at the distance of 45 cm, while the background noise SPL_0 originating from the temperature stabilizer reached approximately 52 dB(C) measured in the time instant when no scan sequence was executed. Next, for three directions of 30°, 90°, and 150°, the noise SPL values measured with the examined person lying in the MRI scanning area were about 10 dB lower when compared with using the water phantom. The obtained noise SPL values were roughly inversely proportional to the effective weights of the male and female testing persons lying on the bottom plastic holder of the permanent magnet and gradient coils. On the other hand, the noise in the neighbourhood of the whole-body MRI device TMR96 achieved its maximum SPL of about 80 dB(C) using the SE scanning sequence and its minimum mean value of 62 dB(C) with no sequence running (the background noise generated mainly by the ventilators inside the cage) as documented by the numerical results in Table 1 and the detailed directional pattern in Figure 4b. In summary, it holds that the maximum SPL was observed for the sound level meter located at the point PB on the patient's bed level and the minimum at the point P0. Evaluations of other authors are usually aimed at high-field MRI systems. Sound noise of various pulse sequences was compared for two whole-body MRI scanners by Cho et al. [25] with the rest value 79.5 dB(C) for the 1.5-T scanner and 68.6 dB(C) for the 2-T scanner. The highest sound pressure level of about 103 dB(C) was observed during the gradient echo sequence with TE = 4 ms, TR = 250 ms in the 1.5-T scanner and TE = 35 ms, TR = 100 ms in the 2-T scanner. Prince et al. [26] investigated acoustic noise in 15 MRI scanners giving a minimum of 82.5 dB(A) for a 0.23-T device using GE sequence, TE = 5 ms, TR= 525 ms and a maximum of 118.4 dB(A) for a 3-T device using the same sequence and TE, but TR = 3000 ms.

The vibration recording experiment was arranged to map basic points on the plastic cover as well as on the surface of the patient's bed. In the case of the TMR96 device, the maximum vibration energy (expressed by RMS and/or from the first cepstral coefficient) was attained for the sensor placement on the patient's bed almost at the top of the plastic cover (point PB)—see the mean values in Table 2. As regards the spectral features, the mean values of the vibration frequencies $F_{V1,2}$ are the highest at P3 position (120°) and the lowest at the point P-3 (left bottom part of the plastic cover with the minimal vibration energy). The obtained results of the supplementary spectral properties are in good correlation with the basic ones—as documented by the visualization in Figure 6. Investigation of spectral differences between two mostly used MR scan sequences (SE/GE types) confirms our assumption that the GE sequence has more structured noise and the SE sequence generates more compact vibration with higher energy in the final effect, larger spread, and lower dispersion of $F_{V1,2}$ frequencies as shown by the graphical results in Figure 5. Due to different construction of the open-air and the whole-body MRI devices, different software tools of their control systems, different types of used phantoms, etc., it was practically impossible to use the identical MR sequences. Only similar types of sequences with similar choice of basic parameters (TE, TR, orientation, etc.) could be applied. Consequently, the analyzed vibration signals had slightly different spectral features—see histograms in Figure 8. This general assumption was confirmed by the results presented in the form of spectrograms and periodograms. On the other hand, as documented by visualization of waveforms of the picked-up vibration signals in Figure 7a, the TMR96 device produces higher vibration levels with higher energy (signal$_{RMS}$). This is in accordance with the basic physical law—greater scan volume in this device results in higher intensity of applied current in the gradient coils in spite of lower basic magnetic field (0.1 T vs. 0.178 T applied in the MRI Opera). As mentioned in the Section 2.1, the influence of different masses (volumes) in the scanning area on the intensity as well as on the spectral properties of the produced acoustic noise was analyzed in our previous research [17] using the MRI Opera device. In near future we would like to carry out similar experiments and measurements also with the TMR96 device.

In the last comparison experiment, we analyzed how the vibrations induced by the pulse current in the gradient coil travel through the holder of the MRI device, and how the actual position of the pick-up microphone corresponds with the one calculated from the determined time delay between the electrical excitation and the subsequently generated acoustic noise signals. As documented by the histogram in Figure 9a, the MRI device Opera has different time delay values determined from the positive and negative peaks of the compared signals. It means that there exist two maxima from which the final time delay was calculated as the median value. It is in agreement with the fact that the positive peaks have higher magnitude than the negative ones. This effect can be caused by the construction of the plastic cover of the gradient coils. The documentary photo in Figure 1a shows that the surface is not planar but slightly convexly curved. Hence, the mechanical force is different for positive and negative impulses originated from the gradient coils—in the case of negative ones the vibration acts against the force of the mechanical stiffness of the curved plate. In the measurement inside the TMR96 device, the sensors were mounted not on the plastic cover surface representing the front part of the whole MRI, but directly on the back part of the gradient coil surface. Though the measured surface was also curved, only one maximum of the time delay was observed in this case, see the histogram in Figure 9b. The obtained results of the backward comparison of the determined distance between the microphone picking up the noise and the origin of the vibration (sensor positions P0 for the MRI Opera and P3 for the TMR96) confirm our assumption that the distance calculated from the determined time delay values was always higher—see the bottom set of graphs in Figure 9. The detected increase of about 4–6 cm in the actual distance corresponds to the increase of the time interval by the delay during which the vibration is generated as a consequence of the excitation impulse in the gradient coil.

The results of the experiments will help to describe the process of the gradient coil electric excitation, the subsequent mechanical vibration, and the resulting acoustic noise generation in the MRI device scanning area and its vicinity. Additional measurement and analysis are necessary for better knowledge of these acoustic noise conditions. In the case of the MRI Opera, there is need for more information about the contribution of the upper gradient coil (and its plastic holder) to the resulting acoustic noise. Therefore, in near future we plan to perform parallel measurement of the vibration signal on the surface of both plastic holders. As regards the TMR96 device, the process of noise and vibration generation inside the scanning tube of the whole-body tomograph must be known. Thus, the measurement with the vibration sensor mounted in the place of the second and third gradient coils must be also performed for detailed mapping of the vibration in the whole 360° angle around the gradient coils. Critical parts (possible loose mounting to the main mass of the resistive magnet) can be found by this method, subsequently repaired, and/or some damping material might be inserted for mechanical suppression of the generated vibration and noise.

Acknowledgments: This work was supported by the Slovak Scientific Grant Agency project VEGA 2/0001/17, the Ministry of Education, Science, Research, and Sports of the Slovak Republic VEGA 1/0905/17, and within the project of the Slovak Research and Development Agency Nr. APVV-15-0029.

Author Contributions: J.P. conceived and designed the measurement and recording experiments, carried out analysis and statistical processing of the data, and evaluated all the results. A.P. cooperated in the vibration measurement with both types of MRI devices, and participated in collection of the noise, vibration, and voice signal database. I.F. reviewed the paper and provided some advice. A.P. read and corrected the English of the manuscript.

Conflicts of Interest: The authors declare no conflict of interest. The founding sponsors had no role in the design of the study; in the collection, analyses, or interpretation of data; in the writing of the manuscript, and in the decision to publish the results.

References

1. Wellard, R.M.; Ravasio, J.P.; Guesne, S.; Bell, C.; Oloyede, A.; Tevelen, G.; Pope, J.M.; Momot, K.I. Simultaneous magnetic resonance imaging and consolidation measurement of articular cartilage. *Sensors* **2014**, *14*, 7940–7958. [CrossRef] [PubMed]
2. He, Z.; He, W.; Wu, J.; Xu, Z. The novel design of a single-sided MRI probe for assessing burn depth. *Sensors* **2017**, *17*, 526. [CrossRef] [PubMed]
3. Panych, L.P.; Madore, B. The physics of MRI safety. *J. Magn. Reson. Imaging* **2018**, *47*, 28–43. [CrossRef] [PubMed]
4. Mainka, A.; Platzek, I.; Mattheus, W.; Fleischer, M.; Müller, A.S. Three-dimensional vocal tract morphology based on multiple magnetic resonance images is highly reproducible during sustained phonation. *J. Voice* **2017**, *31*, 504.e11–504.e20. [CrossRef] [PubMed]
5. Kuortti, J.; Malinen, J.; Ojalammi, A. Post-processing speech recordings during MRI. *Biomed. Signal Process. Control* **2018**, *39*, 11–22. [CrossRef]
6. Freitas, A.C.; Ruthven, M.; Boubertakh, R.; Miquel, M.E. Real-time speech MRI: Commercial Cartesian and non-Cartesian sequences at 3T and feasibility of offline TGV reconstruction to visualise velopharyngeal motion. *Phys. Med.* **2018**, *46*, 96–103. [CrossRef] [PubMed]
7. Sun, G.; Li, M.; Rudd, B.W.; Lim, T.C.; Osterhage, J.; Fugate, E.M.; Lee, J.H. Adaptive speech enhancement using directional microphone in a 4-T MRI scanner. *Magn. Reson. Mater. Phys. Biol. Med.* **2015**, *28*, 473–484. [CrossRef] [PubMed]
8. Vahanesa, C.; Reddy, C.K.; Panahi, I.M. Improving quality and intelligibility of speech using single microphone for the broadband fMRI noise at low SNR. In Proceedings of the IEEE International Conference of the Engineering in Medicine and Biology Society (EMBC), Orlando, FL, USA, 16–20 August 2016; pp. 3674–3678.
9. Han, L.; Shen, Z.; Fu, C.; Liu, C. Design and implementation of sound searching robots in wireless sensor networks. *Sensors* **2016**, *16*, 1550. [CrossRef] [PubMed]
10. Ding, H.; Soon, I.Y.; Yeo, C.K. Over-attenuated components regeneration for speech enhancement. *IEEE Trans. Audio Speech Lang. Process.* **2010**, *18*, 2004–2014. [CrossRef]
11. Přibil, J.; Přibilová, A.; Frollo, I. Analysis of acoustic noise and its suppression in speech recorded during scanning in the open-air MRI. In *Advances in Noise Analysis, Mitigation and Control*; Ahmed, N., Ed.; InTech: Rijeka, Croatia, 2016; pp. 205–228, ISBN 978-953-51-2674-4.
12. Přibil, J.; Přibilová, A.; Frollo, I. Mapping and spectral analysis of acoustic vibration in the scanning area of the weak field magnetic resonance imager. *J. Vib. Acoust. Trans. ASME* **2014**, *136*, 051005. [CrossRef]
13. Tayong, R.; Dupont, T.; Leclaire, P. Experimental investigation of holes interaction effect on the sound absorption coefficient of micro-perforated panels under high and medium sound levels. *Appl. Acoust.* **2011**, *72*, 777–784. [CrossRef]
14. Zhao, X.; Wang, X.; Yu, Y. Enhancing low-frequency sound absorption of micro-perforated panel absorbers by combining parallel mechanical impedance. *Appl. Acoust.* **2018**, *130*, 300–304. [CrossRef]

15. Gai, X.L.; Xing, T.; Li, X.H.; Zhang, B.; Wang, F.; Cai, Z.N.; Han, Y. Sound absorption of microperforated panel with L shape division cavity. *Appl. Acoust.* **2017**, *122*, 41–50. [CrossRef]

16. Moelker, A.; Wielopolski, P.A.; Pattynama, M.T. Relationship between magnetic field strength and magnetic-resonance-related acoustic noise levels. *Magn. Reson. Mater. Phys. Biol. Med.* **2003**, *16*, 52–55. [CrossRef] [PubMed]

17. Přibil, J.; Přibilová, A.; Frollo, I. Influence of the human body mass in the open-air MRI on acoustic noise spectrum. *Acta IMEKO* **2016**, *5*, 81–86. [CrossRef]

18. Liang, Z.P.; Lauterbur, P.C. *Principles of Magnetic Resonance Imaging: A Signal Processing Perspective*; Wiley-IEEE Press: New York, NY, USA, 1999; ISBN 978-0-780-34723-6.

19. Winkler, S.A.; Alejski, A.; Wade, T.; McKenzie, C.A.; Rutt, B.K. On the accurate analysis of vibroacoustics in head insert gradient coils. *Magn. Reson. Med.* **2017**, *78*, 1635–1645. [CrossRef] [PubMed]

20. Fraden, J. *Handbook of Modern Sensors. Physics, Designs, and Applications*, 4th ed.; Springer: New York, NY, USA, 2010; ISBN 978-1-4419-6466-3.

21. E-Scan Opera. *Image Quality and Sequences Manual. 830023522 Rev; A*, Esaote S.p.A.: Genoa, Italy, 2008.

22. TNMR Reference Manual, Hardware Reference Manual, DSPect User Guide. Available online: http://www.tecmag.com/support_contact/pulse_sequences/ (accessed on 10 October 2010).

23. Andris, P.; Dermek, T.; Frollo, I. Simplified matching and tuning experimental receive coils for low-field NMR measurements. *Measurement* **2015**, *64*, 29–33. [CrossRef]

24. Andris, P.; Frollo, I. Asymmetric spin echo sequence and requirements on static magnetic field of NMR scanner. *Measurement* **2013**, *46*, 1530–1534. [CrossRef]

25. Cho, Z.H.; Park, S.H.; Kim, J.H.; Chung, S.C.; Chung, S.T.; Chung, J.Y.; Moon, C.W.; Yi, J.H.; Sin, C.H.; Wong, E.K. Analysis of acoustic noise in MRI. *Magn. Reson. Imaging* **1997**, *15*, 815–822. [CrossRef]

26. Prince, D.L.; De Wilde, J.P.; Papadaki, A.M.; Curran, J.S.; Kitney, R.I. Investigation of acoustic noise on 15 MRI scanners from 0.2 T to 3 T. *J. Magn. Reson. Imaging* **2001**, *13*, 288–293. [CrossRef]

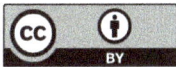

![sensors logo] *sensors*

MDPI

Article

Visible and Extended Near-Infrared Multispectral Imaging for Skin Cancer Diagnosis

Laura Rey-Barroso [1],*, Francisco J. Burgos-Fernández [1], Xana Delpueyo [1], Miguel Ares [1], Santiago Royo [1], Josep Malvehy [2], Susana Puig [2] and Meritxell Vilaseca [1]

[1] Centre for Sensors, Instruments and Systems Development, Technical University of Catalonia, Terrassa 08222, Spain; francisco.javier.burgos@upc.edu (F.J.B.-F.); xana.delpueyo@upc.edu (X.D.); miguel.ares@oo.upc.edu (M.A.); santiago.royo@upc.edu (S.R.); meritxell.vilaseca@upc.edu (M.V.)
[2] Dermatology Department of the Hospital Clinic of Barcelona, IDIBAPS; Barcelona 08036, Spain; jmalvehy@gmail.com (J.M.); susipuig@gmail.com (S.P.)
*   Correspondence: laura.rey.barroso@upc.edu; Tel.: +34-97-739-8905

Received: 15 March 2018; Accepted: 2 May 2018; Published: 5 May 2018

Abstract: With the goal of diagnosing skin cancer in an early and noninvasive way, an extended near infrared multispectral imaging system based on an InGaAs sensor with sensitivity from 995 nm to 1613 nm was built to evaluate deeper skin layers thanks to the higher penetration of photons at these wavelengths. The outcomes of this device were combined with those of a previously developed multispectral system that works in the visible and near infrared range (414 nm–995 nm). Both provide spectral and spatial information from skin lesions. A classification method to discriminate between melanomas and nevi was developed based on the analysis of first-order statistics descriptors, principal component analysis, and support vector machine tools. The system provided a sensitivity of 78.6% and a specificity of 84.6%, the latter one being improved with respect to that offered by silicon sensors.

Keywords: InGaAs camera; multispectral imaging; infrared; skin cancer; melanoma

---

1. Introduction

Due to the uncontrolled growth of abnormal cells in skin cancer, chromophores such as melanin, hemoglobin, and water might differ among tumors of different etiologies; thus, skin cancer lesions can be identified clinically when a lesion changes its color, increases its size or thickness, and gets an unusual texture or its outline becomes irregular [1,2]. In this context, multispectral imaging systems, which provide precise quantification of spectral, colorimetric, and spatial features, have been employed over the last few years to analyze spectral and colorimetric properties of the skin reliably and non-invasively [3,4]. Specifically, they have also been used to improve the detection of skin cancer, especially melanoma, which is the most aggressive and lethal form.

In 2005, Tomatis et al. [5] developed an automated multispectral imaging system for the diagnosis of pigmented lesions. The device consisted of a spectrophotometer with a light source, a monochromator, and a bundle of optical fibers coupled to a probe head. The spectral range from 483 nm to 950 nm was covered with 15 spectral bands. A region-growing algorithm segmented the lesions and extracted descriptors to be used as input for setting and testing a neural network classifier.

Some years later, Kuzmina et al. [6] used a multispectral system that incorporated halogen lamps and filters from 450 nm to 950 nm with a spectral bandwidth of 15 nm. They observed that wavelengths closer to the infrared (IR) range penetrate deeper into the skin, resulting in decreased contrast due to higher light scattering. However, in the case of melanomas the contrast at 950 nm was found to be much higher, indicating considerably deeper structural damage.

In 2012, Bekina et al. [7] analyzed lesions under a multispectral system with four different spectral bands, each one to obtain information from specific structures of the skin: 450 nm for superficial layers, 545 nm for blood distribution, 660 nm for melanin detection, and 940 nm for the evaluation of deeper skin layers. Then, a ratio was calculated between the intensities of green light (545 nm), where the hemoglobin absorption is high, and red light (660 nm), where it is low. It was proven that pathological tissues showed higher values of this index than the surrounding skin as a consequence of having higher blood content. The same authors developed a similar system [8] that consisted of a multispectral imaging system with a CCD imaging sensor and a liquid crystal tunable filter (LCTF) (with spectral bands from 450 nm to 950 nm in steps of 10 nm) (Nuance EX), a spectral optimized lens, and internal optics. The illumination system was a ring of halogen lamps with a polarizer orthogonal to the camera in order to remove the artifacts caused by light reflection. In order to differentiate between melanoma and nevi, a new parameter was suggested based on skin optical density differences at three wavelengths: 540 nm, 650 nm, and 950 nm.

Additionally, Jakovels et al. [9] used principal component analysis (PCA) of multispectral imaging data in the wavelength range from 450 nm to 950 nm for distant skin melanoma recognition, which resulted in clear separation between malignant melanomas and pigmented nevi.

Delpueyo et al. [10] also proposed a light-emitting diodes (LEDs)-based multispectral imaging system with eight different wavelengths (414–995 nm) but using the analysis of the spatial distribution of color and spectral features through descriptors based on the first-order statistics of the histogram to improve the detection of skin cancer lesions, specifically melanomas and basal cell carcinomas.

Recently, Kim et al. [11] have investigated the potential of mobile smartphone-based multispectral imaging for the quantitative diagnosis and management of skin lesions. The authors miniaturized a spectral imaging system so that it could be attached to a smartphone, allowing users to obtain ten images sequentially within a range of wavelengths from 440 nm to 690 nm, with one white-light image. The results suggested that smartphone-based multispectral imaging and analysis had great potential as a healthcare tool for quantitative mobile skin diagnosis.

Despite the fact that sensitivity and specificity obtained with the former multispectral imaging systems based on silicon imaging sensors have reached similar values to those obtained by experienced dermatologists through dermoscopy [10,12], they have not yet superseded histological examination. In fact, this continues to be the clinical gold standard, providing diagnostic confirmation after surgical excision of the tumor.

Digital cameras based on silicon have a spectral response in the visible (VIS) up to the near-infrared (NIR) (900 nm–1000 nm). However, multispectral, extended, near-infrared (exNIR) optical imaging is nowadays available thanks to new indium gallium arsenide (InGaAs) cameras with high quantum efficiency within 900 nm–1600 nm. This has sparked interest among biologists in this relatively unexplored spectral region also known as "the second near-infrared window" (900 nm–1400 nm) [13].

Going further than 900 nm into the exNIR enables deeper in vivo optical imaging as photons at these wavelengths penetrate deeper into living tissue [14]; this could be a hint to explore further this spectral region as a means of improving skin cancer diagnosis and prognosis, as it may release information about how tissues are damaged due to ultraviolet radiation, water content, and other factors that might be different in benign and malignant lesions. For instance, due to the increased absorption of water in this spectral range, spectral images in the exNIR can provide information about the presence of angiogenesis, a tumorous growth of blood vessels around the malignant lesion.

In fact, the near-infrared region has been widely utilized in the past decade, and a number of clinical imaging applications have already been developed [15].

In this study, we investigate the possibilities of a multispectral imaging system based on an InGaAs camera and light-emitting diodes (LEDs) for the detection of skin cancer, especially melanomas, in the exNIR range, specifically from 995 nm to 1613 nm. Although InGaAs sensors tend to be noisier than CMOS or CCD sensors and the deeper scattering at exNIR wavelengths can reduce image contrast, we consider that the study of this unexplored spectral range can bring very interesting results to the scientific community.

2. Experimental Setup and Clinical Measurements

The device developed to perform exNIR multispectral imaging of skin cancer is depicted in Figure 1b,c. It integrates a 16-bit depth InGaAs camera (Hamamatsu C10633-23, Hamamatsu Photonics, Shizuoka, Japan) with spectral sensitivity from 900 nm to 1600 nm, readout speed of 50 fps, and 320 × 256 pixels together with a Kowa LM12HC-SW 1.4/12.5 mm short-wave infrared (SWIR) lens with high transmission from 800 nm to 2000 nm (Kowa Company, Ltd., Aichi, Japan). Additionally, a LED-based light source was built on a cylinder of polyvinyl chloride (PVC) including high power Surface Mounted Displays (SMD) LEDs with peak wavelengths at 995 nm, 1081 nm, 1214 nm, 1340 nm, 1486 nm, and 1613 nm (Figure 2b); they were selected in accordance with the absorption curves of the principal chromophores of the skin, such as bilirubin, hemoglobin, and water, especially taking into account their most representative minimums and maximums, and the spectral bands with considerable differences among them allowing characterization of the tissue constituents [10]. The tip of the cylinder is a cone with an opening of 20 mm × 20 mm and a diffuser. Four LEDs per spectral band were included in the light source with a separation of 90° among them to ensure a uniform illumination over the skin; a total amount of 24 LEDs was finally placed on the ring. All parts were assembled in a handheld configuration with a trigger to start the acquisition. A base was also designed and constructed to hold the multispectral system when it was not being used. It incorporated a calibrated reference at the bottom that consisted of the Neutral 5 gray color of an X-Rite ColorChecker® (Grand Rapids, MI, USA) with level of reflectance similar to that of the skin in the exNIR range. The degradation of the reference over time was controlled by visual inspection and spectrally by means of a spectrometer. If the reference showed dirty areas or scratches or its reflectance spectrum presented variations up to 5% with respect to the spectrum when it was brand new, it was replaced.

The exNIR system was used together with another multispectral imaging system previously built [10] for capturing reflectance and color features in the VIS and NIR ranges (Figure 1a). In this case, the camera integrated in the multispectral head is a 12-bit depth DMK 23U445 with a 1/3″ CCD sensor of Sony ICX445ALA with 1280 × 960 pixels of resolution and readout speed of 30 fps; it represented an advantage over the spatial resolution of the exNIR camera, which limited the performance of the analysis in this spectral range. The lens coupled was a Schneider-Kreuznack Cinegon with spectral sensitivity from 400 nm to 1000 nm and a working distance from infinite to 20 mm, which allowed focusing the skin lesions at a distance of 40 mm with a field of view of 15 mm × 20 mm. As in the previous case, sequential multiplexed illumination is used by means of a ring of 32 LEDs (four per wavelength) with the following peak wavelengths: 414 nm, 447 nm, 477 nm, 524 nm, 671 nm, 735 nm, 890 nm, and 995 nm (Figure 2a). For each wavelength, the forward current of the LEDs was tuned to obtain a constant temporal behavior in terms of radiance. The final currents used for each wavelength were selected, taking into account a compromise between emission stability and the exposure time needed to make use of the whole dynamic range of the cameras: from 0 to 4095 digital levels in the case of the VIS-NIR system and from 0 to 65,533 in the case of the exNIR system. In general, measurements of radiance over time showed that LEDs needed at least two seconds to stabilize, and therefore this delay was added when any LED was switched on (Figure 3). Infrared LEDs used in the exNIR device showed a much more stable behavior than those in the VIS-NIR range; for this reason, the two-second delay was not implemented in this system. Despite that, the spectral assessment in the exNIR was less accurate than in the VIS-NIR, because exNIR LEDs presented a wider Full Width at Half Maximum (FWHM). In consequence, the information captured at each spectral band and then associated with the wavelength peak of each LED includes a broader range of data coming from more wavelengths.

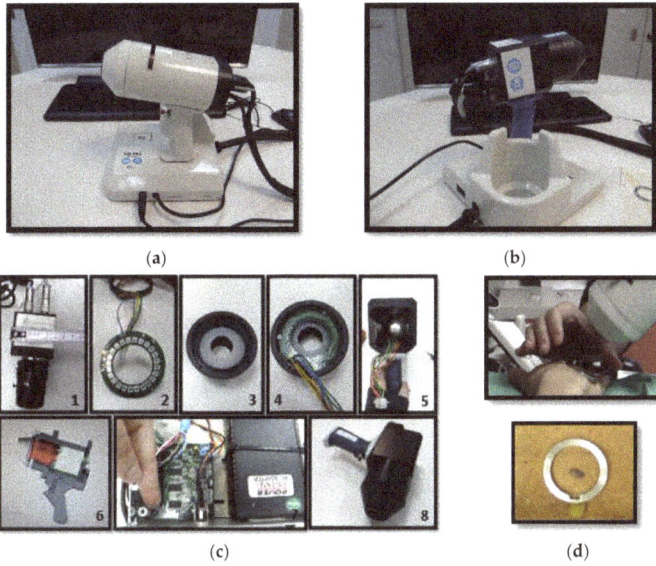

Figure 1. (**a**) General view of the previously developed handheld VIS-NIR multispectral device. (**b**) General view of the handheld exNIR multispectral device. (**c**) Components of the exNIR imaging system: 1—InGaAs camera, 2—Ring of LEDs, 3—Tip of PVC cone, 4—Ring of LEDs placed at the tip. 5—Handheld case, 6—AutoCad design, 7—Electronic control, and 8—Handheld case with camera inside. (**d**) Clinical measurement and metallic ring, which is glued to the patient's skin for the tip of both systems to place them in the same position and parallel to the skin, without making any contact.

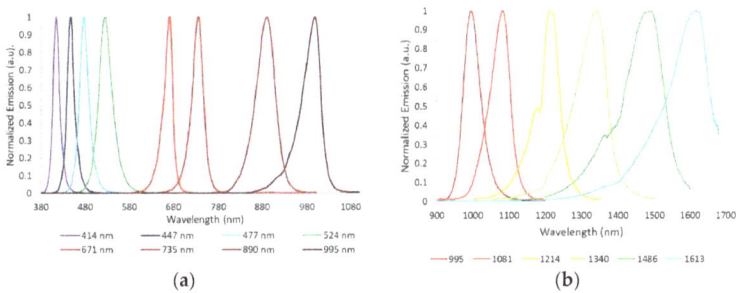

Figure 2. Normalized spectral emission of the LEDs in (**a**) the VIS-NIR and (**b**) exNIR ranges.

A user-friendly acquisition software was built based on Borland Builder C++ to be used for physicians in a clinical environment. The software controls individually and synchronously the emission of the LEDs and the acquisition of spectral images. The software interface asks for a daily calibration to guarantee accurate measurements at all wavelengths along LEDs lifecycle. It involves the acquisition of images of the neutral reference (Neutral 5) at each spectral band and at ten different exposure times to adapt the dynamic range of the system to every skin phenotype, thus avoiding saturated or noisy areas. This set of calibration images is used later for calculating the reflectance images from the raw spectral images (see next section). Then, a measurement over the actual skin lesion can be taken, and the system will make a sequence of acquisitions at every spectral band. In the case of the multispectral system with LEDs in the VIS and NIR ranges, eight images are obtained, while for the one in the exNIR, six images of a lesion are taken. Each one is acquired with a given exposure time, chosen from a learning table among the ten exposure times previously used to take images of the reference. The exposure times are chosen by an algorithm with a target averaged digital level (DL) for each image that is about half of the dynamic range of the camera; in this way, saturated images are avoided. This active exposure time selection also contributes to compensating variations of LEDs' power output due to their lifecycle. Another advantage of this algorithm is that it allows the evaluation of all kinds of skin, from brighter to darker ones. A set of dark current images also needs to be acquired by just making another calibration in a room in dark conditions, to take into account the straylight caused by internal reflections and noise sensed by the camera at the time of calculating the reflectance curve of a pixel area; the same ten exposure times previously used are applied. The straylight was measured sequentially switching on the LEDs, as during the calibration with the reference, in order to remove from the image the reflections caused by the inner surface of the PVC painted cone. Environmental illumination barely affects the measurement, because the tip of the devices is fully covered by the metallic ring and the patient's skin. One lesion is fully analyzed when sequentially measured with the VIS-NIR and the exNIR multispectral imaging systems. Apart from the additional spectral information from 414 nm to 995 nm, the use of the VIS-NIR system allows to locate with higher accuracy some lesions that present blurry boundaries in the IR.

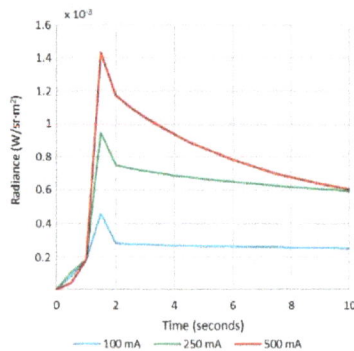

Figure 3. Radiance (W/sr·m²) of the 414 nm LEDs at different forward currents measured every second over 10 s.

As a pilot study, the VIS-NIR and exNIR multispectral systems were used to analyze 39 nevi and 14 melanomas from Caucasian patients at the Hospital Clínic i Provincial de Barcelona (Barcelona, Spain). Patients could be seated or lying down on the hospital bed while capturing.

All of them provided written informed consent before any examination and ethical committee approval (Spanish Agency of Drugs and Clinical Products, document number 7576) was obtained. The study complied with the tenets of the 1975 Declaration of Helsinki (Tokyo revision, 2004). The lesions were diagnosed by dermatologists (SP and JM) using a commercial dermoscope and the confocal laser scanning microscope VivaScope® 1500 from MAVIG GmbH (Munich, Germany). When malignancy was suspected, the lesion was excised and a histological analysis was carried out.

3. Data Processing

The images from the multispectral systems were processed through a graphical user interface (GUI) built in Matlab R2015a (The MathWorks Inc., Natick, MA, USA). It has different functions to make internal calibration algorithms and also to compute reflectance spectra that can be used to compare subtle differences between benign and malignant lesions. In order to calculate the reflectance images, the corresponding calibration images from the reference and dark current images are selected by the program. Then, for a given exposure time and wavelength, being different the exposure time for each wavelength, the reflectance at each pixel (i, j) is calculated as follows:

$$R_{Lesion}(i, j) = k\frac{I(i, j) - I_D(i, j)}{I_N(i, j) - I_D(i, j)}, \tag{1}$$

where $R_{Lesion}(i, j)$ is the spectral reflectance image; $I(i, j)$, $I_N(i, j)$, and $I_D(i, j)$ contain the DLs of the raw, neutral gray reference and dark current images, respectively; and k is the calibrated reflectance of the neutral gray reference, given by the manufacturer.

Since the purpose was to obtain information about the lesions themselves and not from the whole reflectance images, which also contain spectral information about the surrounding healthy skin, every lesion was segmented. The segmentation of lesions from the IR images was a challenge, because in many cases they were hardly distinguishable from the surrounding skin because of the decreased contrast due to higher scattering at these wavelengths. In order to overcome this, two different algorithms of segmentation were used for each multispectral system.

For the images of the lesion in the exNIR range, manual segmentation coupled with previous image registration was used. In this case, the corresponding images of the lesion taken in the VIS range were correlated to those captured by the exNIR multispectral system in order to overcome the constraint of the second device. This could be easily done by means of a mathematical transformation of the images matrices, since skin lesions were measured by both systems at the same position and in the same orientation thanks to a metallic ring were the tip of both systems could be attached to the patient's skin (Figure 1d). The metallic ring was glued to the patient's skin by means of a medical adhesive ring that was different for every patient; this combination prevents the systems from touching the skin. Afterwards, when the corresponding images were shown together, one on top of the other, manual segmentation was performed over the images in the exNIR range (Figure 4a).

The algorithm used for the images in the VIS-NIR range consisted of searching the DL threshold to establish those pixels belonging to the patient's lesion (foreground) and those to the surrounding healthy skin (background). The DL threshold was calculated with the Otsu's method, which maximizes the between-class variance of the lesion and the skin pixel values based on the intensity of the histogram [16]. A binary image is created according to the threshold, and pixels below are transformed into zeros and above into ones. This binary image can be used as a mask to be applied to all the spectral images and obtain the DLs corresponding to the pixels of the lesion. However, Otsu's method is based on a global threshold that can only be used in lesions that are clearly different from the skin. In order to solve skin inhomogeneity, reflectance images were divided into four subimages, allowing different thresholds adapted to the local characteristics to be calculated (Figure 4b). The image used for performing VIS-NIR segmentation was taken at 414 nm, since this spectral band enhanced the detection of melanin, and therefore it extended the contour of the lesion to its real size.

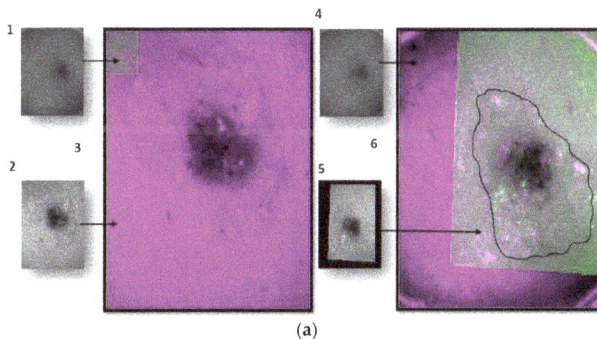

(a)

Figure 4. *Cont.*

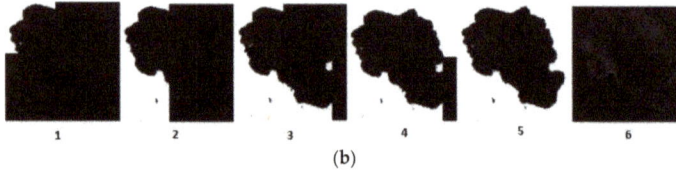

(b)

Figure 4. Steps of the segmentation algorithm for both multispectral imaging systems. (**a**) Example of how the segmentation is done for a lesion taken with the exNIR system: (1) Reflectance image taken with the exNIR device. (2) Reflectance image taken with the VIS-NIR camera. (3) Reflectance images from both cameras superimposed. Here, it can be seen how both systems take images at different resolutions, rotated with respect to each other a certain angle. (4) Reflectance image of the exNIR imaging system. (5) Reflectance image from the VIS-NIR system, to which a mathematical operation for correlation has been applied. (6) These last images were superimposed. (**b**) Example of how the segmentation is done for a lesion taken with the VIS-NIR imaging system: images correspond to the implementation of the Otsu method for each subimage. A mask for each of them is calculated in (1–4), and they are put together to form the (5) final mask for segmentation. (6) is the result of segmenting the lesion.

Different parameters to discriminate between benign and malignant lesions were also calculated based on spectral features additionally to the reflectance images (Equation (1)). To avoid the influence of the patient's healthy skin, another set of reflectance images were calculated by subtraction of the mean reflectance value of the patient's skin from the reflectance images of the segmented lesion (Equation (2)). This was proposed as an empirical approach to improve the results, if possible, due to the different penetration depths of wavelengths owing to the different absorption of structures inside the tissue; however, in multispectral technology, images contain a mixture of light coming from not only a specific depth inside the tissue but also from the preceding layers due to backscattering.

Another two set of images were also computed by taking the logarithm of the latter ones, in order to obtain information in terms of absorbance, too.

$$R_{Lesion-Skin}(i,j) = k\frac{I_{lesion}(i,j) - I_D(i,j)}{I_N(i,j) - I_D(i,j)} - mean\left(k\frac{I_{skin}(i,j) - I_D(i,j)}{I_N(i,j) - I_D(i,j)}\right),$$ (2)

At a second stage, a statistical analysis over the former images was carried out as a first approach to characterize the spatial features based on the histogram of the lesions and obtain further information for the classification algorithm. This analysis was envisaged to provide information about the distribution of digital levels at each spectral band and all over the sample rather than only taking into account the traditional statistical descriptors: mean (μ), maximum (*max*), minimum (*min*), and standard deviation (σ). Accordingly, first order statistics descriptors such as the energy (*En*), the entropy (*Ep*), and the third central moment (μ_3) were obtained from the histogram of the segmented lesion in terms of the spectral reflectance and absorbance; these parameters have been shown to provide useful information about human features such as the iris pattern [17]. They are defined as follows:

$$E_n = \sum_{i=0}^{N-1} P(i)^2,$$ (3)

$$E_p = -\sum_{i=0}^{N-1} P(i)^2 \log\left[P(i)^2\right],$$ (4)

$$\mu_3 = \sum_{i=0}^{N-1} (i-\mu)^3 P(i)^2,$$ (5)

where $P(i)$ is the value (frequency) of the intensity element i (bin) of the histogram and N is the number of levels that the histogram is divided into.

Energy is a numerical descriptor of uniformity that ranges between 0 and 1, reaching the maximum value for a constant image [18]. In regards to entropy, it is a well-known statistical measure of randomness, uncertainty, or disorder in image values, with 0 being the minimum value for a constant image and $\log^2(N)$ the maximum [18]. The third central moment or skewness, μ_3, refers to the skewness of the histogram about its mean; it has a range of values between -1 and 1, positive for histograms skewed to the right, negative for the ones skewed to the left, and 0 for symmetric ones [18]. According to all this, these descriptors can be used to account for reflectance distribution features of skin lesions besides the more classical averaged spectral information obtained from traditional multispectral imaging systems.

4. Classification Algorithm

In order to determine which of the former statistical descriptors related with reflectance and absorbance values were useful to discriminate between malignant and benign tumors, as well as reflectance/absorbance minus the average of the healthy skin, scatter plots with the values for every lesion analyzed were evaluated. In total, there were 392 scatter plots, 224 from the VIS-NIR system and 168 from the exNIR. A Matlab-based classification algorithm was then used to find the best ones. The algorithm included the definition of upper and lower thresholds on the scatterplots that were experimentally set to delimit the area where benign lesions were prone to lay down. The lesions that fell outside the thresholds for at least one parameter were considered to be malignant (i.e., melanomas).

The classification algorithm worked as follows: after setting the thresholds of all parameters, they were ordered according to the number of malignant lesions that they allowed to classify. Accordingly, the first parameter on the list was such allowing the greatest number of malignant lesions to be classified, the second one was such allowing the second greatest number, and so forth. The algorithm then started from the first of the list alone and calculated the corresponding sensitivity, i.e., the percentage of malignant lesions classified as such. The second parameter of the list was then chosen to perform the classification together with the first one, and the sensitivity was computed again. If the second parameter did not allow for the improvement of the classification with at least one more malignant lesion detected, it was discarded as it was considered to be redundant. Otherwise, it was included. Next, the third parameter on the list was added to the first two, and the sensitivity was calculated again, repeating the described process until the addition of more parameters did not improve the sensitivity of malignant lesions.

Thresholds were not set to include all nevi or all melanomas, because preliminary tests showed large values of false positives and false negatives, which would considerably increase the complexity of the algorithm.

After choosing the best statistical descriptors as those allowing more melanomas to be classified as melanomas, a Principal Component Analysis (PCA) [19] was carried out to automatize and enhance the performance of the classification algorithm by avoiding the use of experimental thresholds manually selected.

At first, the matrix of data was standardized. This was done by subtracting the mean and dividing by the standard deviation of every descriptor as follows:

$$Descriptor_{norm} = \frac{Descriptor_{Lesion} - mean(Descriptor)}{stdv(Descriptor)}, \tag{6}$$

Then, Singular Value Decomposition (SVD) [19] was performed over the matrix containing the d best descriptors to detect melanomas for every of the 53 lesions (Y_{dx53}). SVD represents an expansion of the original data in a coordinate system in which the covariance matrix is diagonal. This operation is performed with the *svd* Matlab function obtaining the matrices U_{dxd}, whose columns correspond to nonzero singular values form a set of orthonormal basis vectors for the range of

Y; D_{dx53}, whose diagonal values are the square roots of the eigenvalues; and V_{53x53}, where the columns are the eigenvectors of the standardized data matrix. V therefore contains the principal directions to form a base in which the variance between classes is maximized and D the coefficients by which these eigenvectors are multiplied, to obtain the data coordinates transformed into the base of principal directions.

The initial data could be reproduced from the following matrices as follows:

$$\hat{Y}(i,j) = U(i,j)\cdot D(i,j)\cdot V^t(i,j),\tag{7}$$

The first principal components (PCs) can then be calculated as follows:

$$PC_1(i,j) = D(1,1)\cdot V(i,1),\tag{8}$$

$$PC_2(i,j) = D(2,2)\cdot V(i,2),\tag{9}$$

$$PC_3(i,j) = D(3,3)\cdot V(i,3),\tag{10}$$

Many PCs as descriptors originally available are obtained, although the first three PCs are those that are known to contain the higher variability among data (in descendent order).

PCs were represented one against the others, as it is shown in the next section with the aim of transforming the actual descriptors to another coordinate axes where the different classes, nevi, and melanomas are thought to be represented as separate as possible. Additionally, a decision boundary using a Support Vector Machine (SVM) training algorithm was implemented to classify nevi and melanomas [19]. It looks for a hyperplane that separates the space of descriptors into two classes with the maximum margin. This maximum margin is the distance from the decision surface to the closest data point and determines the margin of the classifier. This method of construction necessarily means that the decision function for an SVM is fully specified by a (usually small) subset of the data that defines the position of the separator. These points are referred to as the support vectors; in a vector space, a point can be thought of as a vector between the origin and that point. In the end, the different positions of the separator form the decision boundary from which sensitivity and specificity values can be established. Sensitivity corresponds to the true positive rate defined as the proportion of melanomas that lay inside the boundaries, correctly identified as such; specificity relates to the true negative rate defined as the proportion of nevi that lay outside the boundaries.

5. Results and Discussion

Figure 5 shows the mean reflectance ($\pm\sigma$) of the whole set of melanomas and nevi measured, separately. The mean reflectance of melanomas in the VIS-NIR and exNIR ranges is lower than that of nevi, being that of nevi, which is especially higher from 995 nm to 1350 nm than for melanomas. This wavelength range, often called second near-infrared window, corresponds to that in which radiation can penetrate deeper into the tissue (longer wavelengths are highly absorbed by water) and thus can inform about deeper structures, which could be notably different between nevi and melanomas.

This behavior agreed with a previous study in which the average reflectance of the nevi was found to be higher with respect to the melanoma population in the VIS range [10], although the standard deviation of the data that was analyzed made it quite entangled.

Figure 6 depicts representative reflectance images of a nevus and a melanoma for all the spectral range evaluated (414 nm–1613 nm). It can be seen that nevi are usually more homogeneous at all wavelengths, while melanomas grow deeper in the skin as it was found in IR images. Our results correlate with those found by Zhang et al. [20], who identified a strong absorption between 1400 nm and 1450 nm, and also beyond this range, due to the presence of water in tissue, causing a contrast decrease of spectral images. They also evaluated the spectral behavior of tissues for different thicknesses but ex-vivo samples were used; therefore, an accurate comparison with our findings cannot be performed, since we carried out in-vivo measurements.

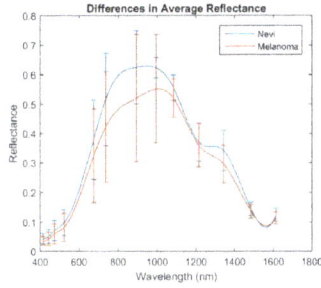

Figure 5. Averaged spectral reflectance curves (±σ) of nevi and melanomas in the VIS-NIR and exNIR ranges.

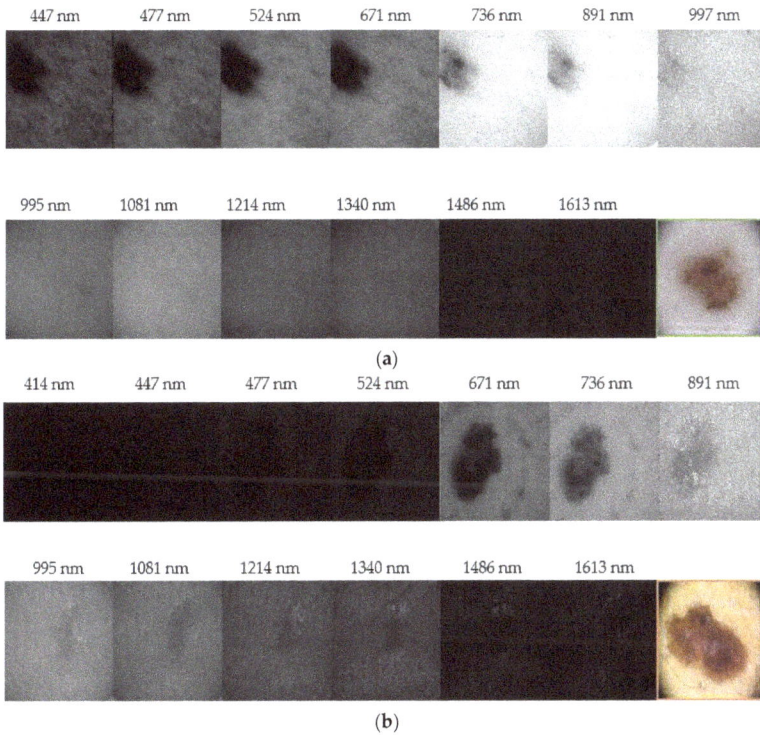

Figure 6. Reflectance images obtained with the systems in the VIS-NIR and exNIR ranges: (**a**) nevus and (**b**) melanoma. (**a**) shows that nevi are usually more homogeneous at all wavelengths. Furthermore, the IR light, which penetrates deeper in the skin, shows that melanomas generally grow deeper in (**b**). Color images were taken with a dermoscope.

In the end, the number d of best statistical descriptors exhibiting a more accurate classification of lesions that the Matlab algorithm retrieved was eight, corresponding to seven different spectral bands:

- Minimum of the spectral reflectance (minus the average of the healthy skin) at 414 nm.
- Spectral absorbance in terms of the standard deviation at 477 nm.
- Spectral absorbance in terms of the energy at 477 nm.

- Spectral reflectance in terms of energy at 524 nm.
- Spectral reflectance in terms of the skewness at 671 nm.
- Spectral reflectance in terms of the mean at 995 nm.
- Spectral absorbance (minus the average of the healthy skin) in terms of standard deviation at 1214 nm.
- Minimum of the spectral absorbance at 1613 nm.

Table 1 shows these parameters, how the total sensitivity is increased when a new selected parameter is added to the set in the iterative algorithm, and where the experimental thresholds were set in order to obtain the highest possible values of sensitivity.

Table 1. Best statistical descriptors, corresponding experimental upper and lower thresholds, and total cumulative sensitivity.

Parameter	Upper Threshold	Lower Threshold	Cummulative Sensitivity
Min. of the reflectance at 414 nm (minus skin)	0.8	−0.33	36%
Absorbance in terms of σ at 477 nm	0.082	0.039	43%
Absorbance in terms of the energy at 477 nm	0.125	0.046	50%
Reflectance in terms of energy at 524 nm	0.28	0.03	64%
Reflectance in terms of the skewness at 721 nm	1.8×10^{-3}	−2	71.5%
Reflectance in terms of the mean at 995 nm	0.55	0.4	83%
Absorbance (minus skin) in terms of σ at 1214 nm	0.082	0.04	91%
Minimum of the absorbance at 1613 nm	1.95	1.18	100%

Combinations of more parameters did not produce better discrimination between nevi and melanomas, taking into account the manual experimental thresholding defined in the scatterplots.

Figure 7a shows two representative histograms of a nevus (left) and a melanoma (right) from which the statistical descriptors were computed; they correspond to reflectance images at 1214 nm. The averaged spectral reflectance (μ); the standard deviation (σ); and corresponding Ep, En, and μ_3 are also shown. It can be seen that the En is lower, and the Ep and μ_3 are higher for the melanoma. It means that they are characterized by less uniform images, with a higher disorder in terms of reflectance and a histogram more skewed than that of the nevus. However, it can be appreciated that the μ of the melanoma is higher than that of the nevus. Figure 7b depicts a scatter plot of the spectral absorbance minus the average of the healthy skin in terms of standard deviation at 1214 nm. It can be observed that the experimental thresholding was not accurate enough to separate melanomas and nevus.

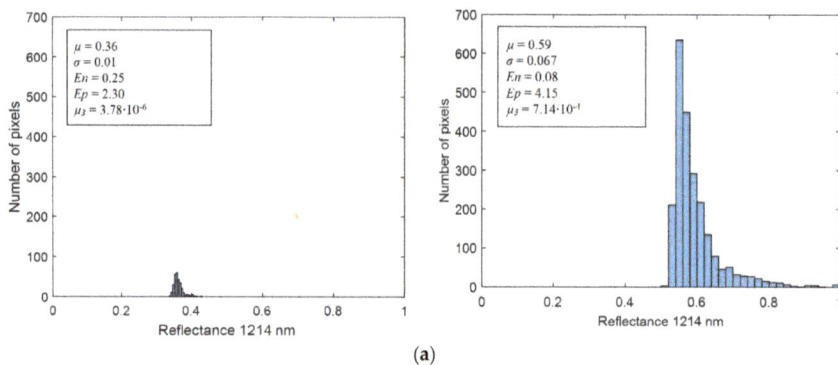

(a)

Figure 7. *Cont.*

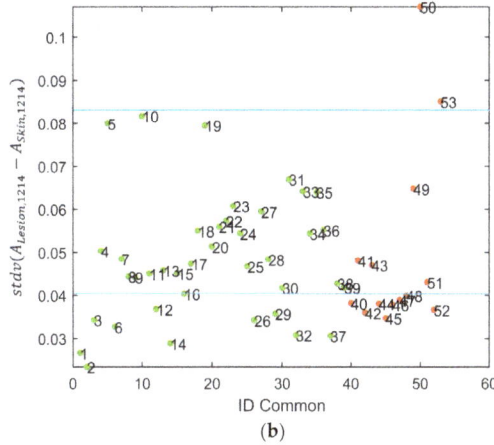

Figure 7. (**a**) Reflectance histogram at 1214 nm including the mean (μ), standard deviation (σ), energy (*En*), entropy (*Ep*), and skewness or third central moment (μ_3) values of a nevus (left) and a melanoma lesion (right). (**b**) Scatter plot of the spectral absorbance minus the average of the healthy skin in terms of standard deviation at 1214 nm in which manual thresholds have been identified.

In this preliminary study, the first three PCs were found to contain most of the variability among data (98.3%); PC1 explained 73.3%, while PC1 and PC2 explained 83.3% of the variability. Figure 8 shows the PCs plotted against each other to obtain the best descriptor's space to separate the two types of lesions, as well as the decision boundaries established using a SVM. As it can be seen, the standardization of the descriptors used and the posterior PCA showed to be useful for separating away benign and malignant lesions.

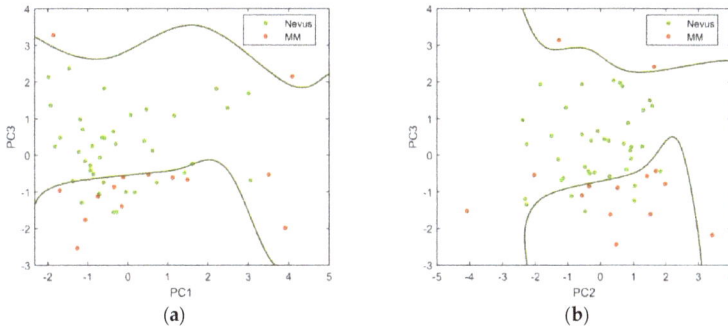

Figure 8. (**a**) PC3 vs. PC1 and (**b**) PC3 vs. PC2 descriptors for nevi (green markers) and melanoma (orange markers) are represented.

Among all the PCs evaluated, those that produced more precise classifications were the PC3 vs. PC1 (sensitivity = 85.7% and specificity = 76.9%) and the PC3 vs. PC2 (sensitivity = 78.6% and specificity = 84.6%).

Delpueyo et al. found sensitivity and specificity values of 87.2% and 54.5%, respectively, when using only the VIS-NIR device for the analysis of 290 nevi and 95 melanomas [10]. Even though the sensitivity values were similar or slightly lower than when using only the VIS-NIR device [10], the specificity was clearly increased so that exNIR information seems to be relevant for the classification between benign and malignant lesions.

In fact, the detection of malignant lesions at early stages, when they can still be controlled and successfully excised, is crucial when dealing with skin cancer, and this is the reason why dermatologists are more concerned with increasing sensitivity than specificity. However, many of the multispectral systems used for detection of skin cancer in the VIS range generate a large number of false positives and, consequently, a large number of unnecessary biopsies [21,22]. Therefore, the inclusion of longer wavelengths seems to be helpful in order to improve the specificity values reached at the time of the study.

6. Conclusions

In this pilot study, a novel exNIR multispectral imaging system for skin cancer diagnosis has been presented. The preliminary analysis of melanomas and nevi from 995 nm to 1613 nm considering spectral and spatial descriptors showed the potential of this technique, particularly for the information obtained from deeper layers of the skin by the use of IR light. In order to improve its performance, the data collected was combined with that provided by a VIS-NIR multispectral imaging system developed in a previous study. The evaluation of lesions from 414 nm to 1613 nm offered an exhaustive spectral assessment of skin lesions.

In addition, the combination of the selected as best parameters for classification, the experimental thresholding, and the use of PCA and SVM enhanced the accuracy of the initial discrimination methodology, leading to similar values of sensitivity but increased ones for specificity. Therefore, exNIR spectral information seems to be relevant for the diagnosis of skin cancer, particularly when nevi and melanomas are taken into account.

The developed methodology was limited by some factors that should be considered for future improvements of the system. Firstly, the resolution of the InGaAs sensor was rather low, limiting the performance of this device. Secondly, the selection of exNIR LEDs was a challenge due to the current state of the art of solid-state technology within this spectral range and the limited availability of wavelengths; their wider FWHMs also contributed to a less accurate spectral reconstruction. Thirdly, the need of the VIS-NIR images for the segmentation of the lesions captured with the exNIR system was also a restriction of this system. Finally, the field of view (FOV) of both systems was another limitation, since only image lesions smaller than 20 mm could be acquired.

The set of lesions was large enough to train the SVM with accurate results but was not to check with other lesions how good the decision boundaries were to separate nevi from melanoma. Future work will be focused on increasing the sample set. Also, combining spectral and 3D data available from a former study [10,23] will increase noticeably the morphological and textural information of lesions and hopefully improve the sensitivity and specificity values. Moreover, usage of the proposed methodology may benefit from conjoint use with the VIS-NIR and exNIR modality to maximize specificity. However, a solution to address the course of action in case of conflict between categorization within the two ranges would be needed. Alternative algorithms considering not only the detection of melanomas but the rate of true positives and true negatives should also be investigated.

Author Contributions: L.R.-B. and X.D. performed the experiment and analyzed the data; F.J.B.-F. contributed to technical aspects of the experiment; J.M. and S.P. coordinated the clinical assessments; M.V. conceived the experiment; F.J.B.-F., M.V., M.A., and S.R. carried out the experiments; and L.R.-B., F.J.B.-F., and M.V. wrote the paper.

Funding: This research was supported by the Spanish Ministry of Economy and Competitiveness under the grant DPI2014-56850-R, DPI2017-89414-R, and by the European Union through the project DIAGNOPTICS 'diagnosis of skin cancer using optics' (ICT PSP seventh call for proposals 2013).

Conflicts of Interest: The authors declare no conflict of interest.

Ethical Statements: All subjects gave their informed consent for inclusion before they participated in the study. The study was conducted in accordance with the Declaration of Helsinki, and the protocol was approved by the Ethics Committee of Research of the Hospital Clínic i Provincial de Barcelona and the Spanish Agency of Medicines and Medical Devices (537/1S/EC).

References

1. Guy, G.P.; Ekwueme, D.U. Melanoma Treatment Costs: A systematic review of the literature, 1990–2011. *Am. J. Prev. Med.* **2012**, *43*, 537–545. [CrossRef] [PubMed]
2. Stern, R.S. Prevalence of a History of Skin Cancer in 2007: Results of an incidence-based model. *Arch. Dermatol.* **2010**, *146*, 279–282. [CrossRef] [PubMed]
3. Pladellorens, J.; Pintó, A.; Segura, J.; Cadevall, C.; Antó, J.; Pujol, J.; Vilaseca, M.; Coll, J. A Device for the Color Measurement and Detection of Spots on the Skin. *Skin Res. Technol.* **2008**, *14*, 65–70. [CrossRef] [PubMed]
4. Jolivot, R.; Benezeth, Y.; Marzani, F. Skin Parameter Map Retrieval from a dedicated Multispectral Imaging System Applied to Dermatology/Cosmetology. *J. Biomed. Imaging* **2013**, *2013*, 1–15. [CrossRef] [PubMed]
5. Tomatis, S.; Carrara, M.; Bono, A.; Bartoli, C.; Lualdi, M.; Tragni, G. Automated Melanoma Detection with a Novel Multispectral Imaging System: Results of a prospective study. *Phys. Med. Biol.* **2005**, *50*, 1675–1687. [CrossRef] [PubMed]
6. Kuzmina, I.; Diabele, I.; Jakovels, D.; Spigullis, J.; Valeine, L.; Kapsotinsh, J.; Berzina, A. Towards Non-Contact Skin Melanoma Selection by Multispectral Analysis. *J. Biomed. Opt.* **2011**, *16*, 060502. [CrossRef] [PubMed]
7. Bekina, A.; Diebele, I.; Rubins, U.; Zaharans, J.; Dejarbo, A.; Sigulis, J. Multispectral assessment of skin malformations using a modified video-microscope. *Latv. J. Phys. Tech. Sci.* **2012**, *49*, 4–8. [CrossRef]
8. Diebele, I.; Kuzmina, I.; Lihachev, A.; Kapsotinsh, J.; Dejarbo, A.; Valiene, L.; Spigulis, J. Clinical evaluation of melanomas and common nevi by spectral imaging. *Biomed. Opt. Express* **2012**, *3*, 467–472. [CrossRef] [PubMed]
9. Jakovels, D.; Lihacova, I.; Kuzmina, I.; Sigulis, J. Evaluation of Skin Melanoma in Spectral Range 450–950 nm Using Principal Component Analysis. In Proceedings of the European Conference on Biomedical Optics, Munich, Germany, 24 June 2013; Volume 8803. [CrossRef]
10. Delpueyo, X.; Vilaseca, M.; Royo, S.; Ares, M.; Rey-Barroso, L.; Sanabria, F.; Puig, S.; Malvehy, J.; Pellacani, J.; Noguero, F.; et al. Multispectral imaging system based on light-emitting diodes for the detection of melanomas and basal cell carcinomas: A pilot study. *J. Biomed. Opt.* **2017**, *22*, 065006. [CrossRef] [PubMed]
11. Kim, S.; Cho, D.; Kim, J.; Kim, M.; Youn, S.; Jang, J.E.; Je, M.; Lee, D.H.; Lee, B.; Farkas, D.L.; et al. Smartphone-based multiespectral imaging: System development and potential for mobile skin diagnosis. *Biomed. Opt. Express* **2016**, *7*, 005294. [CrossRef] [PubMed]
12. Langley, R.G.; Walsh, N.; Sutherland, A.E.; Propperova, I.; Delaney, L.; Morris, S.F.; Gallant, C. The diagnostic accuracy of in vivo confocal scanning laser microscopy compared to dermoscopy of bening and malignant melanocytic lesions: A prospective study. *Arch. Dermatol.* **2007**, *215*, 365–372. [CrossRef]
13. Salo, D.; Kim, D.; Cao, Q.; Berezin, M.Y. Multispectral imaging/deep tissue imaging: Extended near-infrared: A new window on in vivo bioimaging. *BioOpt. World* **2014**, *7*, 22–25.
14. Mourant, J.R.; Fuselier, T.; Boyer, J.; Johnson, T.M.; Bigio, I.J. Predicrions and measurements of scattering and absorption over broad wavelength ranges in tissue phantoms. *Arch. Dermatol.* **2007**, *215*, 365–372. [CrossRef]
15. Godoy, S.E.; Ramirez, D.A.; Myers, S.A.; von Winckel, G.; Krishna, S.; Berwick, M.; Padilla, S.; Sen, P.; Krishna, S. Dynamic infrared imaging for skin cancer screening. *Infrared Phys. Technol.* **2015**, *70*, 147–152. [CrossRef]
16. El-Baz, A.; Jiang, X.; Suri, J.S. *Biomedical Image Segmentation*, 1st ed.; CRC Press: Boca Raton, FL, USA, 2017; pp. 249–271. ISBN 9781482258554.
17. Herrera, J.A.; Vilaseca, M.; Düll, J.; Arjona, M.; Torrecilla, E.; Pujol, J. Iris color and texture: A comparative analysis of real irises, ocular prostheses, and colored contact lenses. *Color Res. Appl.* **2011**, *36*, 373–382. [CrossRef]
18. Martinez, W.L.; Martinez, A.R.; Solka, J.L. *Exploratory Data Analysis with Matlab*, 3rd ed.; Chapman and Hall CRC Press: New York, NY, USA, 2017; Part II; ISBN 9781498776066.
19. Ritter, G.; Wilson, J. Image Features and Descriptors. In *Handbook of Computer Vision Algorithms in Image Algebra*, 2nd ed.; CRC Press: Boca Raton, FL, USA, 2000; pp. 299–305. ISBN 0849300754.

20. Zhang, H.; Salo, D.; Kim, D.M.; Komarov, S.; Tai, Y.C.; Berezin, M.Y. Penetration depth of photons in biological tissues from hyperspectral imaging in shortwave infrared in transmission and reflection geometries. *J. Biomed. Opt.* **2016**, *21*, 126006. [CrossRef] [PubMed]

21. Monheit, G.; Cognetta, A.B.; Rabinovitz, H.; Gross, K.; Martini, M.; Grichnik, J.M.; Mihm, M.; Prieto, V.G.; Googe, P.; King, R.; et al. The performance of MelaFind: A prospective study. *Arch. Dermatol.* **2011**, *147*, 188–194. [CrossRef] [PubMed]

22. Burroni, M.; Sbano, P.; Cevenini, G.; Risulo, M.; Dell'Eva, G.; Barbini, P.; Miracco, C.; Fimiani, M.; Adreassi, L.; Rubegni, P. Dysplastic naevus vs. in situ melanoma: Digital dermoscopy analysis. *Br. J. Dermatol.* **2005**, *152*, 679–684. [CrossRef] [PubMed]

23. Ares, M.; Royo, S.; Vilaseca, M.; Herrera, J.A.; Delpueyo, X.; Sanabria, F. Handheld 3D Scanning System for In-Vivo Imaging of Skin Cancer. In Proceedings of the 5th International Conference on 3D Body Scanning Technologies, Lugano, Switzerland, 21–22 October 2014. [CrossRef]

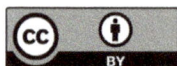

![sensors logo] *sensors*   MDPI

Article

Evaluation of Laser-Assisted Trans-Nail Drug Delivery with Optical Coherence Tomography

Meng-Tsan Tsai [1,2,3], **Ting-Yen Tsai** [1], **Su-Chin Shen** [4,5], **Chau Yee Ng** [3,5], **Ya-Ju Lee** [6], **Jiann-Der Lee** [1,7] and **Chih-Hsun Yang** [3,5,*]

1   Department of Electrical Engineering, Chang Gung University, Taoyuan 33302, Taiwan;
    mengtsan@gmail.com (M.-T.T.); trendy1991818@gmail.com (T.-Y.T.); jdlee@mail.cgu.edu.tw (J.-D.L.)
2   Medical Imaging Research Center, Institute for Radiological Research, Chang Gung University and Chang
    Gung Memorial Hospital at Linkou, Taoyuan 33302, Taiwan
3   Department of Dermatology, Chang Gung Memorial Hospital, Linkou 33305, Taiwan;
    charlene870811@gmail.com
4   Department of Ophthalmology, Chang Gung Memorial Hospital, Linkou 33305, Taiwan;
    suchin@adm.cgmh.org.tw
5   College of Medicine, Chang Gung University, Taoyuan 33302, Taiwan
6   Institute of Electro-Optical Science and Technology, National Taiwan Normal University,
    Taipei 11677, Taiwan; yajulee@ntnu.edu.tw
7   Department of Neurosurgery, Chang Gung Memorial Hospital, LinKou 33305, Taiwan
*   Correspondence: dermadr@hotmail.com; Tel.: +886-3-328-1200 (ext. 2215)

Academic Editor: Dragan Indjin
Received: 19 October 2016; Accepted: 7 December 2016; Published: 12 December 2016

Abstract: The nail provides a functional protection to the fingertips and surrounding tissue from external injuries. The nail plate consists of three layers including dorsal, intermediate, and ventral layers. The dorsal layer consists of compact, hard keratins, limiting topical drug delivery through the nail. In this study, we investigate the application of fractional CO_2 laser that produces arrays of microthermal ablation zones (MAZs) to facilitate drug delivery in the nails. We utilized optical coherence tomography (OCT) for real-time monitoring of the laser–skin tissue interaction, sparing the patient from an invasive surgical sampling procedure. The time-dependent OCT intensity variance was used to observe drug diffusion through an induced MAZ array. Subsequently, nails were treated with cream and liquid topical drugs to investigate the feasibility and diffusion efficacy of laser-assisted drug delivery. Our results show that fractional CO_2 laser improves the effectiveness of topical drug delivery in the nail plate and that OCT could potentially be used for in vivo monitoring of the depth of laser penetration as well as real-time observations of drug delivery.

Keywords: drug delivery; nail; optical coherence tomography; fractional laser; laser ablation

1. Introduction

The nail is a modified form of stratum corneum, with a thick laminated keratinized structure overlying the nail bed and matrix. However, the thick structure limits drug delivery to the nail bed, which is problematic when it comes to treating nail diseases such as onychomycosis. The nail plate is composed of 25 sheets of keratinized cells that can be divided into dorsal, intermediate, and ventral layers. Compared with the intermediate layer, the dorsal and ventral layers are thinner. The dorsal and ventral layers consist of harder skin-type keratin with lipids. In contrast, the intermediate layer is composed of hair-type keratin with few lipids, making the intermediate layer more flexible. Therefore, the dorsal layer forms a barrier for drug delivery [1–4]. To improve the efficiency of drug delivery through the nail, a new strategy is to produce micropores on the nail to remove the dorsal layer [5,6]. Therefore, the development of permeation-enhanced techniques for skin has become an important area of study to improve drug delivery. Recently, transdermal drug delivery became a new route of drug and vaccine administration, providing the advantages of avoiding the first-pass metabolism, sustained therapeutic action, and better patient compliance [7,8]. Strategies to bypass the tightly packed stratum corneum, the rate-limiting step in transdermal drug penetration, will facilitate topical medication delivery deep into the skin. Several methods have been developed to improve transdermal drug delivery, including chemical enhancers [9,10], nanocarriers [11,12], microneedles [13,14], sonophoresis [15,16], and iontophoresis [17,18]. The biocompatibility and biotoxicity of chemical enhancers and nanocarriers are important issues. For microneedles, although new biodegradable polymers reduce the risk of microneedles retained in skin tissue, these materials are not able to produce sufficient mechanical strength to penetrate the skin barrier. On the contrary, metallic microneedles can easily penetrate the skin barrier but may cause allergic reactions. Both ultrasound and iontophoresis to facilitate drug delivery have been proposed in previous studies, but accurate control of the treatment depth remains a challenging issue.

The development of laser techniques has promoted various applications, in particular for therapies and biomedical imaging. In therapeutic applications, lasers offer an excellent solution in clinical medicine because they result in less bleeding, reduced infections, and minimized incision areas [19]. With a pulsed high-energy laser, the biological tissue can be coagulated, and even ablated, which enables skin tightening, hemangioma treatment, and the removal of unwanted hair and blood vessels [20–24]. Ablative fractional lasers are primarily used to treat photodamaged skin, deep rhytides and scarring. Current fractional laser systems for dermatology include carbon dioxide (CO_2, 10,600 nm) and erbium-doped yttrium aluminum garnet (Er:YAG, 2940 nm) lasers. The fractional CO_2 laser produces deep vertical holes down to the dermis to assist the delivery of topically applied drugs into the skin. Recently, this approach was used in the treatment of fungal nail diseases [25]. The micro-channel array created by a fractional CO_2 laser creates tiny pores on the skin surface that enhance the penetration of topically applied drugs. Penetration-enhanced techniques for skin and nails are rapidly developing, enabling significant increases in the efficiency of disease treatment.

Currently, various optical imaging approaches to monitor transdermal drug delivery have been proposed, such as confocal laser scanning microscopy (CLSM) [26], two-photon microscopy (TPM) [27], infrared microscopic imaging (IMI) [28], and Raman microscopy (RM) [28]. Although both CLSM and TPM can provide cellular-level resolution, their imaging depth is limited to hundreds of micrometers, which is not deep enough to observe drug diffusion beneath the skin surface. Moreover, CLSM or TPM need extra fluorescent labeling. Compared to CLSM and TPM, IMI provides a wider imaging field, but skin specimens must be carefully prepared before imaging, and IMI cannot be used for in vivo imaging. The imaging depth of RM is limited when used for studies on drug delivery. The thickness of nails ranges from hundreds of micrometers to several millimeters, making the approaches mentioned earlier unsuitable for investigating drug delivery via nails. Moreover, these methods do not acquire depth and time-resolved information of the dynamics of drug diffusion from the nail surface to the nail bed. Therefore, in this paper, we propose the use of optical coherence tomography (OCT) to investigate the dynamics of transdermal drug delivery.

OCT uses backscattered tissue signals to reconstruct the 2D/3D morphology of biological tissue [29–31]. Compared to ultrasound imaging, OCT provides higher resolutions in both the transverse and depth directions (up to 1–10 μm). Moreover, OCT can probe deeper tissue structures than of microscopic techniques such as confocal microscopy, TPM, and harmonic generation microscopy [32–34]. Besides this deeper imaging depth, OCT imaging is noninvasive, has a high imaging speed, and can be used for internal hollow organ scanning with concomitant use of an endoscope. Various functional OCT with different purposes have been developed including optical coherence angiography [35,36], polarization-sensitive OCT for the measurement of tissue birefringence [37,38], and optical coherence elastography [39,40]. In previous studies, we have demonstrated that the photothermolysis of human skin induced by an ablative laser can be monitored with OCT [41]. Furthermore, preliminary OCT results have proven the feasibility of laser-assisted therapy [42]. In this study, we investigate the time-dependent variation of OCT intensity during the diffusion process of drug particles. Additionally, we also estimate the time-dependent speckle variance (SV) [43–46] of OCT intensity, observe in vivo laser-assisted drug delivery, and evaluate the diffusion ability of different drug preparations (liquid and cream drugs) in nails treated with fractional CO_2 laser. Finally, we evaluate the relative diffusion velocities of cream and liquid drugs in the nail by estimating the center-of-mass locations of time-dependent SV.

2. Experiment Method and Setup

The experiments in this study were approved by the Chang Gung Medical Foundation Institutional Review Board (No. 101-2921A3) and were conducted in the outpatient clinic of the Department of Dermatology of Chang Gung Memorial Hospital, Taipei, Taiwan. The volunteers were subjected to irradiance by a fractional CO_2 laser (UltraPulse Encore Active FXTM; Lumenis, Santa Clara, CA, USA) under various exposure energies of 20, 30, 40, and 50 mJ. The average power and the pulse width of the used CO_2 laser are 330 W and 0.15 ms, respectively. Single laser pulse induced each MAZ on the nail plate. The maximum output energy was up to 50 mJ. The fingernails of the volunteers were exposed to laser energies of 20, 30, 40, and 50 mJ. Fingernails were scanned by the OCT system after laser exposure to discern induced photothermolysis. Liquid or cream topical drugs (Sulconazole Nitrate) were then applied to the exposed region of the fingernail, and we scanned the nail continuously with OCT. The liquid drug we used was an Exelderm solution consisting of Sulconazole nitrate with a concentration of 1%, and the cream drug we used was Exelderm cream composed of Sulconazole nitrate with a concentration of 1%. The Exelderm solution is a solution of propylene glycol, poloxamer 407, polysorbate 20, butylated hydroxyanisole, and purified water, with sodium hydroxide. Exelderm cream is in an emollient cream base, which consists of propylene glycol, stearyl alcohol, isopropyl myristate, cetyl alcohol, polysorbate 60, sorbitan monostearate, glyceryl stearate and PEG-100 stearate, ascorbyl palmitate, and purified water with sodium hydroxide. Additionally, previous reports have demonstrated that propylene glycol is a drug load enhancer and that sodium hydroxide is an uptake rate enhancer [47]. Before OCT measurement, the finger was immersed into the ultrasonic cleaner to remove the dust in microthermal ablation zones (MAZs) for 5 min and then dried in air for 30 min.

In this study, a swept-source OCT (SS-OCT) system was set up for in vivo fingernail scanning. The setup of the SS-OCT system is similar to that of a previous study [42]. A swept source (HSL-20, Santec Corp., Aichi, Japan) at 1.3 µm was used as the light source of the OCT system with a scanning spectrum of 110 nm. The longitudinal and transverse resolutions are approximately 7 and 5 µm, respectively. The physical scanning range is $3 \times 3 \times 3$ mm^3. The maximum imaging depth of this OCT system is approximately 3 mm. Because the light source can provide a scan rate of 100 kHz, the corresponding frame rate of the OCT system was set to 100 frames/s. Unconscious motion by the volunteer during the OCT measurement was reduced using a specially designed mount fabricated by a 3D printer to fix the finger stably. Moreover, to investigate the feasibility of laser-assisted drug diffusion, the drug was rubbed on the nails and scanned with OCT. We record sequential 2D OCT images before and after the drug application.

3. Results and Discussion

Fractional laser ablation causes tissue vaporization, producing a microthermal ablation zone (MAZ) array. However, the induced MAZ penetration depth is hard to predict because of differences in the optical properties of biological tissues. To investigate the induced photothermolysis on the nail, four fingernails of a 26-year-old volunteer were sequentially exposed to fractional CO_2 laser with exposure energies of 50, 40, 30, and 20 mJ. The four treated nails were then scanned in vivo by the OCT system to acquire 3D microstructural images. Figure 1 shows the OCT results of four fingernails after exposure to these laser energies. Figure 1a–h represent the top view of the 3D OCT images and the representative cross-sectional images of four nails, respectively, which were obtained after laser exposures to energies of 50, 40, 30, and 20 mJ. Laser exposure induced MAZs as indicated by white arrows in Figure 1. Figure 1a–d demonstrate the increased size and penetration depth of MAZs corresponding to the increasing exposure energy. Based on the OCT results, the penetration depth and the diameter of the induced MAZ corresponding to exposure energy can be estimated. The average penetration depths of Figure 1a–d are 372, 321, 290, and 255 μm, respectively. Additionally, the average diameters of Figure 1a–d are 203, 183, 171, and 137 μm, respectively. The results show that an exposure energy of 50 mJ provides a deeper penetration depth while sparing the nail bed. Therefore, we chose 50 mJ as the optimal exposure energy to induce MAZ on the nails in the following experiments.

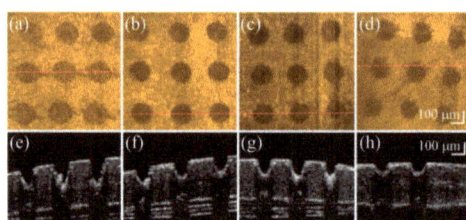

Figure 1. In vivo (**a–d**) top-view and (**e–h**) representative cross-sectional OCT images of four fingernails after fractional laser exposures to (from left to right) energies of 50, 40, 30, and 20 mJ. The red-dash lines in (**a–d**) indicate the corresponding locations of (**e–h**).

To understand the influence on the OCT intensity of the unexposed and exposed nail regions after the drug application, a fingernail of one 22-year-old male volunteer was exposed to a fractional CO_2 laser with an exposure energy of 50 mJ. In this case, only one-half of the fingernail was exposed, while the other half was spared. The finger was later fixed on the specially designed mount for motion reduction and scanned with OCT. We compare the difference of drug delivery between untreated nail and the laser-treated nail by treating both sides with liquid drug preparation and scanned with OCT. The scanning range covered both regions of the nail, and the changes before and after drug application were recorded. We analyze the intensity variation of OCT signal beneath the nail surface. A segmentation algorithm proposed in our previous study was used to explore the OCT signal beneath the nail surface [48,49]. Figure 2 shows the time-series 2D OCT images obtained at the same location of the fingernail. Figure 2a is the OCT image obtained before liquid drug application, where the left part is the untreated nail structure and the right part represents the laser-treated nail with MAZs. Figure 2b–l were obtained at various times after the liquid drug application. In Figure 2b, the strongly scattered spots, which are indicated by the white arrows, are a result of the aggregation of drug particles.

Figure 3 shows the averaged A-scan profiles of the unexposed and treated regions, as marked by the yellow and white lines in Figure 2a. Here, the A-scan represents a one-dimensional scan along the depth direction, representing the relationship between the backscattered intensity and the depth. For both lines, 11 adjacent A-scans, corresponding to a transverse range of 50 μm, were chosen for the acquisition of an averaged A-scan profile. Thus, Figure 3a represents the averaged A-scan profiles of the yellow line in Figure 2 obtained at 0, 2.0, 4.0, 6.0, 8.0, and 10.0 s after the drug application. In contrast, Figure 3b plots the averaged A-scan profiles of the white line in Figure 2 obtained at 0, 2.0, 4.0, 6.0, 8.0, and 10.0 s after the drug application. The yellowish region in Figure 3 represents the nail layer, and the greenish region indicates the tissue beneath the nail bed. In Figure 3a, the time-series of averaged A-scan profiles illustrate that there is no significant change in the backscattered intensity, especially in the yellowish region. In comparison to the results of Figure 3a, after the drug application, changes in the backscattered intensity of the yellowish region in Figure 3b was observed, marked by the black arrows. Our results show that the changes in OCT backscattered intensity can be used to identify the drug's diffusion. However, because the vessels exist in the soft tissue of skin beneath the nail bed (the greenish region), which also result in OCT intensity variation, it is hard to tell whether these changes are due to the diffusion of drug particles or the motion of red blood cells in the soft tissue layer. Therefore, in this study, we focus on investigating the intensity variation of the nail plate.

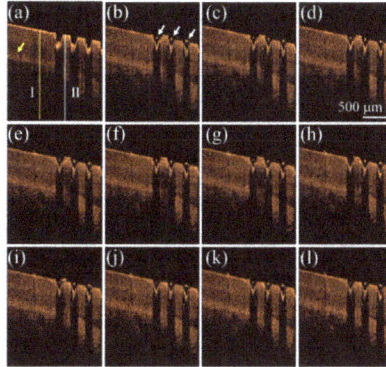

Figure 2. Time-series 2D OCT images obtained at the same location of the fingernail after 50 mJ fractional laser exposure. OCT images obtained (**a**) before the liquid drug application and at (**b**) 0 s; (**c**) 0.2 s; (**d**) 0.4 s; (**e**) 0.6 s; (**f**) 0.8 s; (**g**) 1.0 s; (**h**) 2.0 s; (**i**) 4.0 s; (**j**) 6.0 s; (**k**) 8.0 s; and (**l**) 10.0 s after the liquid drug application. The white arrows indicate that the stronger OCT backscattered signal resulted from the aggregation of drug particles. The yellow arrow indicates the nail bed. The yellow and white lines indicate the locations for estimation of the averaged A-scan profiles of the unexposed and treated regions.

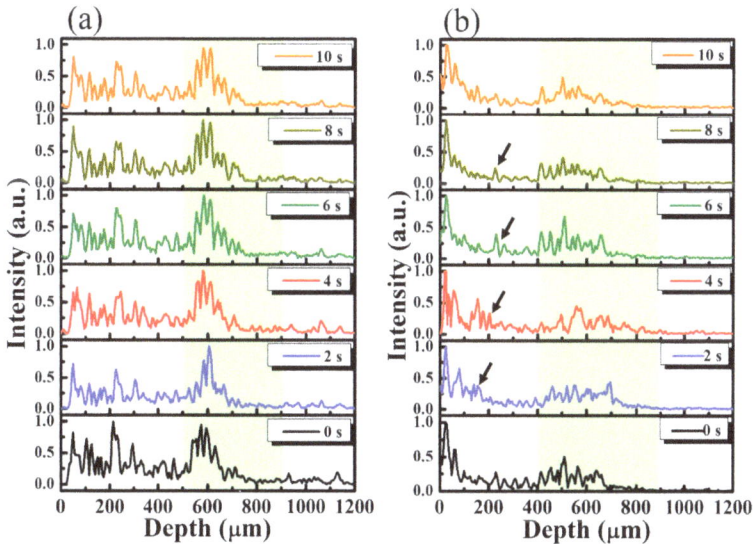

Figure 3. (**a**) Averaged A-scan profiles of the yellow line (the unexposed region) in Figure 2 and (**b**) the averaged A-scan profiles of the white line (the exposed region) in Figure 2 obtained at time points of 0, 2.0, 4.0, 6.0, 8.0, and 10.0 s after the drug application. The black arrows indicate the variation in OCT backscattered intensity after the drug application.

According to the results in Figure 3, the diffusion of drug particles results in the variation of OCT backscattered intensity. Therefore, to quantitatively evaluate the intensity variation, the SV between the time-series OCT images was estimated. First, the OCT image obtained at the point of the drug application was used as a reference, and the OCT images obtained at various time points after the drug application were then individually compared with the reference image to acquire a corresponding SV image. Therefore, an SV image at time t after the drug application can be estimated as

$$SV_{t_n}(x,z) = \frac{\left\{I_{t_0}(x,z) - \frac{1}{2}[I_{t_0}(x,z) + I_{t_n}(x,z)]\right\}^2 + \left\{I_{t_n}(x,z) - \frac{1}{2}[I_{t_0}(x,z) + I_{t_n}(x,z)]\right\}^2}{2} \quad (1)$$

where x, z are the pixel locations in the transverse and longitudinal directions, respectively [43,44], and t_0 and t_n represent the start of the drug application and the nth time point after the drug application, respectively. In our previous study, although SV can be used to observe the diffusion of water through fingernails after fractional laser exposure, it was found to be difficult to further investigate the depth-resolved drug diffusion because of the shadowing effect resulting from particle diffusion [46]. Thus, to reduce the shadowing effect, Equation (1) can be revised as

$$SVR_{t_n}(x,z) = SV_{t_n}(x,z) \times e^{\frac{1}{\gamma} \sum_{i=1}^{z} SV_{t_n}(x,i)} \quad (2)$$

where γ is an attenuation coefficient. To reject the contribution of speckle noise, we set the threshold SV value to 0.05, using the time-series 2D images to estimate the SV values before the drug application.

Subsequently, liquid and cream drugs were tested to study the feasibility of drug diffusion through MAZs. We repeat the same experiment protocol of Figure 2. First, the fingernails of one 24-year-old male volunteer were exposed to a fractional CO_2 laser with an exposure energy of 50 mJ. During OCT scanning, the finger was fixed on the specially designed mount to reduce motion artifacts, and the same location of fingernail was continuously scanned by the OCT system to obtain a time series of 2D OCT images. The liquid drug preparation was then applied to the nail surface and the nail was continuously scanned for 60 s. To compare the intensity variance before and after the drug application, a 2D OCT image was obtained at the beginning of the drug application as the reference image, and time-series OCT images were recorded after the drug application to estimate the SV images. Finally, the OCT image and corresponding SV image at each time point were merged into an SV-OCT image.

Figure 4a shows a 2D OCT image of the nail after fractional laser exposure with an exposure energy of 50 mJ, and Figure 4b–l represent time-series SV-OCT images obtained after the liquid drug application. To indicate the corresponding location of the SV signal in the nail, the OCT structural image and SV image were merged. The OCT structural intensity is shown in the gray scale, and the SV signal is shown in the red scale. Here, the occurrence of the SV signal indicates the location of intensity variance due to the moving particles, but the SV value is not proportional to the particle concentration. Strong backscattered spots, which are indicated by the white arrows in Figure 4b, moved with time, as shown in Figure 4b–l. These strong backscattered spots are a result of the aggregation of drug particles. The thickness of the liquid drug on the nail surface gives a redundant optical path difference, which will probably cause SV estimation errors. Therefore, a segmentation algorithm proposed in our previous study was performed before SV estimation [46]. Based on this segmentation algorithm, the nail surface can be detected, allowing the nail surfaces of the time-series OCT images to be realigned with the nail surface of the reference image. Since the blood flow in the soft tissue beneath the nail layer also causes time-dependent variations in OCT backscattered intensity, it is difficult to differentiate the SV contributions of the drug diffusion and the vessels in the soft tissue layer. Therefore, only SV signals in the nail structure are presented in this study; nevertheless, observations of the drug diffusion in the nail layer enable us to identify whether the drug particles have reached the nail bed. In Figure 4c, the SV signal began to occur around the boundaries of the induced MAZs, and the area of SV distribution then increased with time. After 10 s, the SV signal could be observed in the whole nail region.

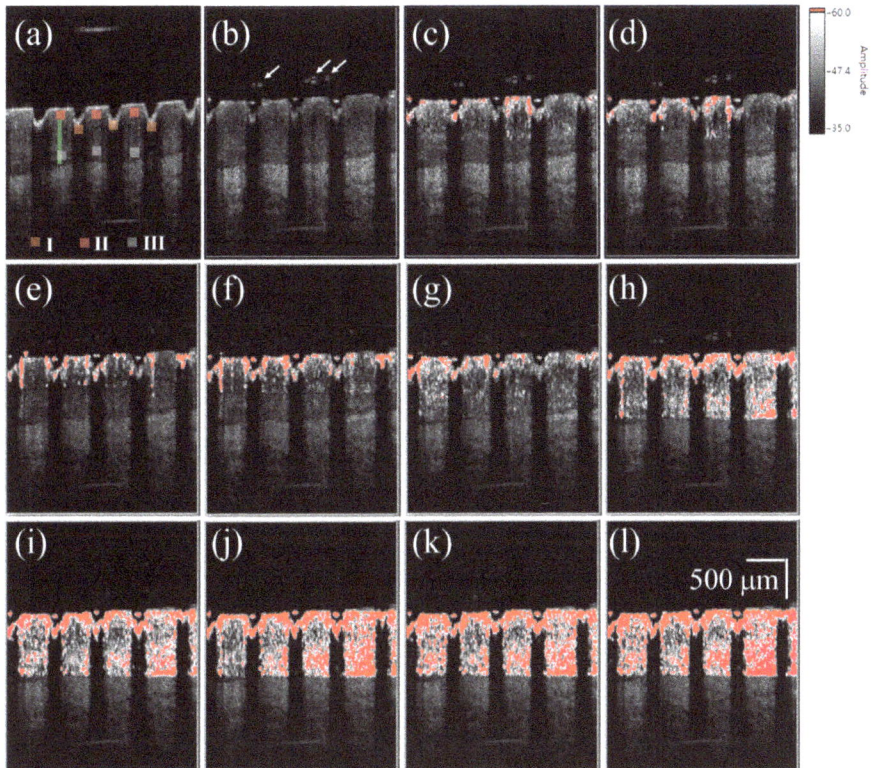

Figure 4. (a) 2D OCT image of the nail after 50 mJ laser exposure. Time-series SV-OCT images of the treated nail obtained after the liquid drug application at (**b**) 0 s; (**c**) 0.2 s; (**d**) 0.4 s; (**e**) 0.6 s; (**f**) 0.8 s; (**g**) 1.0 s; (**h**) 2.0 s; (**i**) 4.0 s; (**j**) 6.0 s; (**k**) 8.0 s; and (**l**) 10.0 s. The white arrows indicate the stronger backscattered signal, resulting from the drug particles. The scalar bar in (**l**) represents a length of 500 μm in length.

To investigate the diffusion of the cream drug in the fingernail, the same finger in the experiment of Figure 4 was utilized again and the same experimental procedure was repeated on the next day of the liquid drug experiment. To avoid the accumulation of drug particles in the nail, the nails were immersed into the ultrasound cleaner to remove the unwanted depositions in the MAZs before each experiment. Additionally, in our method, we used the B-scan obtained in the beginning of the drug application as the reference image to estimate the SV. Therefore, the effect induced by the residual drug can be greatly reduced. The cream drug preparation was then rubbed onto the nail surface and simultaneously scanned by the OCT system for 60 s. Figure 5a shows a 2D OCT image of the treated nail obtained before the cream drug application, where the induced MAZ forms an inverted pyramid shape. Figure 5b–l are the time-series SV-OCT images obtained at various time points after the cream drug application. White color represents the tissue structure, and the red color indicates the existence of an SV signal. After the drug application, the cream drug preparation occupied the MAZs, causing a stronger backscattered intensity in the MAZ region. From Figure 5b–d, we can see that the SV signal only existed on the nail surface, and gradually occurred in the nail structure as time increased. After 10 s, SV was observed in the entire nail structure. This SV is a result of the time-dependent variation of OCT intensity due to the diffusion of drug particles. Again, only SV signals in the nail layer are presented. Additionally, a comparison of Figures 4 and 5 suggests that the SV signals found in the MAZ of Figure 5 were absent in the MAZ of Figure 4. This is because the MAZs in Figure 5 were occupied by the cream drug particles. After applying the segmentation algorithm, an intact nail surface was found in Figure 5, and the MAZs in Figure 5 were included in the SV estimation. However, in the OCT images obtained from the experiment with the liquid drug after processing the segmentation algorithm, the MAZs were not included in the SV estimation.

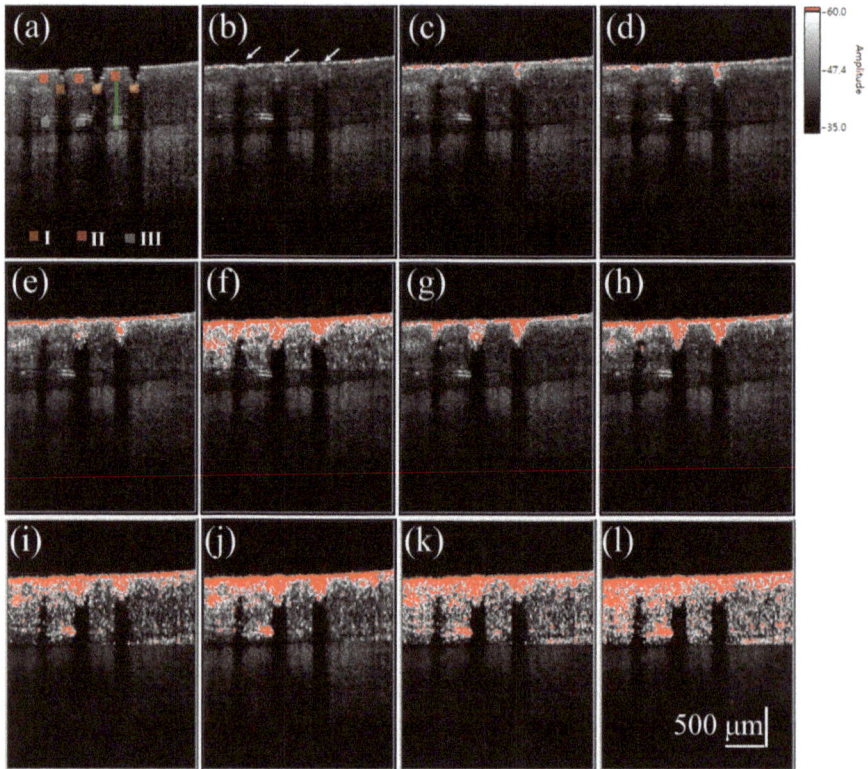

Figure 5. (a) 2D OCT image of the nail after fractional laser exposure with an exposure energy of 50 mJ. Time-series SV-OCT images of the nail obtained at (**b**) 0 s; (**c**) 0.2 s; (**d**) 0.4 s; (**e**) 0.6 s; (**f**) 0.8 s; (**g**) 1.0 s; (**h**) 2.0 s; (**i**) 4.0 s; (**j**) 6.0 s; (**k**) 8.0 s; and (**l**) 10.0 s after the cream drug application. The white arrows indicate that the MAZs were filled with the cream drug. The scalar bar in (l) represents a length of 500 μm in length.

For the study of drug particles diffusion behavior in nail layers, three regions (Regions I, II, and III in Figures 4 and 5) were selected for analysis. Three orange squares located at the tip regions of the MAZs in Figures 4 and 5 (Region I) were averaged, as were the three red squares located at the upper nail regions in Region II and the three white squares located in the middle of the two MAZs (Region III). For each region, the summation of the SV values of three colored square was averaged to acquire an averaged summation result at various time points. Figure 6a,b show the averaged summations of SV values of Regions I, II, and III in Figures 4 and 5, respectively. From Figure 6a, we see that the averaged summation of the SV values in Region I increased after the drug application, reaching a saturation level after approximately 15 s. The results for Regions II and III in Figure 6a indicate that the averaged SV summation started to increase after 1 s. In comparison, Figure 6b shows the same trend for region I, but the summations only start to increase after 2 s in Regions II and III. Figure 6 show that MAZs effectively improve the drug diffusion through the nail layer. Three regions in each depth range (indicated by red, orange and white squares in Figures 4a and 5a) are selected to estimate the average summation of SV values. The standard deviation of the three regions at the same depth range is shown in Figure 6.

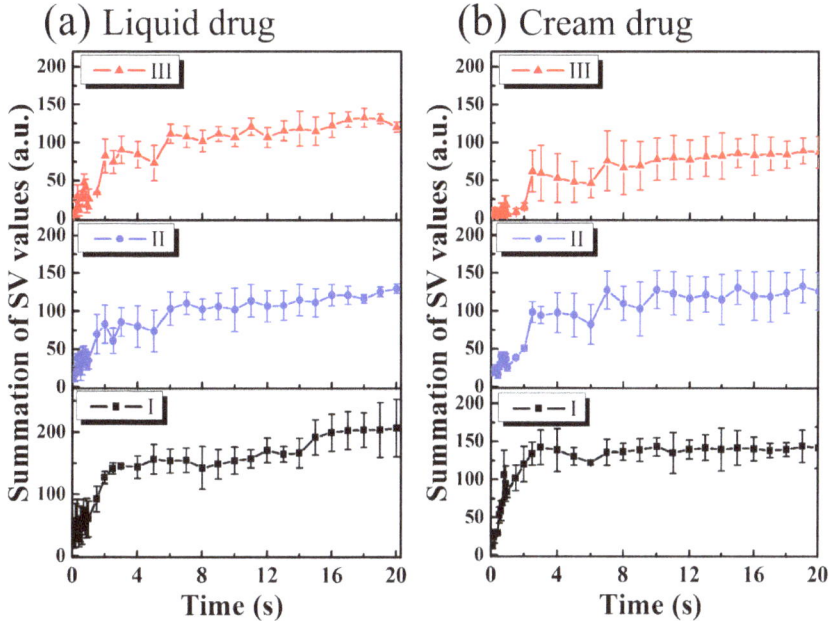

Figure 6. (a) Averaged summation of SV values of Regions I, II, and III indicated by the squares in Figure 4 as a function of time; (b) Averaged summation of SV values of Regions I, II, and III indicated by the squares in Figure 5 as a function of time.

4. Conclusions

In this study, we demonstrated that using a fractional ablative laser produces MAZ arrays on fingernails that facilitate drug delivery. However, the induced depth of photothermolysis is difficult to predict. Therefore, we used OCT for in vivo evaluation of photothermolysis on nail induced by the fractional CO_2 laser. In addition, we propose a method here for in vivo observations of drug diffusion through the induced MAZs based on the evaluation of the time-dependent OCT intensity. In this study, the exposure energy for producing microthermal ablation zones in nails was set to be 50 mJ, which is the maximum output energy of the CO_2 laser. From OCT scanning results, 50 mJ laser energy can induce an averaged penetration depth of more than 370 μm in nails, making drug particles easily penetrate the nail barrier and reach the skin tissue beneath the nail. These results suggest that OCT could serve as a potential tool for in vivo observations of drug diffusion.

Acknowledgments: This research was supported in part by the Ministry of Science and Technology (MOST) and Chang Gung Memorial Hospital, Taiwan, Republic of China, under grants MOST104-2221-E-182A-004-MY2, MOST104-2221-E-182-027-MY2, MOST105-2221-E-182-016-MY3, CMRPD2F0131, and CMRPD2B0033.

Author Contributions: Meng-Tsan Tsai and Chih-Hsun Yang designed the experiments; Ting-Yen Tsai and Ya-Ju Lee performed the experiments; Meng-Tsan Tsai, Su-Chin Shen, Chau Yee Ng, Chih-Hsun Yang, and Jiann-Der Lee analyzed the data; Meng-Tsan Tsai, Chau Yee Ng and Chih-Hsun Yang wrote the paper.

Conflicts of Interest: The authors declare no conflict of interest.

References

1. Gupchup, G.V.; Zatz, J.L. Structural characteristics and permeability properties of the human nail: A review. *J. Cosmet. Sci.* **1999**, *50*, 363–385.
2. Repka, M.A.; O'Haver, J.; See, C.H.; Gutta, K.; Munjal, M. Nail morphology studies as assessments for onychomycosis treatment modalities. *Int. J. Pharm.* **2002**, *245*, 25–36. [CrossRef]
3. Shivakumar, H.; Juluri, A.; Desai, B.; Murthy, S.N. Ungual and transungual drug delivery. *Drug Dev. Ind. Pharm.* **2012**, *38*, 901–911. [CrossRef] [PubMed]
4. Gupta, A.K.; Paquet, M. Improved efficacy in onychomycosis therapy. *Clin. Dermatol.* **2013**, *31*, 555–563. [CrossRef] [PubMed]
5. Elkeeb, R.; AliKhan, A.; Elkeeb, L.; Hui, X.; Maibach, H.I. Transungual drug delivery: Current status. *Int. J. Pharm.* **2010**, *384*, 1–8. [CrossRef] [PubMed]
6. Chiu, W.S.; Belsey, N.A.; Garrett, N.L.; Moger, J.; Price, G.J.; Delgado-Charro, M.B.; Guy, R.H. Drug delivery into microneedle-porated nails from nanoparticle reservoirs. *J. Control. Release* **2015**, *220*, 98–106. [CrossRef] [PubMed]
7. Prausnitz, M.R.; Langer, R. Transdermal drug delivery. *Nat. Biotechnol.* **2008**, *26*, 1261–1268. [CrossRef] [PubMed]
8. Wong, T.W. Electrical, magnetic, photomechanical and cavitational waves to overcome skin barrier for transdermal drug delivery. *J. Control. Release* **2014**, *193*, 257–269. [CrossRef] [PubMed]
9. Man, G.; Elias, P.M.; Man, M.-Q. Therapeutic benefits of enhancing permeability barrier for atopic eczema. *Dermatol. Sin.* **2015**, *33*, 84–89. [CrossRef]
10. Hu, L.; Man, H.; Elias, P.M.; Man, M.-Q. Herbal medicines that benefit epidermal permeability barrier function. *Dermatol. Sin.* **2015**, *33*, 90–95. [CrossRef]
11. Merino, V.; Escobar-Chávez, J.J. *Current Technologies to Increase the Transdermal Delivery of Drugs*; Bentham Science Publishers: Sharjah, United Arab Emirates, 2010.
12. Goswami, S.; Bajpai, J.; Bajpai, A. Designing gelatin nanocarriers as a swellable system for controlled release of insulin: An in vitro kinetic study. *J. Macromol. Sci. A* **2009**, *47*, 119–130. [CrossRef]
13. Van der Maaden, K.; Jiskoot, W.; Bouwstra, J. Microneedle technologies for (trans) dermal drug and vaccine delivery. *J. Control. Release* **2012**, *161*, 645–655. [CrossRef] [PubMed]
14. Tsioris, K.; Raja, W.K.; Pritchard, E.M.; Panilaitis, B.; Kaplan, D.L.; Omenetto, F.G. Fabrication of silk microneedles for controlled-release drug delivery. *Adv. Funct. Mater.* **2012**, *22*, 330–335. [CrossRef]
15. Smith, N.B. Perspectives on transdermal ultrasound mediated drug delivery. *Int. J. Nanomed.* **2007**, *2*, 585–594.
16. Azagury, A.; Khoury, L.; Enden, G.; Kost, J. Ultrasound mediated transdermal drug delivery. *Adv. Drug Del. Rev.* **2014**, *72*, 127–143. [CrossRef] [PubMed]
17. Bounoure, F.; Skiba, M.L.; Besnard, M.; Arnaud, P.; Mallet, E.; Skiba, M. Effect of iontophoresis and penetration enhancers on transdermal absorption of metopimazine. *J. Dermatol. Sci.* **2008**, *52*, 170–177. [CrossRef] [PubMed]
18. Escobar-Chavez, J.J.; Merino, V.; López-Cervantes, M.; Rodriguez-Cruz, I.M.; Quintanar-Guerrero, D.; Ganem-Quintanar, A. The use of iontophoresis in the administration of nicotine and new non-nicotine drugs through the skin for smoking cessation. *Curr. Drug Disc. Technol.* **2009**, *6*, 171–185. [CrossRef]
19. Jelínková, H. *Lasers for Medical Applications: Diagnostics, Therapy and Surgery*; Elsevier: Amsterdam, The Netherlands, 2013.
20. Stafford, R.J.; Fuentes, D.; Elliott, A.A.; Weinberg, J.S.; Ahrar, K. Laser-induced thermal therapy for tumor ablation. *Crit. Rev. Biomed. Eng.* **2010**, *38*, 79–100. [CrossRef] [PubMed]
21. Longo, C.; Galimberti, M.; De Pace, B.; Pellacani, G.; Bencini, P.L. Laser skin rejuvenation: Epidermal changes and collagen remodeling evaluated by in vivo confocal microscopy. *Laser Med. Sci.* **2013**, *28*, 769–776. [CrossRef] [PubMed]
22. Chung, S.H.; Mazur, E. Surgical Applications of femtosecond lasers. *J. Biophotonics* **2009**, *2*, 557–572. [CrossRef] [PubMed]
23. Garvie-Cook, H.; Stone, J.M.; Yu, F.; Guy, R.H.; Gordeev, S.N. Femtosecond pulsed laser ablation to enhance drug delivery across the skin. *J. Biophotonics* **2016**, *9*, 144–154. [CrossRef] [PubMed]

24. Lee, W.-R.; Shen, S.-C.; Al-Suwayeh, S.A.; Yang, H.-H.; Yuan, C.-Y.; Fang, J.-Y. Laser-assisted topical drug delivery by using a low-fluence fractional laser: Imiquimod and macromolecules. *J. Control. Release* **2011**, *153*, 240–248. [CrossRef] [PubMed]

25. Lim, E.-H.; Kim, H.-R.; Park, Y.-O.; Lee, Y.; Seo, Y.-J.; Kim, C.-D.; Lee, J.-H.; Im, M. Toenail onychomycosis treated with a fractional carbon-dioxide laser and topical antifungal cream. *J. Am. Acad. Dermatol.* **2014**, *70*, 918–923. [CrossRef] [PubMed]

26. Stumpp, O.F.; Bedi, V.P.; Wyatt, D.; Lac, D.; Rahman, Z.; Chan, K.F. In vivo confocal imaging of epidermal cell migration and dermal changes post nonablative fractional resurfacing: Study of the wound healing process with corroborated histopathologic evidence. *J. Biomed. Opt.* **2009**, *14*, 024018. [CrossRef] [PubMed]

27. Hanson, K.M.; Behne, M.J.; Barry, N.P.; Mauro, T.M.; Gratton, E.; Clegg, R.M. Two-photon fluorescence lifetime imaging of the skin stratum corneum pH Gradient. *Biophys. J.* **2002**, *83*, 1682–1690. [CrossRef]

28. Xiao, C.; Moore, D.J.; Rerek, M.E.; Flach, C.R.; Mendelsohn, R. Feasibility of tracking phospholipid permeation into skin using infrared and Raman microscopic imaging. *J. Investig. Dermatol.* **2005**, *124*, 622–632. [CrossRef] [PubMed]

29. Huang, D.; Swanson, E.A.; Lin, C.P.; Schuman, J.S.; Stinson, W.G.; Chang, W.; Hee, M.R.; Flotte, T.; Gregory, K.; Puliafito, C.A. Optical coherence tomography. *Science* **1991**, *254*, 1178–1181. [CrossRef] [PubMed]

30. Ahmad, A.; Shemonski, N.D.; Adie, S.G.; Kim, H.-S.; Hwu, W.-M.W.; Carney, P.S.; Boppart, S.A. Real-time in vivo computed optical interferometric tomography. *Nat. Photonics* **2013**, *7*, 444–448. [CrossRef] [PubMed]

31. Wu, C.T.; Tsai, M.T.; Lee, C.K. Two-level optical coherence tomography scheme for suppressing spectral saturation artifacts. *Sensors* **2014**, *14*, 13548–13555. [CrossRef] [PubMed]

32. Deka, G.; Wu, W.-W.; Kao, F.-J. In vivo wound healing diagnosis with second harmonic and fluorescence lifetime imaging. *J. Biomed. Opt.* **2013**, *18*, 061222. [CrossRef] [PubMed]

33. Yeh, A.T.; Kao, B.; Jung, W.G.; Chen, Z.P.; Nelson, J.S.; Tromberg, B.J. Imaging wound healing using optical coherence tomography and multiphoton microscopy in an in vitro skin-equivalent tissue model. *J. Biomed. Opt.* **2006**, *9*, 248–253. [CrossRef] [PubMed]

34. Cobb, M.J.; Chen, Y.; Underwood, R.A.; Usui, M.L.; Olerud, J.; Li, X.D. Noninvasive assessment of cutaneous wound healing using ultrahigh-resolution optical coherence tomography. *J. Biomed. Opt.* **2006**, *11*, 064002. [CrossRef] [PubMed]

35. Wang, H.; Baran, U.; Wang, R.K. In vivo blood flow imaging of inflammatory human skin induced by tape stripping using optical microangiography. *J. Biophotonics* **2015**, *8*, 265–272. [CrossRef] [PubMed]

36. Liu, G.; Jia, W.; Sun, V.; Choi, B.; Chen, Z. High-resolution imaging of microvasculature in human skin in vivo with optical coherence tomography. *Opt. Express* **2012**, *20*, 7694–7705. [CrossRef] [PubMed]

37. Sakai, S.; Yamanari, M.; Miyazawa, A.; Matsumoto, M.; Nakagawa, N.; Sugawara, T.; Kawabata, K.; Yatagai, T.; Yasuno, Y. In vivo three-dimensional birefringence analysis shows collagen differences between young and old photo-aged human skin. *J. Investig. Dermatol.* **2008**, *128*, 1641–1647. [CrossRef] [PubMed]

38. Sakai, S.; Yamanari, M.; Lim, Y.; Nakagawa, N.; Yasuno, Y. In vivo evaluation of human skin anisotropy by polarization-sensitive optical coherence tomography. *Biomed. Opt. Express* **2011**, *2*, 2623–2631. [CrossRef] [PubMed]

39. Nguyen, T.-M.; Song, S.; Arnal, B.; Huang, Z.; O'Donnell, M.; Wang, R.K. Visualizing ultrasonically induced shear wave propagation using phase-sensitive optical coherence tomography for dynamic elastography. *Opt. Lett.* **2014**, *39*, 838–841. [CrossRef] [PubMed]

40. Wang, S.; Larin, K.V. Optical Coherence Elastography for Tissue Characterization: A Review. *J. Biophotonics* **2015**, *8*, 279–302. [CrossRef] [PubMed]

41. Tsai, M.-T.; Yang, C.-H.; Shen, S.-C.; Lee, Y.-J.; Chang, F.-Y.; Feng, C.-S. Monitoring of wound healing process of human skin after fractional laser treatments with optical coherence tomography. *Biomed. Opt. Express* **2013**, *4*, 2362–2375. [CrossRef] [PubMed]

42. Yang, C.-H.; Tsai, M.-T.; Shen, S.-C.; Ng, C.Y.; Jung, S.-M. Feasibility of ablative fractional laser-assisted drug delivery with optical coherence tomography. *Biomed. Opt. Express* **2014**, *5*, 3949–3959. [CrossRef] [PubMed]

43. Mariampillai, A.; Standish, B.A.; Moriyama, E.H.; Khurana, M.; Munce, N.R.; Leung, M.K.; Jiang, J.; Cable, A.; Wilson, B.C.; Vitkin, I.A. Speckle variance detection of microvasculature using swept-source optical coherence tomography. *Opt. Lett.* **2008**, *33*, 1530–1532. [CrossRef] [PubMed]

44. Cadotte, D.W.; Mariampillai, A.; Cadotte, A.; Lee, K.K.; Kiehl, T.-R.; Wilson, B.C.; Fehlings, M.G.; Yang, V.X. Speckle variance optical coherence tomography of the rodent spinal cord: In vivo feasibility. *Biomed. Opt. Express* **2012**, *3*, 911–919. [CrossRef] [PubMed]

45. Lee, C.-K.; Tseng, H.-Y.; Lee, C.-Y.; Wu, S.-Y.; Chi, T.-T.; Yang, K.-M.; Chou, H.-Y.E.; Tsai, M.-T.; Wang, J.-Y.; Kiang, Y.-W. Characterizing the localized surface plasmon resonance behaviors of Au nanorings and tracking their diffusion in bio-tissue with optical coherence tomography. *Biomed. Opt. Express* **2010**, *1*, 1060–1074. [CrossRef] [PubMed]

46. Mahmud, M.S.; Cadotte, D.W.; Vuong, B.; Sun, C.; Luk, T.W.; Mariampillai, A.; Yang, V.X. Review of speckle and phase variance optical coherence tomography to visualize microvascular networks. *J. Biomed. Opt.* **2013**, *18*, 050901. [CrossRef] [PubMed]

47. Murthy, S.N.; Vaka, S.R.K.; Sammeta, S.M.; Nair, A.B. Transcreen-N™: Method for rapid screening of trans-ungual drug delivery enhancers. *J. Pharm. Sci.* **2009**, *98*, 4264–4271. [CrossRef] [PubMed]

48. Tsai, M.-T.; Yang, C.-H.; Shen, S.-C.; Chang, F.-Y.; Yi, J.-Y.; Fan, C.-H. Noninvasive characterization of fractional photothermolysis induced by ablative and non-ablative lasers with optical coherence tomography. *Laser Phys.* **2013**, *23*, 075604. [CrossRef]

49. Wijesinghe, R.E.; Lee, S.-Y.; Kim, P.; Jung, H.-Y.; Jeon, M.; Kim, J. Optical Inspection and Morphological Analysis of Diospyros kaki Plant Leaves for the Detection of Circular Leaf Spot Disease. *Sensors* **2016**, *16*, 1282. [CrossRef] [PubMed]

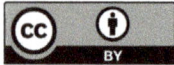

sensors

MDPI

Article

Optical Methods in Fingerprint Imaging for Medical and Personality Applications

Chia-Nan Wang [1,*], **Jing-Wein Wang** [2,*], **Ming-Hsun Lin** [1,*], **Yao-Lang Chang** [1,*] and **Chia-Ming Kuo** [1]

[1]   Industrial Engineering and Management, National Kaohsiung University of Applied Sciences, Kaohsiung 80778, Taiwan; chungys@fotech.edu.tw
[2]   Institute of Photonics and Communications, National Kaohsiung University of Applied Sciences, Kaohsiung 80778, Taiwan
*   Correspondence: cn.wang@kuas.edu.tw (C.-N.W.); jwwang@kuas.edu.tw (J.-W.W.); newfife711365@gmail.com (M.-H.L.); kc88899@gmail.com (Y.-L.C.); Tel.: +886-7-381-4526 (C.-N.W.)

Received: 30 August 2017; Accepted: 20 October 2017; Published: 23 October 2017

Abstract: Over the years, analysis and induction of personality traits has been a topic for individual subjective conjecture or speculation, rather than a focus of inductive scientific analysis. This study proposes a novel framework for analysis and induction of personality traits. First, 14 personality constructs based on the "Big Five" personality factors were developed. Next, a new fingerprint image algorithm was used for classification, and the fingerprints were classified into eight types. The relationship between personality traits and fingerprint type was derived from the results of the questionnaire survey. After comparison of pre-test and post-test results, this study determined the induction ability of personality traits from fingerprint type. Experimental results showed that the left/right thumbprint type of a majority of subjects was left loop/right loop and that the personalities of individuals with this fingerprint type were moderate with no significant differences in the 14 personality constructs.

Keywords: personality traits; fingerprint classification; fingerprint types

---

1. Introduction

Understanding the personality traits of one's self and others contributes to harmonious interpersonal relationships. However, getting to know one's self and others in a short period of time is not an easy task, and inducing the personality traits of others is an even more difficult undertaking. In the Western world, studies on personality traits have a long and broad history [1]. Many related studies have since followed, but the number of proposed personality characteristics has remained high. It was for this reason that Cattell [2] converted these characteristics into 16 types of personality factor questionnaires. Later, Fiske [3] performed a follow-up verification of Cattell's research and derived the "Big Five" personality dimensions. In 1963, Norman [4] verified Cattell's procedures and announced that the five major factors constituted a reasonable method of personality classification.

Research on personality traits is core to many major disciplines, such as medicine, psychology and corporate management, whether for theoretical investigation or practical application [5]. Personality traits stem from a consistent behavioral model and internal processes within each individual, allowing the individual to identify with a consistent behavioral model in different situations. The internal processes of personality traits include emotions, motivation and cognition. Although these processes occur at a deep level, they influence human behavior and feelings [6]. Additionally, other studies have attempted to classify individuals into different personality types [7]. For hundreds of years, the Chinese people have used physiognomy, palmistry (the ridges on the skin of the palm), bone reading and other methods related to physiological features to divulge an individual's personality traits and fortune. To date, however, there are no studies that support a relationship between personality traits and fingerprints, which are an individually unique physiological feature.

Two features of fingerprints that are particularly important: (1) fingerprints do not change with time; and (2) every individual's fingerprints are unique [8]. Due to the above-described two characteristics, fingerprints have long been used for identification purposes [9,10]. Medina-Pérez proposed a new feature representation containing clockwise-arranged minutiae without a central minutia, a new similarity measure that shifted the triplets to find the best minutiae correspondence, and a global matching procedure that selected the alignment by maximizing the amount of global matching minutiae [11]. In comparison with six verification algorithms, the proposed method achieved the highest accuracy in the lowest matching time. Ballan and Gurgen [12] presented a method for fingerprint recognition based on principal component analysis and point patterns (minutiae) obtained from the directional histograms of a fingerprint. This study gave the same performance as that of the uncompressed data, but reduced computation. Yang et al. used fusion to enhance the biometric performance in template-protected biometric systems [13]. They investigated several scenarios (multi-sample, multi-instance, multi-sensor, multi-algorithm and their combinations) on the binary decision level and evaluated the performance and fusion efficiency on a multi-sensor fingerprint database with 71,994 samples. Fingerprint image quality improvement was proposed in [14]. The algorithm consists of two stages. The first stage is decomposing the input fingerprint image into four sub-bands by applying the two -dimensional discrete wavelet transform. At the second stage, the compensated image is produced by adaptively obtaining the compensation coefficient for each sub-band based on the referenced Gaussian template. The method concluded an improved clarity, quality and continuity of ridge structures, and therefore, the accuracy is also increased. Background and the blurred region of fingerprint images are also removed. Bartunek et al. [15] presented several improvements to an adaptive fingerprint enhancement method that is based on contextual filtering. Based on the global analysis and the matched filtering blocks, different forms of order statistical filters were applied. These processing blocks yield an improved and adaptive fingerprint image processing method. Yang et al. [16] proposed a novel and effective two-stage enhancement scheme in both the spatial domain and the frequency domain by learning from the underlying images. They first enhanced the fingerprint image in the spatial domain with a spatial ridge-compensation filter by learning from the images. With the help of the first step, the second stage filter, i.e., a frequency band-pass filter that was separable in the radial and angular frequency domains was employed. The experimental result showed that their algorithm is able to handle various input image contexts and achieves better results compared with some state-of-the-art algorithms over public databases and is able to improve the performances of fingerprint-authentication systems.

Fingerprints are closely related to genetics [17]; however, in the fields of biostatics and psychology, there are currently no studies indicating any relationship between fingerprints and personality traits. Therefore, using fingerprints to induce personality traits is an undeveloped area in scientific research. If the corresponding relationship between fingerprints and personality traits could be determined, this would be an important contribution to science. Since personality traits have a certain degree of stability, continuity and uniqueness and the left/right hand fingerprints of each person are unique, the relationship between these two features is a worthwhile topic for in-depth research. The Big Five personalities have generated substantial interest among personality researchers [3]. The Big Five is a model based on common language descriptors of personality. When factor analysis (a statistical technique) is applied to personality survey data, some words used to describe aspects of personality are often applied to the same person. These five factors are openness to experience (inventive/curious), conscientiousness (efficient/organized), extraversion (outgoing/energetic), agreeableness (friendly/compassionate) and neuroticism (sensitive/nervous).

The purpose in this study is to evaluate the generalizability of Big Five personality factor inventories as inducers of a common set of criteria, criteria representing classes of left and right thumb fingerprints. By assessing people using multiple criterion variables to measure the Big Five personality constructs, the same measure results normally will have the same personality constructs. If the Big Five inventories are all designed to measure equivalent dimensions of personality, then they should show a nontrivial amount of agreement in the variables they are able to induce. Constructing valid measures of personality variables should induce fingerprint classes, assuming those classes have personality determinants. This is especially true of Big Five inventories because those factors are presumed to account for most of the personality-based variation in fingerprints.

This study used classification technology to derive eight fingerprint types and combined these with questionnaire survey results to construct a new "System for Induction of Personality Traits from Fingerprints". Following the research of Costa and McCare [18], this study also summarized 14 personality constructs with Eigen values greater than one from the "Big Five" personality factors. We performed a principal components analysis of the data and found 14 components with Eigen values larger than one. Then, we created 14 scales each comprised of one of the 14 groups of items indicating the 14 components with Eigen values larger than one. The prototype of this system was modified and completed based on the fingerprints and questionnaire feedback of 362 test subjects. This study recruited a separate group of 351 subjects for the live testing of the system. The experimental results showed that the thumbprint types of the left and right hands were correlated with personality traits. Subjects in the left loop/right loop fingerprint category accounted for the largest group (41.8%). The second largest group was the S-type/S-type (twin loop/twin loop) type (13.5%), followed by the eddy/eddy type (12.1%). The personality traits of the latter two groups showed significant differences in some constructs.

Whilst better known in medication, double blind experiments are adopted in this paper. Surveys with questionnaires are used to keep credibility so the chance of observer's bias can be minimized. The framework of the following sections in this paper is as follows: Section 2: research framework and flow figure, expansion of the "Big Five" personality factors into 14 constructs, design of the personality traits questionnaire and the "System for Induction of Personality Traits from Fingerprints"; Section 3: statistical analysis and post-test verification of the survey results on the relationship between personality traits and finger classification; Section 4: conclusions.

2. Research Methods

2.1. Research Framework

The "Big Five" personality factors are advanced global factors that describe human personality, and the 16 personality factors are basic primary factors. This study summarized the questionnaire results after analysis of both global and primary factors. From these data, 14 personality constructs appropriate for describing the personalities of the test subjects were designed. A questionnaire was designed based on the 14 personality constructs. Along with the implementation of the questionnaire survey, an optical fingerprint machine of SecuGen Hamster Plus [19] was used to capture the left/right thumbprints of the test subjects. The fingerprint sensor features smart capture technology and switches on the scanner whenever it detects a finger. Thumb samples of both hands are collected, where 282 participants are mostly university students, and their ages are within the interval from 18 to 50 years old. The biometric data were collected in different periods within 3 months. A new fingerprint classification algorithm was used for fingerprint categorization. After relationship analysis of fingerprint types and the 14 personality constructs, this study compiled a table of associations between the eight fingerprint types and the 14 personality constructs. To verify the accuracy of the association table, this study performed post-testing with different subjects. After the questionnaire survey and fingerprinting had been re-conducted, this study modified the content of the association table. The conclusions of this study were formed after discussion of the pretest and posttest results. Figure 1 illustrates the framework and flow of this research.

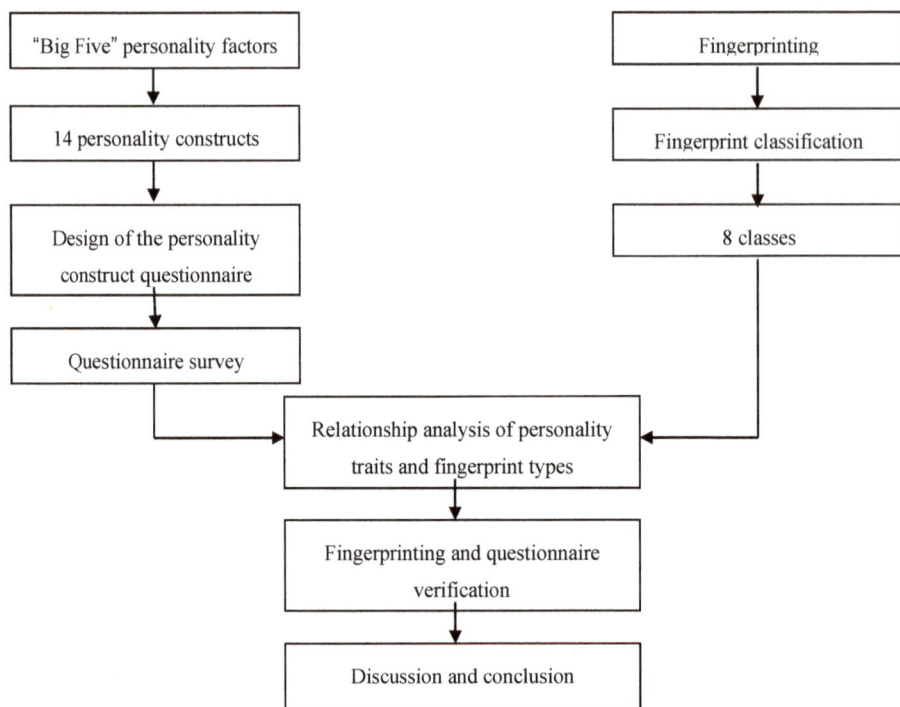

Figure 1. Research framework and flowchart.

2.2. The 14 Constructs of Personality

The "Big Five" personality factors, which have been analyzed and verified by Norman [4], Goldberg [20] and McCrae and Costa [21], are as follows: neuroticism, extraversion, openness, agreeableness and conscientiousness. This study referred to the Big Five personality factors and the 16 personality factors, summarized the questionnaire results according to the personality scores of test subjects and designed a personality trait questionnaire composed of the 14 personality constructs. Neuroticism is the tendency of an individual to experience anxiety or nervousness. This study sub-divided neuroticism into sentimentalism, impulsiveness and strong self-esteem. Extraversion refers to the characteristics and strength of an individual in interpersonal interaction. This study sub-divided extraversion into activeness and passivity. Openness refers to the degree of risk that an individual can accept with regard to new things. This study sub-divided openness into enthusiastic attitude and good money concept. Agreeableness refers to the cognition, affection and attitude displayed by an individual toward various situations or matters. This study sub-divided agreeableness into socially harmonious methods of operation, concern for others' well-being and impatience. Conscientiousness refers to the determination and self-discipline of an individual. This study sub-divided conscientiousness into strong sense of responsibility, slow method of operation, focused attention and strong leadership ability. Table 1 describes the 14 personality constructs in detail.

Table 1. Fourteen constructs of personality.

14 Constructs of Personality	Description of Constructs
Sentimentalism	Emotionally sensitive and easily becomes sentimental; emotionally vulnerable to external stimuli and reveals true feelings.
Impulsiveness	The link that precedes the conversion of one's feelings, perception and thoughts into actions: the desire before the action. The word 'rash' is commonly used to describe such actions that were not previously thought out.
Strong self-esteem	Maintains self-respect and dignity; does not allow discrimination, stigmatization or attack from others.
Liveliness	Refers to the *qi* (energy flow or vitalism) exhibited by an individual; lively people drive the surrounding atmosphere, influence people around them and attract more attention in a group.
Passivity	Always keeps personal opinions and decisions to one's self; does not take the initiative to directly express one's self, but is always waiting for the other person to ask.
Positive attitude	Enthusiasm is a type of outward manifestation of desire; whether the job is actually well done is considered secondary. It is a type of zeal, an attitude of full immersion without distraction.
Good money concept	Ensures that expenditure matches income and avoids debt; considers one's status and position when spending money to select products that are appropriate for one's self.
Socially harmonious method of operation	Behaves appropriately, does not openly offend others, is concerned that matters reach a socially harmonious and satisfactory conclusion.
Concern for others' well-being	Puts one's self in others' shoes and considers others in any situation; an attitude of "not doing unto others what you would not want done unto yourself".
Impatience	Unsettled and irritable behavior when facing situations that require waiting or delay.
Strong sense of responsibility	Fulfills one's obligations regarding any matter; is always aware of possible consequences no matter how great or small the matter and is able to assume one's proper responsibility.
Slow method of operation	Is slow and calm in any situation; gives others the impression of a slow and unconcerned attitude.
Focused attention	Is not easily influenced by the external environment when working or engaging in various matters.
Strong leadership ability	Plays the role of a leader in groups; is good at organizing/assigning tasks and coordinating interpersonal relationships; provides a team with sufficient centripetal force.

2.3. Fingerprint Classification

The actual number of different types of human fingerprints is currently unknown; however, a majority of studies use the five main categories proposed by Henry [22]: Right loop, left loop, tented arch, arch and whorl. This study used an optical fingerprinting machine to capture original images of fingerprints. These original images are often accompanied by deformation caused by problems such as dry, wet, damaged or scarred fingerprints and uneven application of force by the fingerprinting machine when capturing the image. Therefore, enhancement of the images is essential [23]. Fingerprint classification is a coarse level method of partitioning a fingerprint database into smaller subsets, which reduces the search space of a large database. To determine the class of the query fingerprint, only search templates with the same class as the query were used. Inputs are the fingerprint impressions from right and left thumb fingers of an individual. If the size of the database is n and c is the number of classes, the search space without classification is n^2. With fingerprint classification, the search space with classification is n/c. We made an extensive study of the occurrence of fingerprints and indexed them into eight major classes as shown in Figure 2.

After using histogram specification and ridge/valley energy analysis, this study performed energy image projection analysis in eight different directions at an angle of 45° to capture fingerprint regions of interest (ROI). Through the above-described methods, this study classified fingerprint into four categories. They are whorl (plain whorl), S-type (double-loop whorl), eddy (accidental whorl) and balloon (central pocket loop whorl). To accurately trace flow lines to determine fingerprint type, this study used the Poincare index-based modified hierarchical singularity detection algorithm after orientation field estimation to detect the location of singularity. The three-stage pyramid singularity detection algorithm designed by this study can accurately locate the point of singularity through progressively narrowing the detection range. Lastly, after initial type selection had been performed based on the number and type (delta, core point) of the singular points, fingerprint classification was conducted by tracing the flow of the orientation field surrounding the point of singularity and establishing related rules of judgement. This study is interested in finding the exact location of the core point defined by the Henry system and therefore traces the skeletonized ridge curves with 8-adjacency to explore wavelet extrema at one-pixel increments by starting at 10 pixels apart from two sides. The highest extrema in the ridge curve corresponds to the candidate of the core point. We devise two 8-adjacency grids to locate the wavelet extrema. Beginning from two opposite ends and moving toward the center of the sub-region, the black-color pixel of each grid is designated as the central point to trace. Based on this central point, the moving guideline is as follows: if the gray-level of the adjacent pixel is 0, then move toward that pixel, where the number shown in the grid indicates the moving sequence. This method makes it possible to follow the real track of the ridge curve. Whenever a singularity is detected, its location is noted. It is common to have multiple findings of the core point candidate with small vertical displacements, and the area underneath the lowest ridge curve is circumscribed for locating the core point. In the Henry system, the exact core point location can be performed as follows: (a) locate the topmost extrema in the innermost ridge curve, if there is no rod; (b) otherwise, locate the top of the rods. The final eight categories derived are as follows (see Figure 2): right loop, left loop, arch, tented arch, whorl (plain whorl), S-type (double-loop whorl), eddy (accidental whorl) and balloon (central pocket loop whorl).

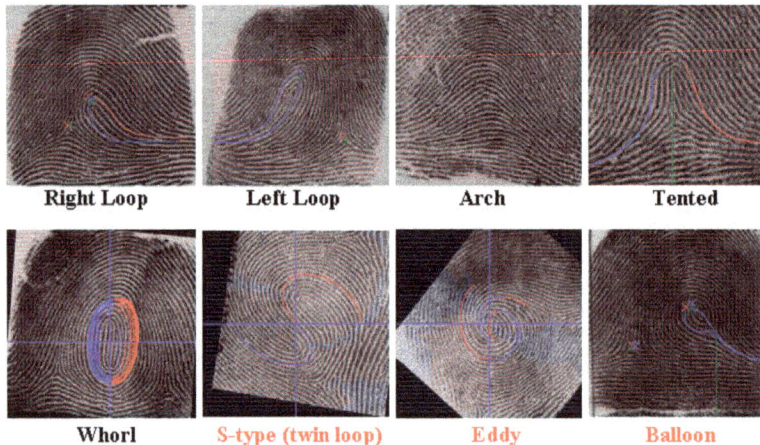

Figure 2. The eight fingerprint types.

2.4. Questionnaire Design and Survey

This study designed a questionnaire with 74 closed questions since there is no measure of personality and fingerprint available. Since the 74 closed questions are many, this study does not provide all question items in this study. The 74 questions followed the 14 different personality constructs [18]. Each construct had at least 3 questions prepared by this study to confirm the results of respondents. However, this study also designed the reliability analysis and validation analysis for verifying the questionnaire design and post-test verification for final result checking. Based on reliability analysis and validation analysis, we confirmed that our questionnaire has the right dimensionality and composition. After factor analysis, the recovered questionnaire data were used to develop 14 personality constructs. The information collected from the questionnaire, along with the left/right thumbprints taken from the test subjects, was used in conjunction with the personality constructs to derive the relationship between fingerprint type and personality traits. A 5-point Likert scale was used for the personality trait questionnaire; 1–5 points were respectively assigned to the options of strongly disagree, disagree, neither agree, nor disagree, agree and strongly agree.

Sampling in this study was conducted via the following steps:

1. Research targets: The use of fingerprints involves personal privacy issues, and the agreement of the respondent with regard to using his/her fingerprints for research is difficult to obtain. Thus, for the sake of convenience in collecting information, this study used non-probability proportional sampling methods and selected the National Kaohsiung University of Applied Sciences at Taiwan as the site for questionnaire distribution. The main respondent targets were students in the Department of Industrial Management, Continuing Education Division.

2. Questionnaire response process: The process of filling out the questionnaires proceeded according to classes (as units) and was arranged according to students' class hours. After the left/right thumbprints of the respondents had been collected into the fingerprint classification system, the questionnaires were filled out.

3. Results: This study distributed 362 questionnaires. After the questionnaires had been collected and any invalid questionnaires removed, the number of valid questionnaires was 282, resulting in a valid recovery rate of 75.4%. After the average value of the questions in each construct had been processed, these data were used for the final score of each respondent.

2.5. Statistical Analysis and Testing

Reliability analysis: This study used Cronbach's α [24] to measure the reliability of the questionnaire. According to the research of DeVellis [25], a reliability coefficient value of 0.7 and up is acceptable. The overall Cronbach's α value for the 74 items in this questionnaire was 0.799, indicating that this questionnaire had high reliability. The Cronbach's α value for the 14 constructs also exceeded 0.7, indicating the reliability of the data. The Cronbach's α value of individual constructs of sentimentalism, impulsiveness, strong self-esteem, liveliness, passivity, positive attitude, good money concept, socially harmonious method of operation, concern for others' well-being, impatience, strong sense of responsibility, slow method of operation, focused attention and strong leadership ability are 0.797, 0.786, 0.793, 0.771, 0.829, 0.770, 0.792, 0.783, 0.764, 0.795, 0.776, 0.808, 0.804 and 0.771, respectively.

Validity analysis: Validity is the degree to which the questionnaire accurately measures what it is intended to measure; in other words, the degree to which it reaches the goals of measurement. This study used factor analysis to obtain the total variance explained by the questionnaire, and this value was used to measure validity. However, Sharma [26] advised against relying solely on the results of Bartlett's test of sphericity to determine whether data are suitable for factor analysis, because the validity of Bartlett's test of sphericity is easily influenced by sample size. Therefore, this study mainly used the Kaiser–Meyer–Olkin (KMO) measure and Bartlett's test of sphericity to determine whether the data were suitable for factor analysis. The KMO coefficient was used to measure whether each variable had sampling adequacy. A KMO coefficient of 0.9 and up was considered upper level, 0.8–0.89 was considered moderate level and lower than 0.5 was an unacceptable level. The KMO and Barlett test results show that KMO = 0.536, indicating that the data in this study were in an acceptable range with regard to sampling adequacy. Bartlett's test of sphericity also reached a level of significance ($p < 0.001$), indicating that the data were suitable for factor analysis. The number of factors in factor analysis could have been determined by the relationship of the 74 questionnaire items. This study used principal component analysis for repeated estimation until the estimation of commonalities converged. Varimax was then used for rotation. The analysis results showed that the Eigen value of 14 questions exceeded 1, and the total explainable variance was 74.75%, surpassing the minimum requirement of 50%. Therefore, this study used these 14 factors as personality constructs.

3. Experimental Results

This study recovered 282 valid questionnaires. Initial results indicated that in left/right hand fingerprint types, the right hand fingerprints did not show arch type; arch type was also not found in some of the left hand fingerprints. Among the fingerprint types, the left loop/right loop type accounted for the largest group of test subjects (118 subjects), followed by the S-type/S-type (38 subjects), eddy/eddy type (34 subjects) and whorl/whorl type (28 subjects). The summary of type numbers is shown in Table 2 and Figure 3. In the questionnaire, 1–5 points each were assigned to the Likert scale options (strongly disagree, disagree, neither agree, nor disagree, agree, strongly agree). This study calculated the mean and standard deviation of each of the 14 personality constructs. Based on the responses on Likert items, this study derived the interrelationship between fingerprint type and personality construct; for details, please see Table 3.

Table 2. Fingerprint type number summary.

Fingerprint Type	Left Loop	Right Loop	Tent	Arch	Whorl	Eddy Loop	S-type	Balloon
Left Loop	2	118	2	0	6	2	6	0
Right Loop	0	0	0	0	2	0	0	0
Tent	0	0	0	0	0	0	0	0
Arch	0	0	0	0	2	0	0	2
Whorl	0	2	0	0	28	2	0	0
Eddy loop	0	4	0	0	10	34	0	0
S-type	0	2	0	0	0	14	38	2
Balloon	0	0	0	0	0	0	0	4

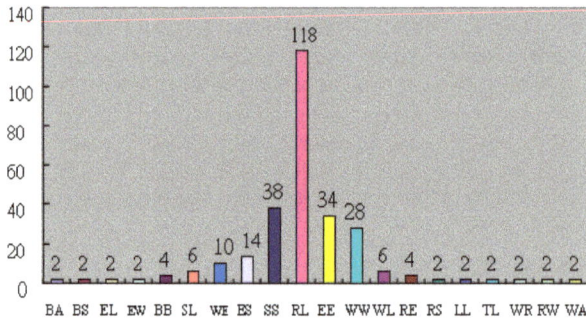

Figure 3. Fingerprint type statistics. BA: Balloon/Arch; BS: Balloon/S-type; EL: Eddy Loop/Left Loop; EW: Eddy Loop/Whorl; BB: Balloon/Balloon; SL: S-type/Left Loop; WE: Whorl/Eddy Loop; ES: Eddy Loop/S-type; SS: S-type/S-type; RL: Right Loop/Left Loop; EE: Eddy Loop/Eddy Loop; WW: Whorl/Whorl; WL: Whorl/Left Loop; RE: Right Loop/Eddy Loop; RS: Right Loop/S-type; LL: Left Loop/Left Loop; TL: Tent/Left Loop; WR: Whorl/Right Loop; RW: Right Loop/Whorl; WA: Whorl/Arch.

Table 3 shows that S-type/right Loop had the highest overall average in the 14 constructs, indicating that subjects with this fingerprint type demonstrated significant inclination in personality traits. The overall average of arch/whorl was the second highest in the 14 constructs, particularly with regard to the traits of "socially harmonious method of operation", "concern for others' well-being", "enthusiastic attitude" and "strong sense of responsibility"; the overall average in terms of these four constructs even exceeded that of S-type/right loop. This indicated that individuals with this fingerprint type have outstanding leadership qualities. Additionally, to summarize the distribution trend of fingerprint type and personality constructs, a sample distributed clustering image of fingerprint type and personality traits is shown in Figure 4, using four of the fingerprint types that accounted for a higher number of subjects and two personality traits. This is a sample distributed chart of personality traits based on fingerprint type, using four of the fingerprint types that accounted for a number of subjects and two personality traits (1–5 points each were assigned to the Likert scale options).

Table 3. Fingerprint types and personality constructs.

Fingerprint Type/Personality	Socially Harmonious Method of Operation	Sentimentalism	Liveliness	Concern for Others' Well-Being	Strong Self-Esteem	Impatience	Impulsiveness	Positive Attitude	Strong Sense of Responsibility	Slow Method of Operation	Passivity	Focused Attention	Strong Leadership Ability	Good Money Concept
Left Loop/Right Loop	△	△	△	△	△	△	△	△	△	△	△	△	△	△
Whorl/Right Loop	X	X	○	△	△	△	X	X	△	X	△	X	X	○
Eddy/Right Loop	X	○	△	△	○	○	○	○	○	○	○	△	○	○
S-type/Right Loop	○	△	X	△	○	○	X	X	X	X	○	X	X	X
Left Loop/Left Loop	○	X	○	△	○	X	○	X	○	X	○	X	X	○
Left Loop/Tent	X	○	○	X	△	△	○	X	X	○	○	X	○	○
Right Loop/Whorl	○	△	X	○	△	△	X	X	X	○	X	X	X	X
Left Loop/Whorl	○	△	△	○	△	△	X	○	△	○	X	○	X	X
Arch/Whorl	△	△	○	△	X	△	△	○	△	X	X	X	○	△
Whorl/Whorl	△	△	X	△	○	△	○	△	△	△	X	X	△	X
Eddy/Whorl	○	△	○	△	○	△	X	△	X	○	X	○	○	○
Left Loop/Eddy	△	△	X	△	○	△	△	△	○	X	△	△	△	X
Whorl/Eddy	X	○	X	△	○	○	X	X	○	△	○	△	△	○
Eddy/Eddy	○	X	○	△	△	△	△	X	X	X	△	X	△	○
S-type/Eddy	△	△	○	X	X	○	○	X	X	△	△	X	△	○
Left Loop/S-type	X	△	X	X	X	△	△	X	△	X	X	X	X	○
S-type/S-type	△	X	△	X	△	○	X	△	△	○	△	△	△	○
Arch/Balloon	△	△	○	X	○	△	X	X	△	X	○	X	△	○
S-type/balloon	△	X	X	X	○	X	X	△	△	X	○	○	△	X
Balloon/Balloon	X	○	X	X	○	X	X	X	X	X	△	X	X	X

△ = within the interval; X = left of the interval (less than 3.6169); ○ = right of the interval (more than 3.8215).

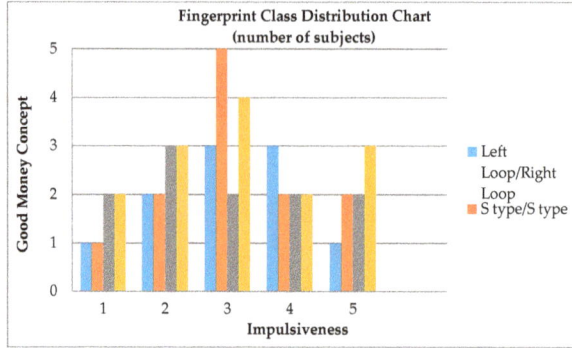

Figure 4. A sample distributed chart of personality traits.

4. Discussions

This study used the statistical concept of interval estimation to determine the personality traits corresponding to different fingerprint types. Using the construct of "socially harmonious method of operation" as an example: this study first calculated the average ($\overline{X} = 3.721$) and standard deviation (S = 0.6307) of this construct in the 282 questionnaires collected and then calculated the 95% confidence interval for the mean: $3.6169 \leq \mu \leq 3.8215$. The researchers then determined whether the average of the personality traits corresponding to each fingerprint type fell within the interval. The results of the interval estimation are shown in Table 3.

4.1. Post-Test Verification I

The purpose of verifying the questionnaire was to test the accuracy level of the system. Verification of the questionnaire consisted of three parts: The first part was a simple personality trait questionnaire consisting of 15 questions; the second part was fingerprinting; and the third part was the test subjects' rating of the accuracy level of the system. The assessment options were extremely inaccurate to extremely accurate (1–10 points). The process of questionnaire verification was as follows: After test subjects had filled in the personality trait questionnaire, their left/right thumbprints were taken. Fingerprint classification was used to determine personality constructs. Test subjects then rated the accuracy level of the system according to their personality construct placement. This study distributed 56 verification questionnaires in total and recovered 45 valid questionnaires, making a recovery rate of 80.34%. Initial results showed that only 12 fingerprint types had been obtained, among which left loop/right loop accounted for the highest proportion. The number summary of fingerprint type is shown in Table 4. Table 4 shows that the left loop/right loop accounted for the highest proportion (14 subjects), followed by eddy/eddy (nine subjects), S-type/S-type (six subjects) and whorl/whorl (five subjects). This study used the concept of interval estimation on the fingerprint type data collected, to determine the relationship between fingerprint type and personality constructs, as shown in Table 5.

Table 4. Fingerprint types number summary and proportions.

Fingerprint Type	Amount	Fingerprint Type	Amount	Fingerprint Type	Amount
Left Loop/Right Loop	14	Left Loop/Whorl	2	S-type/Eddy	1
Whorl/Right Loop	1	Whorl/Whorl	5	Left Loop/S-type	1
Eddy/Right Loop	2	Eddy/Whorl	2	S-type/S-type	6
Left Loop/Tent	1	Eddy/Eddy	9	Balloon/Balloon	1

Table 5. Relationship between fingerprint type and personality traits.

	Socially Harmonious Method of Operation	Sentimentalism	Liveliness	Concern for Others' Well-Being	Strong Self-Esteem	Impatience	Impulsiveness	Positive Attitude	Strong Sense of Responsibility	Slow Method of Operation	Passivity	Focused Attention	Strong Leadership Ability	Good Money Concept
Left Loop/Right Loop	△	△	△	△	△	△	△	○	△	△	△	△	△	×
Whorl/Right Loop	×	×	○	×	×	△	○	×	○	×	△	×	×	○
Eddy/Right Loop	○	△	△	○	×	△	○	×	×	△	×	×	△	○
Left Loop/Tent	○	○	△	×	○	△	○	△	△	△	×	×	△	×
Left Loop/Whorl	△	△	△	×	×	×	○	○	△	×	×	×	○	△
Whorl/Whorl	×	△	△	△	○	○	○	○	×	△	×	△	△	○
Vortex/Whorl	○	△	○	○	○	△	△	○	○	△	○	○	△	△
Vortex/Vortex	○	×	△	△	○	×	△	×	○	△	×	○	△	○
S-type/Eddy	○	○	△	×	×	×	×	△	○	×	×	△	×	×
Left Loop/S-type	△	×	×	△	△	×	△	×	×	△	×	○	△	×
S-type/S-type	△	×	×	△	△	△	△	×	△	△	×	△	△	×
Balloon/Balloon	×	○	△	○	○	△	○	△	×	○	×	×	×	○

Discrepancy between pre-test and post-test shown in the highlighted cell, △ = within the interval; × = left of the interval; ○ = right of the interval.

Table 5 shows that some of the verification questionnaire results regarding personality traits that correspond to fingerprint types differ from the pre-test questionnaire results (Table 3). There are some discrepancies between pre-test and post-test. We amended the legend as the discrepancy between pre-test and post-test shown in the highlighted cell. Possible reasons for these differences are summarized below:

1. Insufficient sample number (subjects): Obtaining test subjects for the post-test verification was difficult, resulting in a small sample number. This may have caused some errors in the process of using interval estimation to determine corresponding personality traits, producing some differences in the results.
2. Insufficient number of samples for different fingerprint types: This study noticed that the number of samples for certain fingerprint types, such as whorl/right loop and left loop/S-type, was very few. The pre-test results and the verification results show that the number of samples obtained for some fingerprint types was very few; this insufficient sample number may have produced error in the process of summarizing results. By contrast, the amount of samples collected in the pre-test and verification processes for certain fingerprint types such as left loop/right loop, whorl/whorl and eddy/eddy, is significantly higher than others. In the verification process, the results of personality traits corresponding to these four fingerprint types were significantly more consistent as compared to other fingerprint types.

This study used the mean confidence interval to determine whether the differences between the pre-test results and those of post-test verification were significant. In view of the individual uniqueness of fingerprints, this study assumed that fingerprint types were mutually independent. Below is a simple explanation using the fingerprint type left loop/right loop and the construct "socially harmonious way of operation":

Pre-test questionnaire: $n_1 = 59$, $\overline{X_1} = 3.65$, $S_1 = 0.665$; verification questionnaire: $n_2 = 14$, $\overline{X_2} = 3.44$, $S_2 = 0.8644$; these data were used for a mean difference test ($\alpha = 0.05$). The resulting mean difference confidence interval was $[-0.2736, 0.6936]$, and the 95% confidence interval included zero; therefore, we can assume that there is no significant difference between the pre-test and post-test results for the fingerprint type left loop/right loop and the construct "socially harmonious method of operation".

4.2. Post-Test Verification II

This study randomly sampled interested participants as subjects for this test. Following the test, participants filled out an accuracy questionnaire on their degree of satisfaction with using fingerprint types to analyze personality traits. There were 306 participants in this test. With the inclusion of the 45 valid questionnaires recovered from Post-Test Verification I, this totals to 351 results for the accuracy survey. The average was 7.1268, and the mode was eight. This means that subjects rated the accuracy of the system developed by this study at more than 70%. The results of the accuracy survey are shown in Table 6. This study used the above data for hypothesis testing. Because researchers wished to determine whether the outcome significantly exceeded the median (5), the null hypothesis was H0: $\mu \leq 6$, and the alternative hypothesis was H1: $\mu > 6$. The test result was 9.7. At the $\alpha = 0.001$ level of significance, the mean was shown to significantly exceed six. Therefore, we can infer that the results obtained from this system were very accurate.

Table 6. Results of the accuracy survey.

Mean	7.126801153	Minimum	1
Standard error	0.116532499	Maximum	10
Standard deviation	2.170759935	Total	2473
Variance	4.712198697	Number of results	351
Mode	8	Median	8

5. Conclusions

Analysis and accurate induction of personality traits is extremely valuable in both daily life and academic research. This study designed 14 personality constructs and implemented the questionnaire survey and fingerprinting through innovative fingerprint classification technology. Through comparison of pre-test and post-test results, this study realized the induction ability of personality traits from fingerprint type. Detailed conclusions are as follows:

1. Validity and reliability analysis showed that personality traits and fingerprint type are statistically correlated. Additionally, more than 70% of subjects were satisfied with the accuracy of the results of personality trait induction.

2. The results of the relationship between personality trait and fingerprint type showed that subjects with the left loop/right loop fingerprint type accounted for the largest proportion and were more moderate in terms of personality traits. In other words, subjects with this fingerprint type did not exhibit any especially prominent personality trait in the 14 constructs. The overall average of S-type/left loop was the highest among the 14 personality constructs, indicating that subjects with this fingerprint type had generally obvious personality traits. Arch/whorl had the second highest overall average in the 14 personality constructs, particularly in the constructs of "socially harmonious method of operation" (5.00), "strong sense of responsibility" (4.83), "enthusiastic attitude" (4.50) and "concern for others' well-being" (4.11). In these four constructs, the overall average of arch/whorl exceeded that of S-type/right loop, indicating that subjects with this fingerprint type had strong leadership qualities.

3. Among the 20 left/right fingerprint types derived from fingerprint classification, four fingerprint types accounted for a majority of subjects. The type accounting for the highest proportion was left loop/right loop (pre-test: 42%, Post-Test Verification I: 34%), followed by eddy/eddy (pre-test: 14.29%, Post-Test Verification I: 12%); S-type/S-type (pre-test 13.74%, Post-Test Verification I: 13%) and whorl/whorl (pre-test: 10.44%, Post-Test Verification I: 10%).

4. In the process of investigating fingerprint type, this study found an additional three fingerprint types apart from the five known types: S-type, eddy and balloon. This is a new discovery in fingerprint classification. With regard to accuracy, the classification accuracy of the eight fingerprint types reached 89.76%.

Research on personality traits, whether in terms of theoretical or practical application, is a key topic in modern research domains. Accurate induction of personality traits is a field of human research that not only urgently requires development, but also offers high practical value in such circumstances as schools selecting suitable students or corporations recruiting suitable personnel. Fingerprints are a unique human biological characteristic. This study is the first to propose a method of using fingerprint type to induce personality traits, as well as to verify the effectiveness of this method. Future research can build on the results of this study and expand research on fingerprint type to other areas, such as the relationship between fingerprint type and learning ability or the industries to which individuals with different fingerprint types are more suited. Moreover, more samples need to be prepared to study in this field to verify the original results and discover new findings.

Acknowledgments: This research was supported in part by MOST 106-2221-E-151-030 from the ministry of Sciences and Technology. The authors also appreciate the support from National Kaohsiung University of Applied Sciences in Taiwan.

Author Contributions: Chia-Nan Wang guided the research direction and found the solutions. Jing-Wein Wang conducted the fingerprint hardware, software and designed the experiments. Ming-Hsun Lin summarized the data and edited the paper. Yao-Lang Chang contributed to software coding. Chia-Ming Kuo worked on the experiment and analyzed the results. All authors contributed to produce the results.

Conflicts of Interest: The authors declare no conflict of interest.

References

1. Barrick, M.R.; Mount, M. The big five personality dimensions and job performance: A meta-analysis. *Pers. Psychol.* **1991**, *44*, 1–26. [CrossRef]
2. Cattell, R.B. The description of personality: Basic trait resolved into clusters. *J. Abnorm. Soc. Psychol.* **1943**, *38*, 476–506. [CrossRef]
3. Fiske, D.W. Consistency of the factorial structures of personality ratings from different source. *J. Abnorm. Soc. Psychol.* **1947**, *44*, 329–344. [CrossRef]
4. Norman, W.T. Toward an adequate taxonomy of personality attributes: Replicated factor structure in peer nomination personality ratings. *J. Abnorm. Soc. Psychol.* **1963**, *66*, 574–583. [CrossRef] [PubMed]
5. Burger, J.M. *Personality*; CENGAGE Learning: Boston, CT, USA, 2015.
6. Hill, C.W.; Jones, G.R.; Schilling, M.A. *Strategic Management Theory: An Integrated Approach*; CENGAGE Learning: Boston, CT, USA, 2015.
7. Kretschmer, E. *Physique and Character*; Dick Press: London, UK, 2007.
8. Edward, H. *Classification and Uses of Finger Prints*; George Rutledge & Sons: London, UK, 1900.
9. Jain, A.; Hong, L.; Bolle, R. On-line fingerprint verification. *IEEE Trans. Pattern Anal. Mach. Intell.* **1997**, *19*, 302–314. [CrossRef]
10. Ratha, N.K.; Bolle, R. *Automatic Fingerprint Recognition Systems*; Springer: New York, NY, USA, 2004.
11. Medina-Pérez, M.A.; García-Borroto, M.; Gutierrez-Rodríguez, A.E.; Altamirano-Robles, L. Improving fingerprint verification using minutiae triplets. *Sensors* **2012**, *12*, 3418–3434. [CrossRef] [PubMed]
12. Ballan, M.; Gurgen, F. On the principal component based fingerprint classification using directional images. *Math. Comput. Appl.* **1999**, *4*, 91–97. [CrossRef]
13. Yang, B.; Busch, C.; Groot, K.; Xu, H.; Veldhuis, R.N.J. Performance evaluation of fusing protected fingerprint minutiae templates on the decision level. *Sensor* **2012**, *12*, 5246–5272. [CrossRef] [PubMed]
14. Wang, J.W.; Le, N.T.; Wang, C.C.; Lee, J.S. Enhanced ridge structure for improving fingerprint image quality based on a wavelet domain. *IEEE Signal Process. Lett.* **2015**, *22*, 390–394. [CrossRef]
15. Bartunek, J.S.; Nilsson, M.; Sallberg, B.; Claesson, I. Adaptive fingerprint image enhancement with emphasis on preprocessing of data. *IEEE Trans. Image Process.* **2013**, *22*, 644–656. [CrossRef] [PubMed]
16. Yang, J.; Xiong, N.; Vasilakos, A.V. Two-stage enhancement scheme for low-quality fingerprint images by learning from the images. *IEEE Trans. Hum. Mach. Syst.* **2013**, *43*, 235–248. [CrossRef]
17. Warman, P.H.; Ennos, A.R. Fingerprints are unlikely to increase the friction of primate fingerpads. *J. Exp. Biol.* **2009**, *212*, 2016–2022. [CrossRef] [PubMed]
18. Costa, P.T.; McCare, R.R. Four ways five factors are basic. *Pers. Individ. Differ.* **1992**, *13*, 653–665. [CrossRef]
19. SecuGen Hamster Plus. Available online: http://secugen.com/products/php.htm (accessed on 3 July 2016).
20. Goldberg, L.R. Language and individual differences: The search for universals in personality lexicons. *Rev. Pers. Soc. Psychol.* **1981**, *2*, 141–165.
21. McCrae, R.R.; Costa, P.T., Jr. *Personality in Adulthood: A Five-Factor Theory Perspective*; Guilford Press: New York, NY, USA, 2003.
22. Henry, E.R. *Classification and Uses of Fingerprints*; Routledge: London, UK, 1990.
23. Wang, J.W. Classification of fingerprint based on traced orientation flow. In Proceedings of the IEEE International Symposium on Industrial Electronics, Bari, Italy, 9–12 December 2010; pp. 1585–1588. [CrossRef]
24. Cronbach, L.J. Coefficient alpha and the internal structure of tests. *Psychometrika* **1951**, *16*, 297–334. [CrossRef]
25. DeVellis, R.F. *Scale Development: Theory and Application*; Sage Publications: London, UK, 2003.
26. Sharma, S. *Applied Multivariate Techniques*; John Wiley and Sons: New York, NY, USA, 1996.

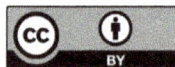

sensors

MDPI

Article

Real-Time External Respiratory Motion Measuring Technique Using an RGB-D Camera and Principal Component Analysis †

Udaya Wijenayake and Soon-Yong Park *

School of Computer Science and Engineering, Kyungpook National University, 80 Daehakro, Bukgu, Daegu 41566, Korea; udaya@vision.knu.ac.kr
* Correspondence: sypark@knu.ac.kr; Tel.: +82-53-950-7575
† This paper is an extended version of our paper published in the Wijenayake, U.; Park, S.Y. PCA based analysis of external respiratory motion using an RGB-D camera. In Proceedings of the IEEE International Symposium on Medical Measurements & Applications (MeMeA), Benevento, Italy, 15–18 May 2016.

Received: 30 May 2017; Accepted: 7 August 2017; Published: 9 August 2017

Abstract: Accurate tracking and modeling of internal and external respiratory motion in the thoracic and abdominal regions of a human body is a highly discussed topic in external beam radiotherapy treatment. Errors in target/normal tissue delineation and dose calculation and the increment of the healthy tissues being exposed to high radiation doses are some of the unsolicited problems caused due to inaccurate tracking of the respiratory motion. Many related works have been introduced for respiratory motion modeling, but a majority of them highly depend on radiography/fluoroscopy imaging, wearable markers or surgical node implanting techniques. We, in this article, propose a new respiratory motion tracking approach by exploiting the advantages of an RGB-D camera. First, we create a patient-specific respiratory motion model using principal component analysis (PCA) removing the spatial and temporal noise of the input depth data. Then, this model is utilized for real-time external respiratory motion measurement with high accuracy. Additionally, we introduce a marker-based depth frame registration technique to limit the measuring area into an anatomically consistent region that helps to handle the patient movements during the treatment. We achieved a 0.97 correlation comparing to a spirometer and 0.53 mm average error considering a laser line scanning result as the ground truth. As future work, we will use this accurate measurement of external respiratory motion to generate a correlated motion model that describes the movements of internal tumors.

Keywords: respiratory motion; radiotherapy; RGB-D camera; principal component analysis (PCA)

---

1. Introduction

Radiotherapy is one of the highly-discussed topics in the modern medical field. It has been widely used in cancer treatments to remove tumors without causing any damages to the neighboring healthy tissues. However, inaccurate system setups, anatomical motion and deformation and tissue delineation errors lead to inconsistencies in radiotherapy approaches. Respiratory-based anatomical motion and deformation largely cause errors in both radiotherapy planning and delivery processes in thoracic and abdominal regions [1,2]. With respiration, tumors in abdominal and thoracic regions can move as much as 35 mm [3–6]. As a consequence, inaccurate respiratory motion estimations directly effect tissue delineation errors, dose miss-calculations, exposure of healthy tissues to high doses and erroneous dose coverage for the clinical target volume [7–11].

Motion encompassing, respiratory gating, breath holding and forced shallow berating with abdominal compression are some of the existing conventional respiratory motion estimation methods [1]. Difficulties in handling patient movements, longer treatment time, patient training and discomfort are some of the most common drawbacks of these methods. On the other hand, real-time tumor tracking techniques have started to gain much attention due to their ability in actively estimating respiratory motion and continuous synchronization of the beam with the motion of the tumor.

Apart from radiotherapy, measurement of the respiration is an important task in pulmonary function testing, which is crucial for early detection of potentially fatal illnesses. Spirometer and pneumotachography are two of the well-known methods of pulmonary function testing. These methods need a direct contact with the patient while measuring and may interfere with the natural respiration. Furthermore, they measure only the full respiratory volume and cannot assess the regional pulmonary function in different chest wall behaviors. Hence, there is a need for a non-contact respiratory measurement technique, which can evaluate not only the complete, but also regional respiration.

In this paper, we investigate the feasibility of using a commercial RGB-D camera as a non-contact, non-invasive and whole-field respiratory motion-measuring device, which will enhance the patient comfort. These low-cost RGB-D cameras can provide real-time depth information of a target surface. We can use this depth information for respiratory motion measurement, but cannot achieve higher accuracy due to a considerable amount of noise in the raw depth data. Therefore, we proposed a technique of making an accurate respiratory motion model using principal component analysis (PCA) and then using that model for real-time respiratory motion measurement. First, we apply hole-filling and bilateral filtering to the first 100 raw depth frames and use that filtered depth data to create a PCA-based motion model. In the real-time respiratory motion-measuring stage, we project each depth frame to the motion model (principal components) and reconstruct back, removing the spatial and temporal noise and holes in the depth data. We can achieve higher motion measurement accuracy by using these reconstructed depth data, instead of raw depth data. The initial result of our proposed method is published in [12].

The results of this study—accurate measurements of external surface motion—can be used to predict the internal tumor motion, which is an important task of radiotherapy systems. Correspondence models that make a relationship between respiratory surrogate signals, such as spirometry or external surface motion, and internal tumor/organ motion have been studied in the literature [13–16]. Neural networks, principal component analysis and b-spline are a few example models that have been used for predicting the internal motion.

This paper is organized as follows. First, a comprehensive review of related works is presented in Section 2. An overview of the proposed method that describes the key steps and how to handle the problems existing in related works is given in Section 3. A detailed description of all of the materials and methods followed in the proposed method is presented in Section 4. The results of the experiments we conducted to evaluate the accuracy of the proposed method are given in Section 5. Finally, Section 6 concludes the paper by discussing the results and issues of the proposed method.

2. Related Work

The Synchrony respiratory tracking system, a subsystem of CyberKnife, is the first technology that continuously synchronizes beam delivery to the motion of the tumor [17]. The external respiratory motion is tracked using three optical fiducial markers attached to a tightly-fitting vest. Small gold markers are implanted near the target area before treatment to ensure the continuous correspondence between internal and external motion. The Calypso, the prostate motion-tracking system integrated into Varian (Varian Medical Systems, Palo Alto, CA, USA), eliminates the need for internal-external motion modeling by implanting three tiny transponders with an associated wireless tracking [18]. The BrainLAB ExacTrac positioning system uses radiopaque fiducial markers, implanted near the target isocenter, with external infrared (IR) reflecting markers [19]. Internal markers are tracked by an X-ray localization system, while an IR stereo camera tracks the external markers. The Xsight Lung

Tracking system (an extension of the CyberKnife system) is a respiratory motion-tracking system of lung lesion that eliminates the need for implanted fiducial markers [20].

Another interesting respiratory motion modeling technique using 4D computed tomography (CT) images was introduced in [21], where PCA is used to reduce the motion artifacts appearing on the CT images and to synthesize the CT images in different respiratory phases. Mori et al. used cine CT images to measure the intrafractional respiratory movement of pancreatic tumors [22]. Yang et al. estimated and modeled the respiratory motion by applying an optical flow-based deformable image registration technique on 4D-CT images that were acquired in cine mode [23]. In contrast to CT, magnetic resonance imaging (MRI) provides lesser ionization and excellent soft tissue contrast that helps to achieve better characterization. Therefore, 4D and cine-MRI images have been widely used for measuring organ/tumor motion due to respiration [24–28]. Apart from that, researchers have been experimenting with ultrasound images for tracking organs that move with respiration [29,30].

Radiography and fluoroscopy imaging techniques such as X-ray, CT and MRI have the problems of higher cost, slow acquisition, low resolution, lower signal-to-noise ratio and especially exposure to an extra dose of radiation [2,21,31,32]. Additionally, some of these systems have the disadvantage of invasive fiducial marker implantation procedures that increase the patient preparation time and treatment time.

To avoid these problems, researchers have proposed optical methods, which mainly consist of cameras, light projectors and markers. With the advantage of non-contact measurement, optical methods have no interference with the natural respiration of the patient. Ferrigno et al. proposed a method to analyze the chest wall motion by using passive markers placed on the thorax and abdomen [33]. Motion measurement is carried out by computing the 3D coordinates of these markers with the help of specially-designed multiple cameras. In [34], the authors proposed a respiratory motion-estimation method based on coded visual markers. They also utilized a stereo camera to calculate the 3D coordinates of the markers and estimated the 3D motion of the chest wall according to the movements of the markers. Yan et al. investigated the correlation between the motion of external markers and an internal tumor target [35]. They placed four infrared reflective markers on different areas of the chest wall and used a stereo infrared camera to track the motion of the markers. Alnowami et al. employed the Codamotion infrared marker-based tracking system to acquire the chest wall motion and applied probability density estimation to predict the respiratory motion [36,37]. Some researchers have investigated respiratory motion evaluation by calculating curvature variance of the chest wall using a fiber optic sensor and fiber Bragg grating techniques [38,39]. Even though the marker-based methods provide higher data acquisition rates and accuracy, the marker attachment procedure is time consuming and results in inconveniences for the patient. Furthermore, a large number of markers is needed to achieve higher spatial resolution.

In contrast to marker-based methods, structured light techniques provide whole-field measurement with high spatial resolution. Structured light systems consist of a projector and camera and emit a light pattern onto the target surface, creating artificial correspondences. The 3D information of the target surface can be found by solving the correspondences on the captured image of the illuminated scene. Aoki et al. proposed a respiratory monitoring system using a near-infrared multiple slit-light projection [40]. Even though they were able to achieve a high correlated respiratory motion pattern to a spirometer, they could not measure the exact respiratory volume or motion due to the variable projection coverage on the chest wall, which is caused by patient movements. Chen et al. solved this problem by introducing active light markers to define the measuring boundary, offering a consistent region for volume evaluation [41]. They also used a projector to illuminate the chest wall with a structured light pattern of color stripes and a camera to capture the height-modulated images. Then, the 3D surface calculated by triangulation is used to derive the respiratory volume information. However, the long baseline and the restriction of the camera plane to be parallel to the reference frame limit the portability of this method. In [31], the authors adopted a depth sensor, which uses a near-UV structured light pattern, along with a state-of-the-art non-rigid registration algorithm to identified the 3D deformation of the chest wall and hence the tumor motion. Time of flight (ToF) is another well-known optical method that has been used by researchers for respiratory motion handling during radiotherapy [42–44].

With the recent advances in commercial RGB-D sensors such as the Microsoft Kinect and ASUS Xtion Pro, these have been used in a broad area of research work. Have a relatively low cost and the fact that these sensors can measure the motion without any markers or wearable devices encourage researchers to use them in respiratory motion analysis. However, the low depth resolution of these sensors, which is about 1 cm at a 2 m distance, restricts the usage mostly for evaluating respiratory functions such as respiratory rate [45–51], where highly accurate motion information is not needed. In the case of radiotherapy, respiratory motion induces tumor movements up to 2 cm in abdominal or thoracic regions and needs less than 1 mm accuracy in motion measurements [52]. Xia and Siochi overcome the low depth resolution of the Kinect sensor by using a translation surface, which magnifies the respiratory motion and reduces the noise of irregular surfaces [53]. A few other researchers utilized RGB-D sensors to acquire 3D surface data of the chest wall and applied PCA to capture 1D respiration curves of disjoint anatomical regions (thorax and abdomen), which is related to the principal axes [32,54]. However, the respiratory motion measurement accuracy of these methods is affected by the patient movements, as they have not provided a proper method for handling these.

3. Overview of the Proposed Method

In this study, we introduce a non-contact, non-invasive and real-time respiratory motion measurement technique using an RGB-D camera, which is small in size and more flexible for handling. Furthermore, we introduce a patient movement-handling method using four dot markers. These four markers define the measurement boundaries of the moving chest wall, providing a consistent region for respiratory motion estimation.

Using the RGB-D camera, we capture continuous depth images of the patient's chest wall at 6.7 fps covering the whole thoracic and abdominal area. Then, we create a respiratory motion model by applying PCA to the first 100 frames, decomposing the data into a set of motion bases that corresponded to principal components (PCs). Before applying PCA, we use an edge-preserving bilateral filter and a hole-filling method to remove the noise and the holes of the first 100 frames.

According to the experimental analysis, we found out that a respiratory motion model can be accurately obtained using the first three principal components. The remaining principal components represent the noise and motion artifact existing in the input data. We start the real-time respiratory motion measurement from the 101st frame, projecting each new depth frame onto the motion model to obtain the low-dimensional representation of the data. To evaluate the motion in metric space, depth images are reconstructed using the projection coefficient. Figure 1 shows the flowchart of the proposed respiratory motion measurement process.

Using an RGB-D camera for respiratory motion measurement has many advantages. First, compared to the CT/MRI techniques, the proposed method prevents patients from being exposed to an extra dose of radiation. The RGB-D camera is a non-contact optical method and has no interference with the natural breathing of the target. Moreover, this can give real-time depth information of the target surface. Therefore, we can provide a comfortable and efficient, but lesser duration, treatment to the patients. Compared to marker-based methods, the RGB-D camera has high spatial resolution and provides depth information of the entire target surface; hence, we can measure not only the entire chest wall motion, but also the regional motions. The RGB-D camera we use in our system provides depth data in 640×480 resolution, and we select a 200×350 ROI providing 70,000 data points for motion measurement, which is much higher than marker-based methods (as an example, [36] used a 4×4 marker grid providing only 16 data points). The smaller size and lower price of the RGB-D cameras facilitate building a more portable and inexpensive respiratory motion measurement system compared to some other optical methods.

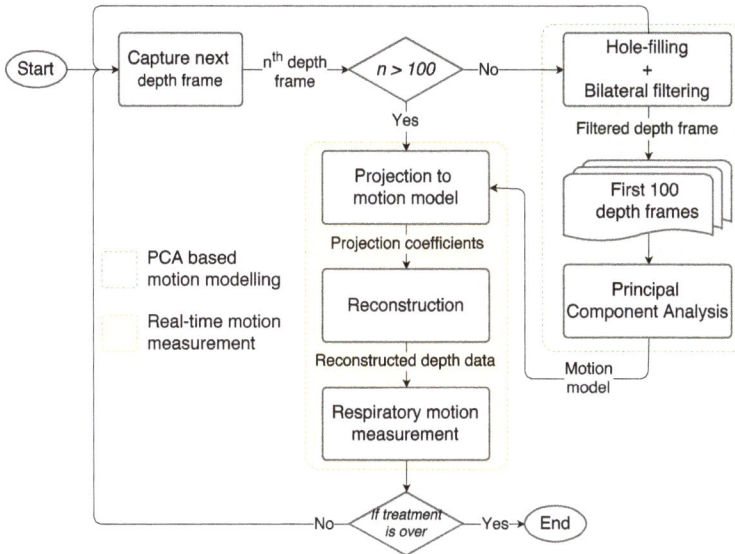

Figure 1. Flowchart of the proposed PCA-based respiratory motion-analyzing system. The first 100 depth frames are used to generate a PCA-based respiratory motion model. Then, that model (principal components) is used for real-time respiratory motion measurement starting from the 101st frame.

However, there is a known problem of low accuracy of the RGB-D cameras. Depth data acquired from low-cost RGB cameras has much noise and many holes that affect the accuracy of motion measurement. Alnowami et al. and Tahavori et al. used depth data acquired from an RGB-D camera for respiratory motion measurement, but could not achieve sub-millimeter level accuracy when it comes to experiments with real persons [55,56]. Using the PCA-based motion model, we increase the motion measurement accuracy by removing the spatial and temporal noise along with the holes in the depth data. When the filtered depth data are used as the input of the PCA-based motion model, we do not need to apply bilateral filtering or hole-filling for each depth frame during real-time motion measurement. Comparing with a laser line scanner, we prove that our method can achieve sub-millimeter accuracy in respiratory motion measurement using a low-cost RGB-D camera.

4. Materials and Methods

4.1. Data Acquisition

We use an Asus Xtion PRO RGB-D camera (consisting of an RGB camera, an infrared camera and a Class 1 laser projector that is safe under all conditions of normal use) to acquire real-time depth data and RGB images of the entire thoracic and abdominal region of the target subjects. The RGB-D camera provides both depth and RGB-D images in 640 × 480 resolution and 30 frames per second. However, due to the process of saving data to disk for later analysis, we could acquire only about 6.7 frames per second. The OpenNI library is used to grab the depth and RGB data from the camera and to convert them to matrix format for later usage. The depth camera covers not only the intended measuring area, but also the background regions. Moreover, the coverage of the chest wall is variable due to the surface motion and the patient movements. However, we should have an anatomically-consistent measuring area during the whole treatment time for delivering the radiation dose accurately.

To handle this problem, we attach four dot markers to define a measuring boundary on the chest wall covering the whole thoracic and abdominal area. Instead of using active LED markers or retroreflective markers, which can interfere with the RGB-D camera, we use small white color circles made of sticker paper.

After obtaining informed consent from all subjects following the institutional ethics, we collected respiratory motion data from ten healthy volunteers. All of the volunteers were advised to wear a skin-tight black color t-shirt and lay down in a supine position. The four markers are attached to the t-shirt, and the RGB-D camera is placed nearly 85 cm above the volunteer as shown in Figure 2. According to the specification of the RGB-D camera, it can provide depth information within an 80 cm to 350 cm range. However, [55] showed that the RGB-D camera gives the best accuracy within the 85 cm to 115 cm range. By keeping the camera closer to the volunteer, we can cover the measuring area with a higher number of pixels, which eventually provides more data points for motion analysis. Analyzing all of these facts, we place the RGB-D camera 85 cm above the patient. Along with the continuous depth frames, visual images are also captured using the built-in RGB camera nearly for a duration of one minute. The RGB images are used only for the purpose of detecting the markers to determine the measuring ROI.

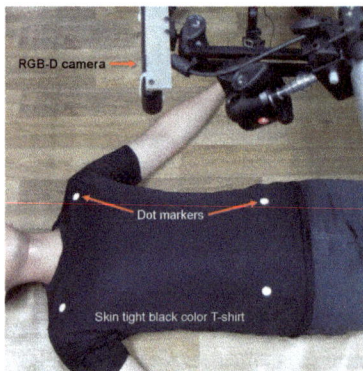

Figure 2. Experimental setup where the patient is laying down in the supine position wearing a skin-tight t-shirt with four white color dot markers. The RGB-D camera is placed nearly 85 cm above the patient.

4.2. Measuring Region

To define the measuring region, we detect the dot markers on the RGB image by applying few image processing techniques. Otsu's global binary thresholding method followed by contour detection and ellipse fitting [57] are applied to identify the center coordinates of each dot marker accurately. Using the intrinsic and extrinsic parameters of the depth and RGB cameras, which are acquired by a calibration process [58,59], depth images are precisely aligned (with sub-pixel accuracy) to the visual (RGB) images. Therefore, the marker coordinates found on visual images can be directly used on depth images to define the ROI, which marks the measuring area. The position, shape and size of the ROI are not consistent throughout all of the depth frames due to the motion of the chest wall and the movement of the patient. In order to make it consistent, the selected ROI on every depth frame is mapped into a predefined size of a rectangular shape using projective transformation [60]. Figure 3 shows the steps followed for detecting the dot markers and creating the rectangular ROI. We use this rectangular ROI for further processing of our proposed method.

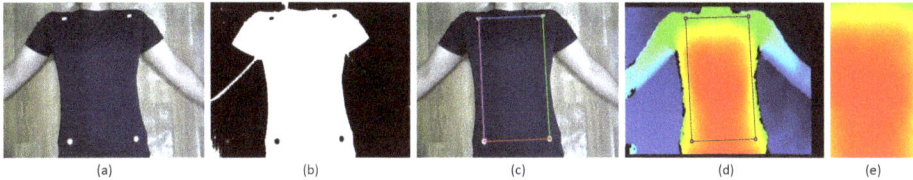

Figure 3. The process of rectangular ROI generation. (**a**) Captured visual image; (**b**) after binarization using Otsu's method; (**c**) defining the measuring area after finding the center coordinates of the four markers; (**d**) identified measuring area projected onto the aligned depth image; (**e**) generated rectangular ROI using perspective transformation.

4.3. Respiratory Motion Modeling Using PCA

4.3.1. Depth Data Pre-Processing

We use the first 100 depth frames to create a respiratory motion model using PCA. Since we use this model for real-time respiratory motion measurement, a precise model should be created using accurate input data. Due to the slight reflection of the t-shirt and device errors, holes can appear in the same spot of the chest wall area for a few continuous depth frames as depicted in Figure 4a. Moreover, there is much noise existing in the raw depth data provided by the sensor. If we directly use these data as the input for PCA without any pre-processing, we will encounter erroneous results as in Figure 4b, where most of the data variation is concentrated in the areas of holes.

To avoid this problem, we first apply a hole-filling technique on depth images using the zero-elimination mode filter. If there are enough non-zero neighbors, this filter replaces pixels with zero depth values with the statistical mode of its non-zero neighbors. Next, we remove noise from depth images using an edge-preserving bilateral filter [61]. Figure 4c shows the PCA result when we use filtered depth data as the input.

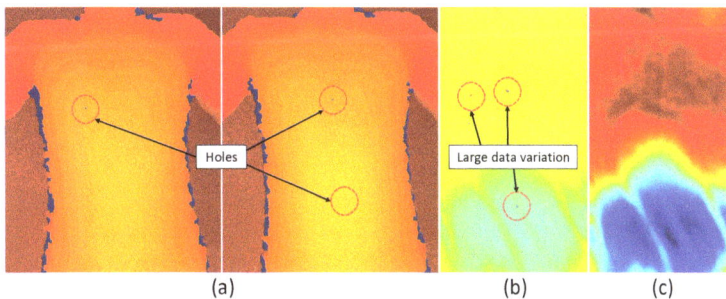

Figure 4. (**a**) Two example depth frames where holes appear in the chest wall region; (**b**) erroneous PCA result (eigenvector) where large data variations appear near the hole regions; (**c**) PCA result after applying hole-filling and bilateral filtering to input depth data.

4.3.2. Principal Component Analysis

After applying filtering to the first 100 depth frames, PCA [62] is applied to make a respiratory motion model that is integrated into the major principal components. By column-wise vectorization of the depth data (d_i) on the selected rectangular ROI, we create an input data matrix D of dimension $m \times n$:

$$D_{m \times n} = \left[\vec{d_1}, \vec{d_2}, \ldots, \vec{d_n} \right],$$

(1)

where n is the total number of depth frames ($n = 100$) and m is number of pixels in the rectangular ROI. First, we subtract the mean vector $\vec{d}$ calculated as:

$$\vec{d} = \frac{1}{n} \sum_{i=1}^{n} \vec{d}_i \qquad (2)$$

from the input data matrix to create a normalized matrix $\hat{D}$:

$$\hat{D} = \left[\vec{d}_1 - \vec{d}, \vec{d}_2 - \vec{d}, \cdots, \vec{d}_n - \vec{d} \right]. \qquad (3)$$

Since $m \gg n$, we use Equation (4) to calculate the $n \times n$ covariance matrix C, reducing the dimensionality of the input data.

$$C = \frac{1}{n-1} \hat{D}^T \hat{D} \qquad (4)$$

The transformation, which maps the high-dimensional input depth data into a low-dimensional PC subspace, is obtained by solving the eigenvalues (λ_j) and eigenvectors ($\vec{\phi}_j$) of the covariance matrix using Equation (5).

$$C\vec{\phi}_j = \lambda_j \vec{\phi}_j \qquad (5)$$

All of the eigenvectors, which correspond to principal components, are then arranged in descending order $\{\vec{\phi}_1, \vec{\phi}_2, \vec{\phi}_3, \cdots, \vec{\phi}_n\}$ according to the magnitude of the eigenvalues ($\lambda_1 \geq \lambda_2 \geq \lambda_3 \geq \cdots \geq \lambda_n$).

Using an experimental analysis, we found out that the first eigenvalue dominates the rest of the eigenvalues and accounts for over 98% of the data variation during regular respiration. However, when the respiration is irregular, three eigenvalues are required to cover 98% of the data variation. Figure 5 depicts the first ten eigenvalues of the covariance matrix calculated from five samples on regular breathing and three samples on irregular breathing. Figure 6 shows three graphs of projection coefficients (explained in Section 4.4.1) corresponding to the first three principal components calculated for regular breathing, while Figure 7 shows examples of irregular breathing. An apparent respiratory motion pattern is visible only on the first PC for regular breathing, while the first three PCs show a respiratory pattern in irregular breathing. Following this analysis, we represent the respiratory motion model W using the first three principal components ($\vec{\phi}_1, \vec{\phi}_2, \vec{\phi}_3$), reducing the dimensionality of input depth data.

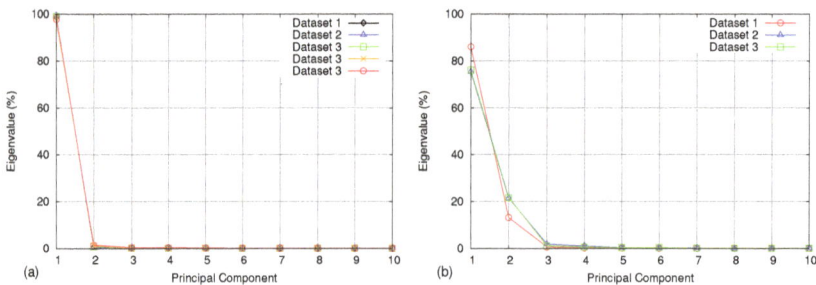

Figure 5. (**a**) Comparison of the first ten principal components using five sets of input data taken during regular breathing and (**b**) three sets of input data taken during irregular breathing. The first principal component is dominant over others and represents over 98% of data variance for regular breathing, while three principal components are needed to cover 98% of data variance for irregular breathing.

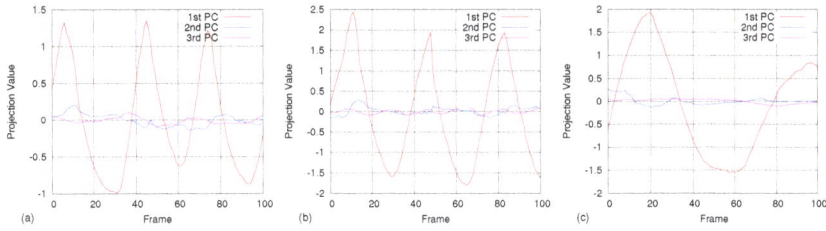

Figure 6. Projection results of 100 depth frames onto the first three PCs. Only the first PC shows a clear respiratory motion pattern for three datasets (**a**,**b**,**c**) taken during regular breathing.

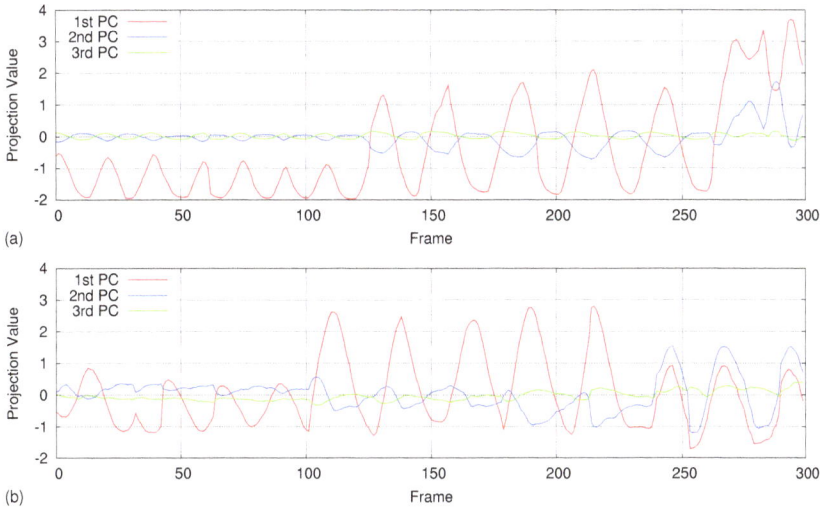

Figure 7. Projection results of 300 depth frames on the first three PCs for irregular breathing. The first two principal components show an apparent respiratory pattern, while the third one also shows a smaller respiratory signal. Graphs (**a**,**b**) represent two datasets.

4.4. Real-Time Respiratory Motion Measurement

After creating a respiratory motion model using the first 100 depth frames, we start the real-time respiratory motion measurement from the 101st frame. The data we use for respiratory motion modeling should cover a few complete respiratory cycles in order to generalize the input data. By following this rule, we can make sure that the motion model represents all of the statuses of the respiratory cycle. After observing all of the experiment datasets, we empirically select 100 as the number of depth frames for PCA-based motion modeling.

4.4.1. Projection and Reconstruction

We project each new depth frame d_i ($i > 100$) onto the motion model $W = \begin{bmatrix} \vec{\phi}_1 & \vec{\phi}_2 & \vec{\phi}_3 \end{bmatrix}$ in order to represent them using the first three principal components. The following equation is used as the projection operation, where $\vec{\beta}_i$ represents the projection coefficients.

$$\vec{\beta}_i = W^T(\vec{d}_i - \vec{\bar{d}}) \tag{6}$$

Even though the calculated projection coefficients represent a clear respiratory motion, we cannot use these directly for measuring the motion as these coefficients are three separate values in the principal component domain instead of the metric domain. Therefore, the following equation is used to reconstruct the depth data $(\hat{\vec{d}}_i)$, which is in the metric domain, from the projection coefficient.

$$\hat{\vec{d}}_i \approx \vec{d} + W\vec{\beta}_i \tag{7}$$

Here, the advantage is that we do not need to apply hole-filling or denoising filters to the depth data that we use for real-time respiratory motion measurement. By reconstructing the depth images using the motion model, we can remove the spatial and temporal noise, as well as the holes in the data. Figure 8 depicts the advantage of applying bilateral filtering and hole-filling to the input depth images for PCA. Figure 8a,b shows the PCA results with and without using filtering on PCA input data, respectively. As shown in Figure 8c,d, if we use the erroneous PC for projection and reconstruction, many holes and much noise will appear on the reconstructed depth data even if there are no holes in the input data. In contrast to that, if we use an accurate PC for projection and reconstruction, we can remove the holes and noise appearing in the input depth data by reconstructing it as shown in Figure 8e,f.

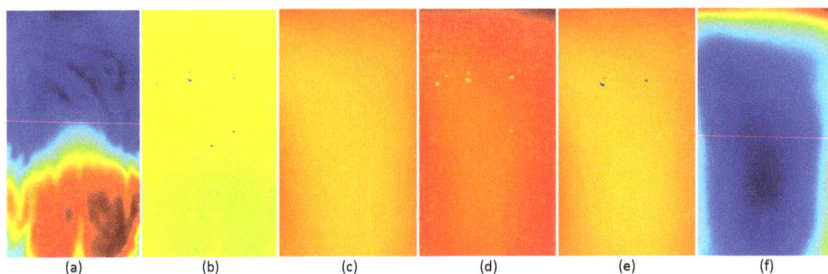

Figure 8. (**a**) PCA result (first eigenvector) using bilateral filtering and hole-filling; (**b**) PCA result (erroneous) without using bilateral filtering and hole-filling; (**c**) example input depth image without any holes; (**d**) reconstruction results of (**c**) using the incorrect PCA results shown in (**b**); (**e**) example input depth image with few holes; (**f**) reconstruction results of (**e**) using the PCA results shown in (**a**).

4.4.2. Motion Measurement

We use these reconstructed depth data for respiratory motion measurements. The rectangular ROI of the reconstructed depth data is further divided into smaller regions as in Figure 9a to separately measure the motion in smaller regions. Average depth values of these smaller regions along with 2D image coordinates and intrinsic camera parameters are used to calculate the 3D (X, Y and Z) coordinates of the mid-points. Then, we use these 3D coordinates to construct a surface mesh model composed of small triangles as in Figure 9b,c, which can be used to represent the chest wall surface and its motion clearly. We define the initial frame (101st frame) as the reference frame and calculate the motion of the remaining frames using the depth difference between the current frame and the reference frame.

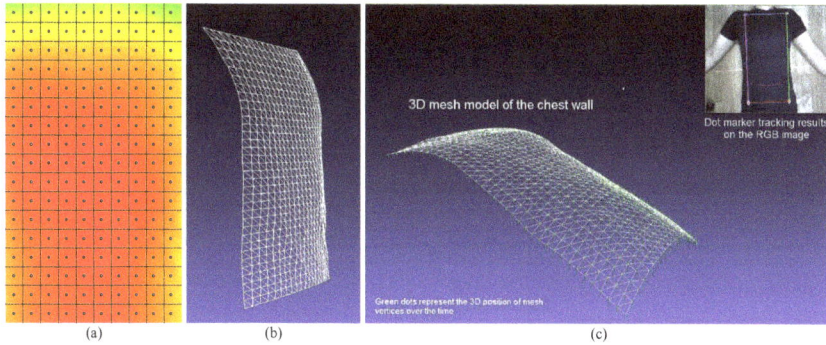

Figure 9. The surface mesh generation process. (**a**) The rectangular ROI of the reconstructed depth is further divided into smaller square ROIs; (**b**) a surface mesh is generated by finding the 3D coordinate of the midpoints of smaller ROIs using the average depth value of the region; (**c**) a selected frame of a video sequence, which shows the motion of the chest wall in a 3D viewer using a mesh model. Green dots represent the 3D position of mesh vertices over time.

4.5. Evaluation of the Accuracy

We propose an experimental setup as shown in Figure 10 for evaluating the accuracy of the proposed method. First, our proposed method is compared with a spirometer, which measures the air flow volume using a mouthpiece device, and then with a laser line scanner, which provides very accurate 3D reconstruction results.

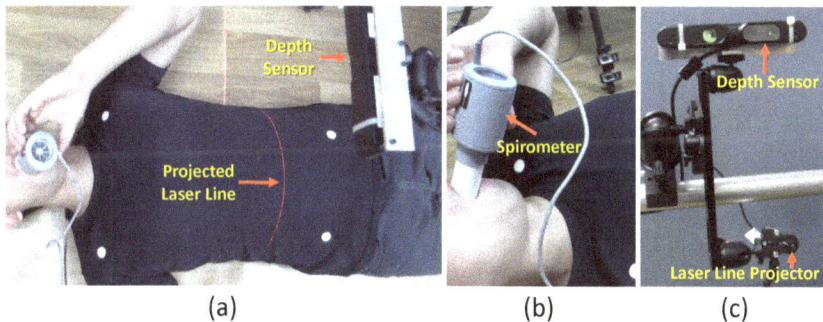

Figure 10. Experimental setup for evaluating the accuracy of the proposed method using a spirometer and a laser line scanner. (**a**) Volunteers are advised to lay down in the supine position and breath only through the spirometer. The RGB-D camera and laser line projector are placed above the volunteer, and the laser line is projected onto the abdomen area. (**b**) CareFusion SpiroUSB^{TM} spirometer. (**c**) The configuration of the RGB-D camera and laser line projector.

4.5.1. Comparison with Spirometer

We compared the respiratory motion pattern generated using the proposed method with a spirometer, which has been used for evaluating the accuracy of RGB-D camera-based respiratory function evaluation methods [41,63,64]. During this experiment, the patient breathed through a calibrated spirometer (SpiroUSB^{TM}, CareFusion) to record the airflow volume while the depth camera captured the chest wall motion simultaneously (see Figure 10a,b). The spirometer provides the air flow volume in liters, not the respiratory motion in millimeters. Therefore, with the help of surface mesh data, we developed a method to measure the volume difference of the current frame compared to a reference frame. We found the volume difference by calculating the sum of the volume of small prisms created by the triangles in the surface mesh of the current frame and their projection on the reference plane as the top and bottom surfaces.

First, these prisms were further divided into three irregular tetrahedrons. Then, the volume of a tetrahedron was calculated using Equation (8), where $a(a_x, a_y, a_z)$, $b(b_x, b_y, b_z)$, $c(c_x, c_y, c_z)$ and $d(d_x, d_y, d_z)$ represent the 3D coordinates of the four vertices.

$$V = \frac{det(A)}{6}, \quad A = \begin{bmatrix} a_x & b_x & c_x & d_x \\ a_y & b_y & c_y & d_y \\ a_z & b_z & c_z & d_z \\ 1 & 1 & 1 & 1 \end{bmatrix} \tag{8}$$

4.5.2. Comparison with Laser Line Scanning

Laser line scanning, which is well known for providing high accuracy (<0.1 mm) [65], is a 3D reconstruction method consisting of a laser line projector and a camera. We used this method to reconstruct a specific position of the chest wall accurately and to compare it with the PCA reconstruction results. The setup for this experiment consists of a laser line projector and the RGB-D camera as shown in Figure 10c. We projected the laser line onto the abdominal area of the target chest wall and captured the illuminated scene using the visual (RGB) camera of the RGB-D sensor. We prepared 15 datasets (D01, D02, ..., D15) from ten healthy volunteers ranging in age from 24 to 32 who participated in the data capturing process. Volunteer information is given in Table 1.

Table 1. Clinical and demographic information of the volunteers who participated in the experiments.

Volunteer	Gender	Age (years)	BMI (kg/m^2)	Datasets
1	M	29	26.4	D01, D02
2	M	32	28.7	D03
3	M	26	27.4	D04, D05
4	M	27	21.5	D06, D07
5	M	25	26.9	D08
6	M	28	26.5	D09
7	M	27	19.3	D10, D11
8	M	24	24.3	D12, D13
9	M	30	20.9	D14
10	M	25	24.0	D15

First, we calibrated the laser line projector and the RGB camera to find the 3D plane equation of the laser line with respect to the camera coordinate system using a checkerboard pattern [65,66]. Then, we separated the measuring area from the rest of the image by defining a rectangular ROI on the RGB images the same as on the depth images. We took the red channel of the RGB image, applied Gaussian smoothing and fit a parabola to each column of the ROI image according to the pixel intensities. Then, by finding the maximum of the parabola, which corresponds to the laser line location, we can identify the 2D image coordinates of it with sub-pixel level accuracy. We projected these image coordinates to the 3D laser plane using the intrinsic camera parameters and calculated the 3D coordinates by finding the ray-plane intersection points. These 3D coordinates are referred to as *laser reconstruction* in the remainder of this paper. Next, we projected the 2D coordinates of the laser line onto the reconstructed depth image $\hat{d}_i$ to identify the 3D coordinates of the laser line according to the proposed PCA-based method and referred to this as *PCA reconstruction*.

The purpose of the proposed method is not to reconstruct the chest wall surface, but to measure the chest wall motion accurately. Therefore, instead of comparing the direct 3D reconstruction results, we compared the respiratory motion; defined as the depth difference between the current frame and reference frame. We chose the 101st frame as the reference frame, as it is the starting frame of real-time respiratory motion measurement. To have a quantitative comparison, we selected five points ($P1, P2, ..., P5$) across the laser line and found the motion error of each point separately for 100 frames. By taking the laser line reconstruction as the ground truth, we calculated the motion error E_{ij} of the j-th point on the laser line of i-th frame ($1 \leq j \leq 5$ and $1 \leq i \leq 100$) using:

$$E_{ij} = \left|(D_{ij}^L - D_{rj}^L) - (D_{ij}^P - D_{rj}^P)\right|,$$ (9)

where D_{ij} is the depth value of the j-th point on the laser line of the i-th frame. L and P represent the laser reconstruction and PCA reconstruction, respectively, while r represents the reference frame.

5. Results

First, we present the accuracy evaluation results of the proposed respiratory motion measurement method compared to the spirometer and laser line scanner. With the use of the spirometer, we examined the respiratory pattern using volume changes. The laser line scanner was used to analyze the motion measurement accuracy of the proposed method. Later, we compared our method with bilateral filtering and then conducted isovolume maneuver to show the advantages of the proposed method over existing ones. Finally, we analyzed how the proposed method works in a condition of longer and irregular breathing. All of these experiments were performed in a general laboratory environment, and the software components were implemented using C++ language with the help of OpenCV and OpenNI libraries.

5.1. Comparison of Respiratory Pattern with Spirometer

Figure 11 depicts the volume comparison graphs of the spirometer and the proposed PCA-based method. The sample rate of the spirometer is lower than the RGB-D camera. Therefore, we applied b-spline interpolation on available spirometer data to generate a smooth motion curve to achieve a similar frame interval as the RGB-D camera.

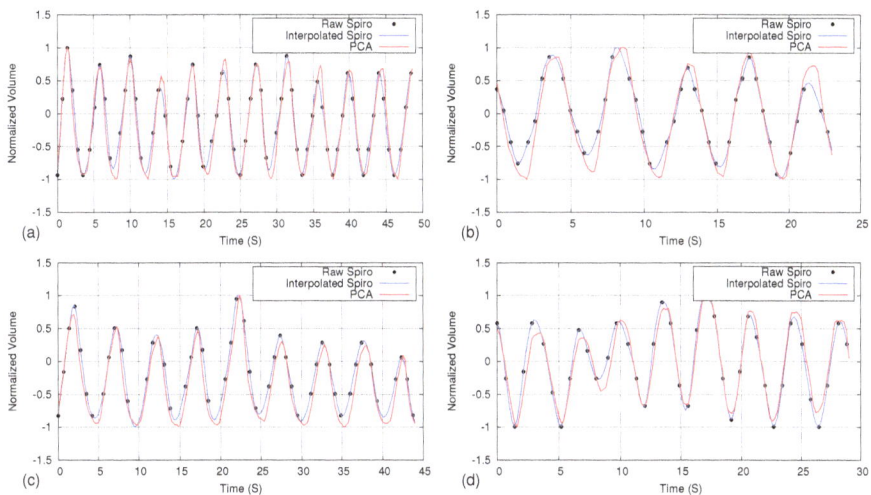

Figure 11. Comparison of respiratory volume measurement (normalized into −1:1 range) using the proposed method (PCA) and a spirometer. Graphs (**a**–**d**) represent the selected four different datasets. Black dots represent the original data points of the spirometer, while the blue line represents the interpolated data.

The magnitude of the respiratory volume is different between the spirometer and the proposed method, as the measuring area and methodology are different. Therefore, we compared the data by normalizing it to a −1:1 range. As shown in Figure 11, the proposed method could generate respiratory motion patterns very similar to the spirometer with a 0.97 average correlation.

5.2. Accuracy Analysis Using Laser Line Scanning

Table 2 gives the motion error results of the five points on the laser line, calculated from 15 datasets. We summarized the data on the table as the average, maximum and standard deviation of the motion error (E_{ij}) over 100 frames. The average motion error of all datasets on all five points is 0.53 ± 0.05 mm. As a qualitative comparison, motion graphs of four datasets calculated on four different points of the laser line are depicted in Figure 12. As a further analysis, we calculated the normalized cross-correlation (NCC) between the PCA motion ($D_{ix}^{P} - D_{rx}^{P}$) and laser line motion ($D_{ix}^{L} - D_{rx}^{L}$) for each x coordinate of the laser line over 100 frames. The graph in Figure 13 shows the NCC results, which was separately calculated for each X-coordinate of the laser line for all 15 datasets. The results indicate a very high correlation between the two motion estimation methods as the average NCC for all of the datasets is 0.98 ± 0.0009.

Table 2. Motion error of the proposed PCA-based method compared to laser line scanning calculated on five locations of the laser line for 15 datasets. All data are given in mm.

Position	Parameters	D01	D02	D03	D04	D05	D06	D07	D08	D09	D10	D11	D12	D13	D14	D15	Average
P1	Average	0.23	0.66	0.18	0.27	0.39	0.36	0.36	0.21	0.83	0.45	0.32	0.36	0.94	0.43	0.55	0.44
	Max.	0.92	2.69	0.66	1.14	0.96	1.41	1.41	0.77	1.91	1.45	1.05	1.47	1.89	1.24	1.51	1.37
	Standard deviation	0.19	0.66	0.13	0.24	0.22	0.32	0.32	0.16	0.47	0.31	0.23	0.29	0.50	0.27	0.38	0.31
P2	Average	0.39	0.34	0.33	0.52	0.22	1.09	0.47	0.47	0.85	0.46	0.30	0.50	0.52	0.97	0.38	0.52
	Max.	1.10	1.34	0.84	1.62	0.66	1.87	1.37	1.31	1.72	1.34	0.79	1.55	1.56	2.51	1.38	1.40
	Standard deviation	0.25	0.31	0.21	0.38	0.16	0.40	0.30	0.33	0.46	0.32	0.19	0.34	0.40	0.66	0.29	0.33
P3	Average	0.31	0.85	0.42	0.50	0.59	0.41	0.44	0.74	0.78	0.70	0.40	0.63	1.04	0.57	0.64	0.60
	Max.	1.09	1.90	1.18	1.29	1.39	1.28	1.59	1.81	1.97	1.83	1.03	1.89	2.55	1.56	1.82	1.61
	Standard deviation	0.25	0.44	0.26	0.32	0.34	0.31	0.34	0.44	0.50	0.46	0.26	0.47	0.65	0.36	0.40	0.39
P4	Average	0.42	0.27	0.28	0.51	0.34	0.40	0.36	0.38	1.18	1.55	0.69	0.50	0.74	0.49	0.41	0.57
	Max.	0.95	1.38	0.77	1.72	0.91	0.90	1.03	1.24	2.45	3.18	1.52	1.52	1.86	1.11	1.02	1.44
	Standard deviation	0.21	0.27	0.19	0.46	0.23	0.24	0.26	0.27	0.71	0.67	0.32	0.43	0.43	0.32	0.24	0.35
P5	Average	0.32	0.43	0.33	0.29	0.51	0.89	0.53	0.70	0.37	0.43	0.38	0.70	0.87	0.63	0.73	0.54
	Max.	0.89	2.23	0.96	1.61	0.97	1.68	1.46	1.59	1.27	1.35	1.02	2.04	2.16	1.63	1.79	1.51
	Standard deviation	0.22	0.49	0.21	0.27	0.23	0.37	0.40	0.40	0.29	0.33	0.25	0.59	0.56	0.37	0.42	0.36

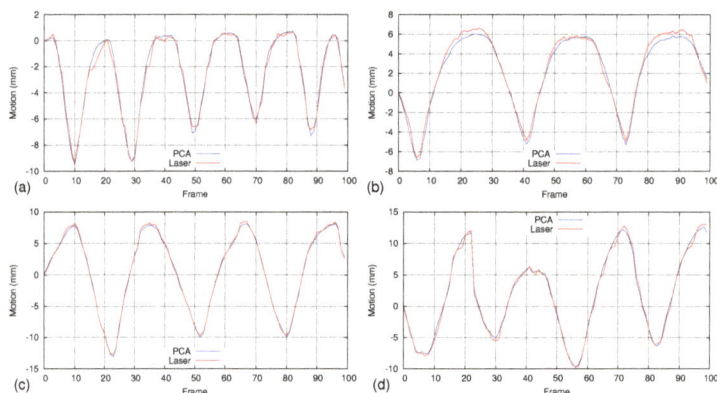

Figure 12. Comparison of respiratory motion measurement using the proposed method (PCA) and laser line scanning. Measurements are taken from different places on the projected laser line. The 101st frame of the dataset is selected as the reference frame, and we measure the motion of remaining frames with respect to it until the 200th frame. Graphs (**a–d**) show the motion measurement results of four different datasets.

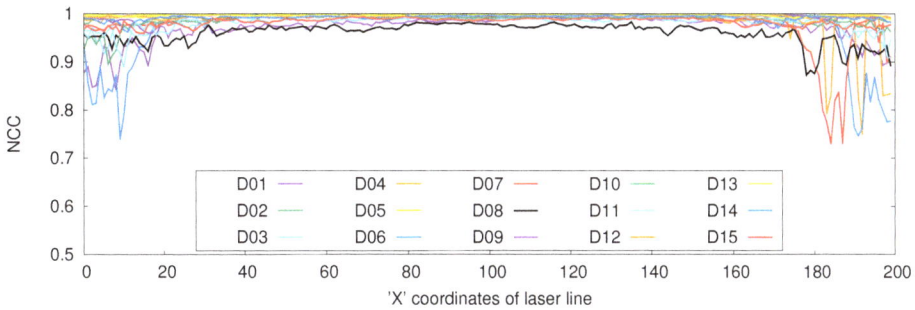

Figure 13. Normalized cross-correlation (NCC) between PCA and laser scanning across 100 frames. NCC is calculated for each point on the laser line along the X-axis separately.

5.3. Comparison with Bilateral Filtering

To show the advantages, we compared our proposed method with bilateral filtering. In our method, hole-filling and bilateral filtering are applied only to the first 100 frames that we used as the input for PCA, and we do not use this during real-time respiratory motion measurements. During this experiment, we measured the respiratory motion by applying bilateral filtering and hole-filling to all frames and without using PCA, and the results are compared with the proposed PCA-based method. Figure 14a shows a part of the motion comparison graph, where the bilateral filtering gives a rough curve with more temporal noise, while the proposed method gives a smoother curve with less temporal noise. The reason is that PCA provides both spatial and temporal filtering, not like bilateral filtering, which provides only spatial filtering.

Furthermore, Figure 14b compares the proposed method and bilateral filtering with a very accurate 3D reconstruction method of laser line scanning (details are given in Section 4.5.2). Considering the laser reconstruction as the ground truth, we calculated the motion error (Equation (9)) of the proposed method and bilateral filtering on a selected location of the chest wall. In the case of the motion comparison provided in Figure 14b, the average error is 0.35 ± 0.06 mm for the proposed method and 0.85 ± 0.08 mm for the bilateral filtering.

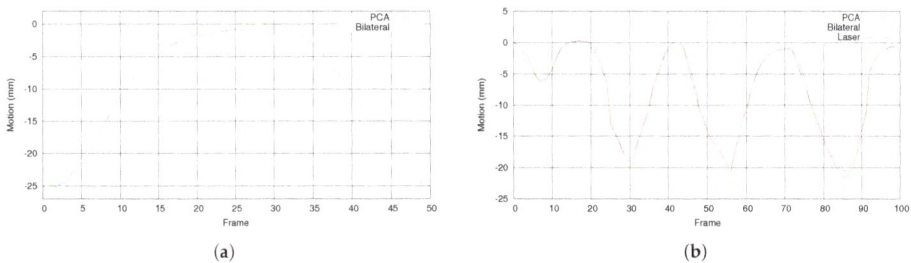

Figure 14. Comparison of the proposed PCA-based method and bilateral filtering. (**a**) A part of the motion comparison graph. The proposed PCA-based method provides a smooth curve, while bilateral filtering gives a rough curve with more temporal noise. (**b**) Comparison of the proposed PCA-based method and bilateral filtering with laser line scanning.

5.4. Isovolume Maneuver

We conducted an isovolume maneuver to emphasize the capability of the regional respiratory motion measurement of the proposed method. During the test, the subjects are advised to hold their breath without air flow, but exchanging the internal volume between thorax and abdomen. Then, we measured the motion of whole chest wall (which is covered by the four dot markers) and the regional motion of thorax and abdomen separately, presented in Figure 15. We used a few additional markers to separate the thorax and abdomen area on the chest wall. Theoretically, there should be no volume changes for the whole chest wall, but as we measure the depth difference in an ROI defined by the markers, which does not cover the entire chest wall area exactly, a motion pattern appears on the whole chest wall. However, opposite phases of the whole thorax and the whole abdomen motion with −0.99 cross-correlation reflecting the volume exchange between them, which we cannot determine using a respiratory volume-measuring devices such as the spirometer.

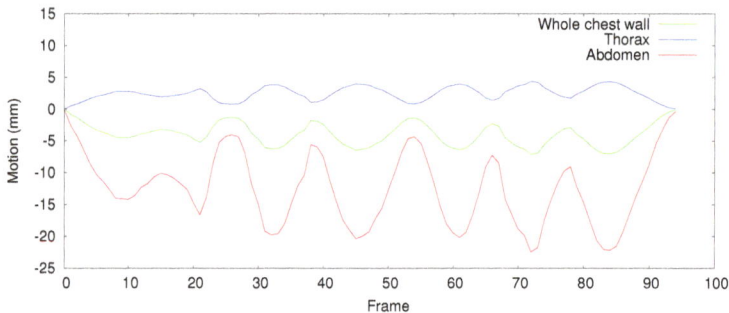

Figure 15. Respiratory motion graph of a volunteer performing the isovolume maneuver. The opposite phase of the whole thorax and the whole abdomen motion reflect the volume exchange between them.

5.5. Handling Irregular Breathing

We analyze how the motion model generated using the first 100 frames affects the accuracy during longer and irregular breathing. For regular respiration that does not have much variation in respiratory rate and volume, only the first principal component is enough to accurately measure the motion. Figure 16 shows two graphs of regular respiratory motion that were calculated over 350 frames compared with the laser line scanning (details are given in Section 4.5.2). Even though we use only the first principal component calculated over 100 depth frames, the average error is about 0.3 mm and 0.8 mm for the two graphs, respectively.

However, during irregular breathing (respiratory rate and amplitude change time to time), accuracy gets lower when we are using only the first principal component as the motion model. As shown in Figure 17, the large difference compared to the laser line scanning proves that only the first principal component is not enough for handling irregular respiratory motions. Therefore, we redo the accuracy analysis including the first three principal components of the motion model and draw the results on the same graph. Using the first three principal components, we could achieve sub-millimeter accuracy (∼0.5 mm) even if the respiratory pattern of the first 100 frames is entirely different from rest of the data.

As a further refinement step for a very long treatment duration, we can update the motion model by recalculating the principal components with a new set of depth data at regular intervals.

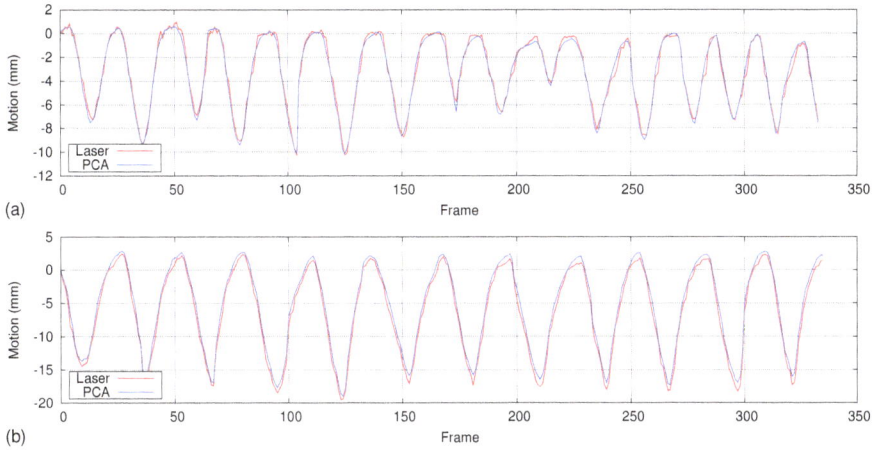

Figure 16. Motion comparison graphs generated for a regular respiratory patterns over a longer duration (350 frames). The first 100 frames are used for PCA, and only the first principal component is used as the motion model. All frames are then used for accuracy analysis. Higher accuracy could be achieved even though only the first PC is used for reconstruction. Graphs (**a**,**b**) show the motion comparison results of two different datasets.

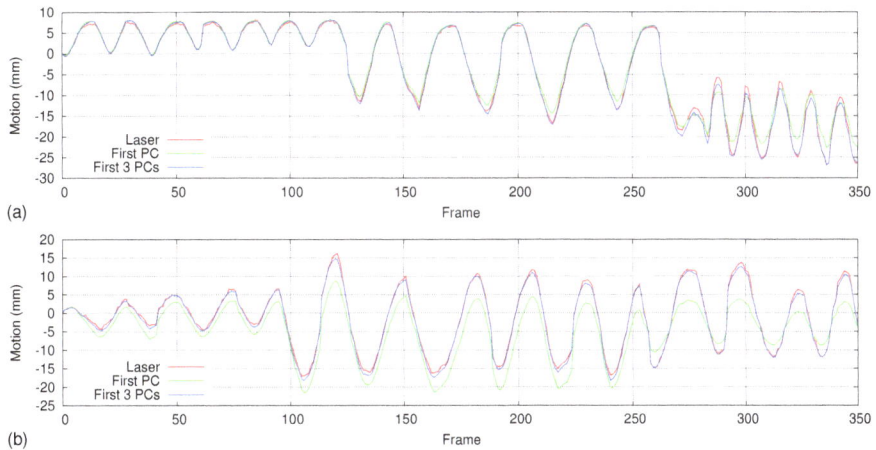

Figure 17. Motion comparison graphs generated for irregular respiratory patterns over a longer duration (350 frames). The first 100 frames are used for PCA, and the first principal component and first three principal components are used as the motion models, respectively. All frames are then used for accuracy analysis. A large difference appears between the laser scanner and PCA method when we are using only the first principal component. Higher accuracy could be achieved when we are using the first three principal components as the motion model. Graphs (**a**,**b**) show the motion comparison results of two different datasets.

6. Discussion and Conclusions

We have proposed a patient-specific external respiratory motion analyzing technique based on PCA. A commercial RGB-D camera was used to acquire the depth data of the target respiratory motion, and PCA was applied to find a motion model corresponding to the respiration. Four dot markers attached to the chest wall were used to define an anatomically-consistent measuring region throughout the measuring period. Using an experimental analysis, we found out that only the first three principal components are sufficient to represent the respiratory motion while the rest of the principal components represent patterns of small perturbations. Therefore, all of the depth data were projected onto the first three principal component and reconstructed removing the spatial and temporal noise existing in the input data.

For the convenience of the volunteers who participated in the laboratory-level experiments, we allowed them to wear a black-colored t-shirt and attached white color dot markers on it. Even though we use a tight-fitting t-shirt, a few wrinkles can appear within the chest wall area and affect the accuracy of the results. Therefore, we recommend not using any clothing that covers the measuring region during the clinical treatment process. We can select dot markers with an apparent color difference with the patient's skin color and directly attach them to the patient's body. Furthermore, it is advisable to attach the dot markers on four locations of the chest wall where there is no compelling motion due to the respiration, such as the end of the collar bones and hip bones.

During respiratory motion modeling using PCA, we used the first 100 depth frames as the input data. The criterion for selecting this number is that input depth data should cover a few complete respiratory cycles. All of our experiment datasets satisfy this criterion within 100 frames. The frame rate during the experiments was about 6.7 fps on average because it takes time for writing/reading data to hard disk frame by frame. However, during real respiratory motion measurement sessions, reading and/or writing data to a hard disk is not necessary; thus, we can achieve a frame rate of around 20 fps. The frame rate was very stable during the experiments with only a 0.4 fps standard deviation.

The accuracy of the proposed method was first evaluated using a spirometer, which has an accuracy level of 3%. Even though the magnitude of the measured volume was different, the spirometer and the proposed method were highly correlated in motion pattern (0.97 average correlation). Second, a laser line scanning technique, which is well known for high accuracy, was used to analyze the motion measurement accuracy of the proposed method. A laser line that was projected onto the abdominal area of the subject was reconstructed using a laser line scanning technique and compared with the proposed PCA reconstruction method. The motion of the projected laser line is measured using the both reconstruction results with respect to a reference frame. We could achieve high correlation (0.98 NCC) between the laser line scanner and the proposed method. Considering the laser scanning results as the ground truth, the measured average motion error of the proposed method is 0.53 mm, which is very comparable to commercial respiratory tracking systems according to Table 3.

Table 3. Accuracy comparison of the proposed method with related respiratory motion tracking methods.

System	Accuracy
Synchrony [17]	<1.5 mm
ExacTrac [19,67]	<1.0 mm
Calypso [18]	<1.5 mm
Yang et al. [23]	1.1 ± 0.8 mm
Chen et al. [41]	4.25 ± 3.49%
Alnowami et al. [55]	3.1 ± 0.6 mm
Proposed Method	0.53 ± 0.25 mm

The proposed method provides not only a high accuracy, but also a very simple system setup, which is very flexible and portable. With the advantage of non-contact measurement, the proposed method has no interference with the patient's respiration and, hence, provides more accurate measurements. Furthermore, the proposed method has the advantage of measuring the motion in a particular location of the chest wall, instead of measuring the motion of the whole chest wall at once.

Finding a motion model that can be used to correlate the external respiratory motion with internal tumor motion has been discussed in the literature [14–16]. Linear, polynomial, b-spline and PCA-based models are a few techniques that have been investigated so far. As future work, we are also planning to work on finding a correlation model, that can be employed to measure internal tumor motion, by using external surface motion as the surrogate input data. Furthermore, we are planning to test the proposed system in a real clinical environment using patients with different demographic and clinical properties.

Supplementary Materials: The Supplementary Materials are available online at http://www.mdpi.com/1424-8220/17/8/1840/s1.

Acknowledgments: This work was supported partly by 'The Cross-Ministry Giga KOREA Project' grant funded by the Korea Government (MSIT) (No.GK17P0300, Real-time 4D reconstruction of dynamic objects for ultra-realistic service), and partly by the Convergence R&D Development Project of the Small and Medium Administration, Republic of Korea (S2392741).

Author Contributions: U.W. developed the software components, conducted the experiments, analyzed the results and drafted the manuscript. S.P. supervised the study and critically revised and finalized the intellectual content of the manuscript.

Conflicts of Interest: The authors declare no conflict of interest.

References

1. Keall, P.J.; Mageras, G.S.; Balter, J.M.; Emery, R.S.; Forster, K.M.; Jiang, S.B.; Kapatoes, J.M.; Low, D.A.; Murphy, M.J.; Murray, B.R.; et al. The management of respiratory motion in radiation oncology report of AAPM Task Group 76. *Med. Phys.* **2006**, *33*, 3874–3900.
2. Ozhasoglu, C.; Murphy, M.J. Issues in respiratory motion compensation during external-beam radiotherapy. *Int. J. Radiat. Oncol. Biol. Phys.* **2002**, *52*, 1389–1399.
3. Hanley, J.; Debois, M.M.; Mah, D.; Mageras, G.S.; Raben, A.; Rosenzweig, K.; Mychalczak, B.; Schwartz, L.H.; Gloeggler, P.J.; Lutz, W.; et al. Deep inspiration breath-hold technique for lung tumors: The potential value of target immobilization and reduced lung density in dose escalation. *Int. J. Radiat. Oncol.* **1999**, *45*, 603–611.
4. Barnes, E.A.; Murray, B.R.; Robinson, D.M.; Underwood, L.J.; Hanson, J.; Roa, W.H.Y. Dosimetric evaluation of lung tumor immobilization using breath hold at deep inspiration. *Int. J. Radiat. Oncol. Biol. Phys.* **2001**, *50*, 1091–1098.
5. Davies, S.C.; Hill, A.L.; Holmes, R.B.; Halliwell, M.; Jackson, P.C. Ultrasound quantitation of respiratory organ motion in the upper abdomen. *Br. J. Radiol.* **1994**, *67*, 1096–1102.
6. Ross, C.S.; Hussey, D.H.; Pennington, E.C.; Stanford, W.; Fred Doornbos, J. Analysis of movement of intrathoracic neoplasms using ultrafast computerized tomography. *Int. J. Radiat. Oncol. Biol. Phys.* **1990**, *18*, 671–677.
7. Langen, K.M.; Jones, D.T.L. Organ motion and its management. *Int. J. Radiat. Oncol. Biol. Phys.* **2001**, *50*, 265–278.
8. Engelsman, M.; Damen, E.M.F.; De Jaeger, K.; Van Ingen, K.M.; Mijnheer, B.J. The effect of breathing and set-up errors on the cumulative dose to a lung tumor. *Radiother. Oncol.* **2001**, *60*, 95–105.
9. Malone, S.; Crook, J.M.; Kendal, W.S.; Zanto, J.S. Respiratory-induced prostate motion: Quantification and characterization. *Int. J. Radiat. Oncol. Biol. Phys.* **2000**, *48*, 105–109.
10. Lujan, A.E.; Larsen, E.W.; Balter, J.M.; Ten Haken, R.K. A method for incorporating organ motion due to breathing into 3D dose calculations. *Med. Phys.* **1999**, *26*, 715–720.
11. Jacobs, I.; Vanregemorter, J.; Scalliet, P. Influence of respiration on calculation and delivery of the prescribed dose in external radiotherapy. *Radiother. Oncol.* **1996**, *39*, 123–128.
12. Wijenayake, U.; Park, S.Y. PCA based analysis of external respiratory motion using an RGB-D camera. In Proceedings of the IEEE International Symposium on Medical Measurements and Applications (MeMeA), Benevento, Italy, 15–18 May 2016; pp. 1–6.
13. Bukovsky, I.; Homma, N.; Ichiji, K.; Cejnek, M.; Slama, M.; Benes, P.M.; Bila, J. A fast neural network approach to predict lung tumor motion during respiration for radiation therapy applications. *BioMed Res. Int.* **2015**, *2015*, 489679. doi:10.1155/2015/489679.
14. McClelland, J.; Hawkes, D.; Schaeffter, T.; King, A. Respiratory motion models: A review. *Med. Image Anal.* **2013**, *17*, 19–42.

15. McClelland, J. Estimating Internal Respiratory Motion from Respiratory Surrogate Signals Using Correspondence Models. In *4D Modeling and Estimation of Respiratory Motion for Radiation Therapy*; Ehrhardt, J., Lorenz, C., Eds.; Springer; Berlin/Heidelberg, Germany, 2013; pp. 187–213.

16. Fayad, H.; Pan, T.; Clément, J.F.; Visvikis, D. Technical note: Correlation of respiratory motion between external patient surface and internal anatomical landmarks. *Med. Phys.* **2011**, *38*, 3157–3164.

17. Seppenwoolde, Y.; Berbeco, R.I.; Nishioka, S.; Shirato, H.; Heijmen, B. Accuracy of tumor motion compensation algorithm from a robotic respiratory tracking system: A simulation study. *Med. Phys.* **2007**, *34*, 2774–2784.

18. Willoughby, T.R.; Kupelian, P.A.; Pouliot, J.; Shinohara, K.; Aubin, M.; Roach, M.; Skrumeda, L.L.; Balter, J.M.; Litzenberg, D.W.; Hadley, S.W.; et al. Target localization and real-time tracking using the Calypso 4D localization system in patients with localized prostate cancer. *Int. J. Radiat. Oncol. Biol. Phys.* **2006**, *65*, 528–534.

19. Jin, J.Y.; Yin, F.F.; Tenn, S.E.; Medin, P.M.; Solberg, T.D. Use of the BrainLAB ExacTrac X-Ray 6D System in Image-Guided Radiotherapy. *Med. Dosim.* **2008**, *33*, 124–134.

20. Fu, D.; Kahn, R.; Wang, B.; Wang, H.; Mu, Z.; Park, J.; Kuduvalli, G.; Maurer, C.R., Jr. Xsight lung tracking system: A fiducial-less method for respiratory motion tracking. In *Treating Tumors that Move with Respiration*; Springer: Berlin/Heidelberg, Germany, 2007; pp. 265–282.

21. Zhang, Y.; Yang, J.; Zhang, L.; Court, L.E.; Balter, P.A.; Dong, L. Modeling respiratory motion for reducing motion artifacts in 4D CT images. *Med. Phys.* **2013**, *40*, 041716.

22. Mori, S.; Hara, R.; Yanagi, T.; Sharp, G.C.; Kumagai, M.; Asakura, H.; Kishimoto, R.; Yamada, S.; Kandatsu, S.; Kamada, T. Four-dimensional measurement of intrafractional respiratory motion of pancreatic tumors using a 256 multi-slice CT scanner. *Radiother. Oncol.* **2009**, *92*, 231–237.

23. Yang, D.; Lu, W.; Low, D.A.; Deasy, J.O.; Hope, A.J.; El Naqa, I. 4D-CT motion estimation using deformable image registration and 5D respiratory motion modeling. *Med. Phys.* **2008**, *35*, 4577–4590.

24. Yun, J.; Yip, E.; Wachowicz, K.; Rathee, S.; Mackenzie, M.; Robinson, D.; Fallone, B.G. Evaluation of a lung tumor autocontouring algorithm for intrafractional tumor tracking using low-field MRI: A phantom study. *Med. Phys.* **2012**, *39*, 1481–1494.

25. Crijns, S.P.M.; Raaymakers, B.W.; Lagendijk, J.J.W. Proof of concept of MRI-guided tracked radiation delivery: Tracking one-dimensional motion. *Phys. Med. Biol.* **2012**, *57*, 7863.

26. Cerviño, L.I.; Du, J.; Jiang, S.B. MRI-guided tumor tracking in lung cancer radiotherapy. *Phys. Med. Biol.* **2011**, *56*, 3773.

27. Cai, J.; Chang, Z.; Wang, Z.; Paul Segars, W.; Yin, F.F. Four-dimensional magnetic resonance imaging (4D-MRI) using image-based respiratory surrogate: A feasibility study. *Med. Phys.* **2011**, *38*, 6384–6394.

28. Siebenthal, M.V.; Székely, G.; Gamper, U.; Boesiger, P.; Lomax, A.; Cattin, P. 4D MR imaging of respiratory organ motion and its variability. *Phys. Med. Biol.* **2007**, *52*, 1547.

29. Hwang, Y.; Kim, J.B.; Kim, Y.S.; Bang, W.C.; Kim, J.D.K.; Kim, C. Ultrasound image-based respiratory motion tracking. *SPIE Med. Imaging* **2012**, 83200N, doi:10.1117/12.911766.

30. Nadeau, C.; Krupa, A.; Gangloff, J. Automatic Tracking of an Organ Section with an Ultrasound Probe: Compensation of Respiratory Motion. In *Medical Image Computing and Computer-Assisted Intervention—MICCAI 2011*; Springer: Berlin/Heidelberg, Germany, 2011; pp. 57–64.

31. Nutti, B.; Kronander, A.; Nilsing, M.; Maad, K.; Svensson, C.; Li, H. *Depth Sensor-Based Realtime Tumor Tracking for Accurate Radiation Therapy*; Eurographics 2014—Short Papers; Galin, E., Wand, M., Eds.; The Eurographics Association: Strasbourg, France, 2014; pp. 10–13.

32. Tahavori, F.; Alnowami, M.;Wells, K. Marker-less respiratory motion modeling using the Microsoft Kinect forWindows. In Proceedings of Medical Imaging 2014: Image—Guided Procedures, Robotic Interventions, and Modeling, San Diego, CA, USA, 15–20 February 2014.

33. Ferrigno, G.; Carnevali, P.; Aliverti, A.; Molteni, F.; Beulcke, G.; Pedotti, A. Three-dimensional optical analysis of chest wall motion. *J. Appl. Physiol.* **1994**, *77*, 1224–1231.

34. Wijenayake, U.; Park, S.Y. Respiratory motion estimation using visual coded markers for radiotherapy. In Proceedings of the 29th Annual ACM Symposium on Applied Computing Association for Computing Machinery (ACM), Gyeongju, Korea, 24–28 March 2014; pp. 1751–1752.

35. Yan, H.; Zhu, G.; Yang, J.; Lu, M.; Ajlouni, M.; Kim, J.H.; Yin, F.F. The Investigation on the Location Effect of External Markers in Respiratory Gated Radiotherapy. *J. Appl. Clin. Med. Phys.* **2008**, *9*, 2758.

36. Alnowami, M.R.; Lewis, E.; Wells, K.; Guy, M. Respiratory motion modelling and prediction using probability density estimation. In Proceedings of the IEEE Nuclear Science Symposuim and Medical Imaging Conference, Knoxville, TN, USA, 30 October–6 November 2010; pp. 2465–2469.

37. Alnowami, M.; Lewis, E.; Wells, K.; Guy, M. Inter- and intra-subject variation of abdominal vs. thoracic respiratory motion using kernel density estimation. In Proceedings of the IEEE Nuclear Science Symposuim and Medical Imaging Conference, Knoxville, TN, USA, 30 October–6 November 2010; pp. 2921–2924.

38. Babchenko, A.; Khanokh, B.; Shomer, Y.; Nitzan, M. Fiber Optic Sensor for the Measurement of Respiratory Chest Circumference Changes. *J. Biomed. Opt.* **1999**, *4*, 224–229.

39. Allsop, T.; Bhamber, R.; Lloyd, G.; Miller, M.R.; Dixon, A.; Webb, D.; Castañón, J.D.A.; Bennion, I. Respiratory function monitoring using a real-time three-dimensional fiber-optic shaping sensing scheme based upon fiber Bragg gratings. *J. Biomed. Opt.* **2012**, *17*, 117001.

40. Aoki, H.; Koshiji, K.; Nakamura, H.; Takemura, Y.; Nakajima, M. Study on respiration monitoring method using near-infrared multiple slit-lights projection. In Proceedings of the IEEE International Symposium on Micro-NanoMechatronics and Human Science, Nagoya, Japan, 7–9 November 2005; pp. 273–278.

41. Chen, H.; Cheng, Y.; Liu, D.; Zhang, X.; Zhang, J.; Que, C.; Wang, G.; Fang, J. Color structured light system of chest wall motion measurement for respiratory volume evaluation. *J. Biomed. Opt.* **2010**, *15*, 026013.

42. Müller, K.; Schaller, C.; Penne, J.; Hornegger, J. Surface-Based Respiratory Motion Classification and Verification. In *Bildverarbeitung für die Medizin 2009*; Meinzer, H.P., Deserno, T.M., Handels, H., Tolxdorff, T., Eds.; Springer: Berlin/Heidelberg, Germany, 2009; pp. 257–261.

43. Schaller, C.; Penne, J.; Hornegger, J. Time-of-flight sensor for respiratory motion gating. *Med. Phys.* **2008**, *35*, 3090–3093.

44. Placht, S.; Stancanello, J.; Schaller, C.; Balda, M.; Angelopoulou, E. Fast time-of-flight camera based surface registration for radiotherapy patient positioning. *Med. Phys.* **2012**, *39*, 4–17.

45. Burba, N.; Bolas, M.; Krum, D.M.; Suma, E.A. Unobtrusive measurement of subtle nonverbal behaviors with the Microsoft Kinect. In Proceedings of the 2012 IEEE Virtual Reality Workshops (VRW), Costa Mesa, CA, USA, 4–8 March 2012; pp. 1–4.

46. Martinez, M.; Stiefelhagen, R. Breath rate monitoring during sleep using near-IR imagery and PCA. In Proceedings of the 21st International Conference on Pattern Recognition (ICPR2012), Tsukuba, Japan, 11–15 November 2012; pp. 3472–3475.

47. Yu, M.C.; Liou, J.L.; Kuo, S.W.; Lee, M.S.; Hung, Y.P. Noncontact respiratory measurement of volume change using depth camera. In Proceedings of the Annual International Conference of the IEEE Engineering in Medicine and Biology Society, San Diego, CA, USA, 28 August–1 September 2012; pp. 2371–2374.

48. Benetazzo, F.; Longhi, S.; Monteriù, A.; Freddi, A. Respiratory rate detection algorithm based on RGB-D camera: Theoretical background and experimental results. *Healthc. Technol. Lett.* **2014**, *1*, 81–86.

49. Bernal, E.A.; Mestha, L.K.; Shilla, E. Non contact monitoring of respiratory function via depth sensing. In Proceedings of the IEEE-EMBS International Conference on Biomedical and Health Informatics (BHI), Valencia, Spain, 1–4 June 2014; pp. 101–104.

50. Al-Naji, A.; Gibson, K.; Lee, S.H.; Chahl, J. Real Time Apnoea Monitoring of Children Using the Microsoft Kinect Sensor: A Pilot Study. *Sensors* **2017**, *17*, 286.

51. Procházka, A.; Schätz, M.; Vyšata, O.; Vališ, M. Microsoft Kinect Visual and Depth Sensors for Breathing and Heart Rate Analysis. *Sensors* **2016**, *16*, 996.

52. Seppenwoolde, Y.; Shirato, H.; Kitamura, K.; Shimizu, S.; van Herk, M.; Lebesque, J.V.; Miyasaka, K. Precise and real-time measurement of 3D tumor motion in lung due to breathing and heartbeat, measured during radiotherapy. *Int. J. Radiat. Oncol. Biol. Phys.* **2002**, *53*, 822–834.

53. Xia, J.; Siochi, R.A. A real-time respiratory motion monitoring system using KINECT: Proof of concept. *Med. Phys.* **2012**, *39*, 2682–2685.

54. Wasza, J.; Bauer, S.; Haase, S.; Hornegger, J. Sparse Principal Axes Statistical Surface Deformation Models for Respiration Analysis and Classification. In *Bildverarbeitung für die Medizin 2012*; Tolxdorff, T., Deserno, M.T., Handels, H., Meinzer, H.P., Eds.; Springer: Berlin/Heidelberg, Germany, 2012; pp. 316–321.

55. Alnowami, M.; Alnwaimi, B.; Tahavori, F.; Copland, M.; Wells, K. A quantitative assessment of using the Kinect for Xbox360 for respiratory surface motion tracking. In Proceedings of the SPIE Medical Imaging. International Society for Optics and Photonics, San Diego, CA, USA, 4 February 2012; p. 83161T-83161T-10.

56. Tahavori, F.; Adams, E.; Dabbs, M.; Aldridge, L.; Liversidge, N.; Donovan, E.; Jordan, T.; Evans, P.; Wells, K. Combining marker-less patient setup and respiratory motion monitoring using low cost 3D camera technology. In Proceedings of the SPIE Medical Imaging. International Society for Optics and Photonics, Orlando, Florida, USA, 21 February 2015; p. 94152I-94152I-7. doi:10.1117/12.2082726.
57. Gonzalez, R.C.; Woods, R.E. *Digital Image Processing*, 3rd ed.; Pearson: New York, NY, USA, 2007.
58. Gui, P.; Ye, Q.; Chen, H.; Zhang, T.; Yang, C. Accurately calibrate kinect sensor using indoor control field. In Proceedings of the 2014 Third International Workshop on Earth Observation and Remote Sensing Applications (EORSA), Changsha, China, 11–14 June 2014; pp. 9–13.
59. Daniel, H.C.; Kannala, J.; Heikkilä, J. Joint Depth and Color Camera Calibration with Distortion Correction. *IEEE Trans. Pattern Anal. Mach. Intell.* **2012**, *34*, 2058–2064.
60. Hartley, R.; Zisserman, A. *Multiple View Geometry in Computer Vision*, 2nd ed.; Cambridge University Press: Cambridge, UK, 2004.
61. Tomasi, C.; Manduchi, R. Bilateral filtering for gray and color images. In Proceedings of the Sixth International Conference on Computer Vision (IEEE Cat. No.98CH36271), Bombay, India, 4–7 January 1998; pp. 839–846.
62. Jolliffe, I. *Principal Component Analysis*; Springer: Berlin/Heidelberg, Germany, 2002.
63. Harte, J.M.; Golby, C.K.; Acosta, J.; Nash, E.F.; Kiraci, E.; Williams, M.A.; Arvanitis, T.N.; Naidu, B. Chest wall motion analysis in healthy volunteers and adults with cystic fibrosis using a novel Kinect-based motion tracking system. *Med. Biol. Eng. Comput.* **2016**, *54*, 1631–1640.
64. Sharp, C.; Soleimani, V.; Hannuna, S.; Camplani, M.; Damen, D.; Viner, J.; Mirmehdi, M.; Dodd, J.W. Toward Respiratory Assessment Using Depth Measurements from a Time-of-Flight Sensor. *Front. Physiol.* **2017**, *8*. doi:10.3389/fphys.2017.00065.
65. Zhou, F.; Zhang, G. Complete calibration of a structured light stripe vision sensor through planar target of unknown orientations. *Imag. Vis. Comput.* **2005**, *23*, 59–67.
66. Dang, Q.; Chee, Y.; Pham, D.; Suh, Y. A Virtual Blind Cane Using a Line Laser-Based Vision System and an Inertial Measurement Unit. *Sensors* **2016**, *16*, 95.
67. Matney, J.E.; Parker, B.C.; Neck, D.W.; Henkelmann, G.; Rosen, I.I. Target localization accuracy in a respiratory phantom using BrainLAB ExacTrac and 4DCT imaging. *J. Appl. Clin. Med. Phys.* **2011**, *12*, 3296.

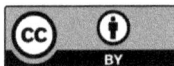

sensors

MDPI

Article

Bio-Photonic Detection and Quantitative Evaluation Method for the Progression of Dental Caries Using Optical Frequency-Domain Imaging Method

Ruchire Eranga Wijesinghe [1,†], **Nam Hyun Cho** [2,3,†], **Kibeom Park** [1], **Mansik Jeon** [1,*] and **Jeehyun Kim** [1]

[1] School of Electronics Engineering, College of IT Engineering, Kyungpook National University, 80, Daehak-ro, Buk-gu, Daegu 41566, Korea; eranga@knu.ac.kr (R.E.W.); pepl10@knu.ac.kr (K.P.); jeehk@knu.ac.kr (J.K.)
[2] Eaton-Peabody Laboratories, Massachusetts Eye and Ear Infirmary(MEEI), 243, Charles Street, Boston, MA 02114, USA; namhyun_cho@meei.harvard.edu
[3] Department of Otology and Laryngology, Harvard Medical School, 243, Charles Street, Boston, MA 02114, USA
* Correspondence: msjeon@knu.ac.kr; Tel.: +82-53-950-7221
† These authors contributed equally to this work.

Academic Editors: Dragan Indjin, Željka Cvejić and Małgorzata Jędrzejewska-Szczerska
Received: 28 September 2016; Accepted: 2 December 2016; Published: 6 December 2016

Abstract: The initial detection of dental caries is an essential biomedical requirement to barricade the progression of caries and tooth demineralization. The objective of this study is to introduce an optical frequency-domain imaging technique based quantitative evaluation method to calculate the volume and thickness of enamel residual, and a quantification method was developed to evaluate the total intensity fluctuation in depth direction owing to carious lesions, which can be favorable to identify the progression of dental caries in advance. The cross-sectional images of the *ex vivo* tooth samples were acquired using 1.3 µm spectral domain optical coherence tomography system (SD-OCT). Moreover, the advantages of the proposed method over the conventional dental inspection methods were compared to highlight the potential capability of OCT. As a consequence, the threshold parameters obtained through the developed method can be used as an efficient investigating technique for the initial detection of demineralization.

Keywords: optical frequency domain imaging (OFDI); optical coherence tomography; dental caries; demineralization; Bio-photonic detection

1. Introduction

Precise structural imaging and quantitative evaluation are critical for the diagnosis of dental caries and research to prevent the formation of initial demineralized regions [1,2]. The depth imaging of enamel, dentin, cavities, pits, and fissures with a high-resolution is particularly important for the study of anatomical and pathological changes of the dental structure [3]. Optical coherence tomography (OCT) is a rapidly advancing optical frequency-domain imaging modality, which can provide non-invasive high-resolution cross-sectional images of dental tissues and various biological tissues [4]. This near-infrared (NIR) biomedical imaging method provides images with high axial and lateral resolutions (i.e., below 8 µm and 15 µm, respectively) [5,6], and, furthermore, OCT has been widely used in different medical applications such as ophthalmology [7,8], dermatology [9], and otolaryngology [10,11]. The methods currently in use for the detection of dental caries such as radiography, microradiography, and X-rays do not provide sufficient resolution, sensitivity, and contrast compared to OCT. Radiography is the most frequently applied inspection method in dentistry with a resolution of 50 μm, which is comparatively lower than the resolution of OCT. Furthermore, radiography is not quantitative, and it is relatively difficult to apply for the initial detection of dental caries [12,13]. Microradiography is another method that can be used to analyze caries quantitatively, but it is hard to apply this method for clinical applications [14]. Other conventional diagnostic methods such as infrared (IR) imaging, dental explorer, and visual inspection are unable to provide more accurate cross-sectional images [15]. Several research groups have determined the mineral loss and the depth of enamel caries using a histology analysis method called transversal microradiography (TMR). However, due to the requirement of a thin sectioning process, applications of the method in dentistry have been scarce [16]. The main drawback of this method is that caries can be detected only at a relatively advanced stage when remineralization is no longer possible, and due to the incapability of obtaining precise quantitative measurements, it is hard to barricade the progression of caries. Thus, owing to the non-invasive and non-destructive imaging capability, and the capability of acquiring precise quantifications such as accurate thickness and volumetric measurements, OCT has gained a significant demand in the medical field as an early diagnosis method. Although OCT has been extensively used as a powerful dental imaging technique, quantitative evaluation of enamel thickness variation, depth dependent intensity fluctuation, and volumetric analysis of enamel residual has not been broadly studied for the initial diagnosis of demineralization.

Especially in dentistry, OCT has been used to produce longitudinal images of dental tissues and caries of an orientation similar to that of the B-scan ultrasound images [17,18]. In these studies, a reduction in enamel reflectivity was observed in areas of dental caries [19]. It is considered that the decrease in reflectivity during demineralization is related to the amount of mineral loss. Few studies have demonstrated that there is two to threefold increase in the scattering coefficient at a wavelength of 1.3 μm [20]. Furthermore, a polarization sensitive OCT (PS-OCT) endoscopic system using a swept source has been implemented as a compact system for dentistry application [21]. Similarly, surface demineralization can be detected using linearly polarized light and measured backscattered signal in two orthogonal axes [22]. Some other OCT techniques have been applied to diagnose dental caries as a result of changes in the optical properties of enamel after undergoing demineralization [23]. The obtained images were quantitatively evaluated by the identification of structures, dimensions, and properties [24]. Moreover, in several review reports and research studies, OCT based dental experiments were demonstrated to verify the stronger optical backscattering signals acquired from the demineralized enamel regions, oral tissue images, caries, periodontal diseases, and oral cancers [25,26]. In addition, infrared light with long wavelengths were used in OCT for clinical applications owing to the high depth penetration [27].

In this paper, we performed an initial *ex vivo* study using a 1.3 μm wavelength laser utilized spectral domain OCT (SD-OCT) system to introduce a quantitative method to calculate the thickness and volume of remaining enamel region (enamel residual). Furthermore, we developed an algorithm to analyze the total intensity fluctuation in depth direction of OCT images, which can be useful to identify the progression of initial caries. As a result, the proposed quantification can be implemented to identify the reduction of enamel region along with the progression of the demineralization. Moreover, the capability of our SD-OCT system to perform the proposed method was validated by obtaining images of *ex vivo* caries with a high resolution and a high depth penetration.

2. Materials and Methods

2.1. Optical Frequency Domain Imaging (OFDI) Technique

The implemented optical frequency domain imaging technique was a customized 1.3 μm SD-OCT system. The speed of the SD-OCT system was 120 frames/s when the image size was 1024×500 pixels, and the average output power of the system was 16 mW. In Figure 1, the broadband light source that was used for light emission is a superluminescent diode (SLED) (Denselight Semiconductors, Singapore) with 1.3 μm central wavelength and 135 nm bandwidth. The axial resolution of the system was 6 µm (in air) and 3.61 µm (in tissue). The transverse resolution of the system was 25 µm. The detector was a 14-bit complementary metal-oxide semiconductor (CMOS) line scan camera (SU-1024LDM Compact; Goodrich, Charlotte, NC, USA) with 1024 pixels. A 50:50 optical fiber coupler was used to split the broadband light beam into the sample and reference arms. A galvanoscanner (GVS002, Thorlabs, Newton, NJ, USA) connected to the sample arm was used to scan the tooth samples. All the samples were scanned with a sufficient cross-sectional scanning range of 1 mm × 1 mm × 1 mm dimensions. A compact spectrometer was designed and contained a collimator, a diffraction grating, an achromatic doublet lens, and a line scan camera. The spectrometer was calibrated to compensate the distortion of the point spread function (PSF), and to improve the signal-to-noise ratio (SNR) up to 110 dB using previous literature reports [28,29]. Further details about the system configuration can be found in Table 1.

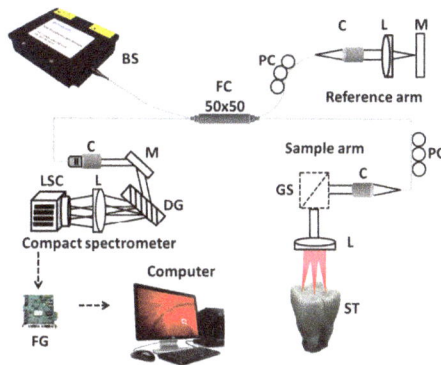

Figure 1. Schematic diagram of the spectral-domain optical coherence tomography (SD-OCT) system. Note the use of the following acronyms in the figure: BS: broadband source, C: collimator, DG: diffraction grating, FC: fiber coupler, FG: frame grabber, GS: galvanoscanner, L: lens, LSC: line scan camera, M: mirror, PC: polarization controller, and ST: sample tooth.

Table 1. The details of the optical frequency domain imaging system.

System Parameters	Specification
Central Wavelength	1310 nm
Spectral bandwidth	135 nm
Axial resolution air/tissue	6 µm/3.61 µm
Transverse resolution	25 µm
Maximum imaging width	8 mm
Maximum imaging depth	>6 mm
Optical power variation	±5%

2.2. Specimen Preparation

For the proposed preliminary study, four types of *ex vivo* tooth samples, including partially demineralized canine tooth sample, partially demineralized pre-molar tooth sample, partially demineralized molar tooth sample, completely demineralized (carious) molar tooth sample, and *in vivo* healthy molar tooth sample were involved in the experiment. All tooth specimens were examined in patients before extraction. The experimented *ex vivo* tooth specimens were extracted after performing early childhood caries (ECC) surgeries for four orthodontic patients at different age groups (10–12 years) of the dental clinic of the Faculty of Dentistry, Kyungpook National University, Daegu, Korea. The details of the experimented volunteers and tooth specimens are illustrated in Table 2. Prior to the OCT inspection, all *ex vivo* tooth specimens were preserved in sterile filtered de-ionized water solution for 24 h at 30 °C to eliminate any possible superficial enamel cracks and maintain a standard smooth surface after the extraction. The experiments were performed in accordance with the guidelines of the Institutional Animal Care and Use Committee of Kyungpook National University (Daegu, Korea) and approvals from the human ethics committees of the Institute for Bio-diagnostics, Kyungpook National University (Daegu, Korea) were obtained prior to sample collection.

Table 2. The details of the experimented tooth specimens.

Experimented Volunteer	Tooth Classification	Inspection Category
11-year-old male	Molar tooth	Healthy
11-year-old female	Molar tooth	Partially demineralized
10-year-old male	Molar tooth	Carious
11-year-old male	Canine tooth	Partially demineralized
12-year-old female	Pre-molar tooth	Partially demineralized

2.3. Intensity Fluctuation Analysis

To evaluate the proposed method precisely, the obtained cross-sectional images were involved in an amplitude scan (A-scan) depth profile analysis to verify the microstructural comparison between healthy, partially demineralized, and carious molar tooth samples. For the A-scan profile analysis, a software-based program was coded using Matlab (Mathworks, Natick, MA, USA) to search the intensity peaks in the depth direction. The acquired 2D OCT image was loaded and a peak search algorithm-based cropped window with 15 intensity signals (A-scan lines) was applied. The developed algorithm detects the maximum intensity in each individual A-scan line to search the peak position, and all the peak positions in all 15 A-scan lines were rearranged while matching the peak intensity index in the A-scans to flatten the region of interest. Owing to the non-flattened region of interest, the maximum intensity index positions vary, and therefore, the index positions with higher intensity values should be rearranged and matched linearly to obtain a flattened image. Finally, all the rearranged and flattened A-scan lines were summed up, averaged, and normalized to obtain a single A-scan depth profile of the region of interest. The applied refractive index of a tooth structure, which affects the depth scale of 2D OCT images was 1.63 [30,31]. Moreover, we performed an additional quantification method to analyze the total intensity fluctuation in deep microstructures according to imaging depth. Thus, an additional automated program was coded using Matlab to analyze the total pixel intensity of each depth range of demodulated 2D OCT images. The analysis was performed for the entire visible depth range of 1 mm, and the total pixel intensity was evaluated for each 250 µm depth range of the cross-sectional image to identify the depth dependent total intensity fluctuation of each tooth specimen category. Then, the entire total pixel intensity of each depth range was summed and averaged for each 2D OCT image. This study was a preliminary observational study, and the data analysis was primarily descriptive. A continuous variation of the optical laser source power was observed, which was compensated afterward. Due to the instability of the laser optical power, the entire intensity of 2D OCT images was compensated by multiplying ±5%.

2.4. Volumetric Analysis

The volumetric measurements of enamel residual was obtained using 2D OCT image based 3D OCT volumetric images by implementing a pixel intensity based automated calculation method, which was performed through a software program coded in Matlab. Figure 2a shows the volumetric calculation algorithm of enamel residual of a single 2D OCT image along with the obtained 3D OCT volumetric image containing 500 2D OCT images (Figure 2c). In the developed algorithm based program, demodulated raw data was loaded and the intensity of the entire cross-sectional region was analyzed. An image window was applied to select the enamel residual region. For the precise selection (filter the region of interest) of the enamel residual region, we approximated the pixel intensity difference between the enamel residual region and other cross-sectional regions, and provided a pre-determined intensity threshold range for a separate evaluation of the enamel residual region.

The entire cross-sectional intensity varies from 0 to 255, and the pre-determined enamel threshold ($TH_{(en)}$) range can be expressed as, $45 \leq TH_{(en)} \leq 255$. The selected threshold range contains the intensity range of the enamel region and excludes the dark black region of the selected image window. The area of a single pixel, which belongs to the selected image window in Figure 2b can be expressed as

$$l_x \times l_y = A_{pix}, \tag{1}$$

where l_x is the pixel size in the x-direction, l_y is the pixel size in the y-direction, and A_{pix} is the area of a single pixel. The pixel sizes in the x-, y-, and z-directions can be expressed as

$$l_x = l_y = 12 \text{ μm, and } l_z = 7 \text{ μm.}$$

The total number of z-direction pixels (B-mode images) is 500 owing to the composition of the 3D OCT image. Therefore, the enamel residual volume (volume of the remaining enamel) of 500 2D OCT images (3D volumetric image) can be calculated as

$$\left(N_1 \times l_x \times l_y\right) \times l_z + \left(N_2 \times l_x \times l_y\right) \times l_z + \left(N_3 \times l_x \times l_y\right) \times l_z + \ldots \left(N_{500} \times l_x \times l_y\right) \times l_z = V_{tot}, \tag{2}$$

where N_i (i = 1, 2, 3, . . . , 500) is the number of image window pixels in each respective window, which satisfies the pre-determined threshold value range, and V_{tot} is the evaluated volume of the enamel residual. $N_1, N_2, \ldots, N_{500}$ represent the sequential number of respective image window pixels. The accuracy of the developed algorithm can be enhanced by providing a precise pre-determined threshold value range to detect the gradual changes of enamel structure as a result of demineralization.

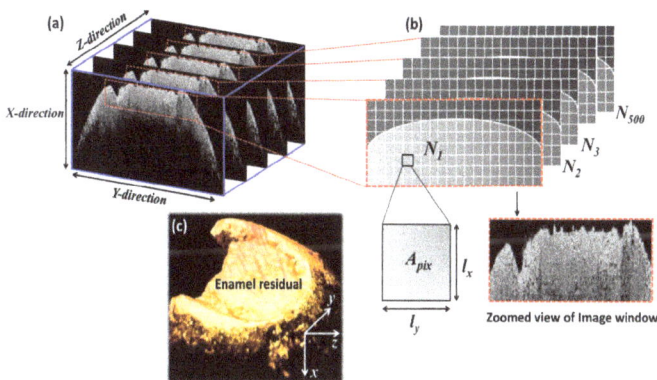

Figure 2. Volumetric evaluation algorithm for enamel residual. (**a**) Sequential 2D OCT images along with the applied image window; (**b**) Detected pixels, which satisfy the applied pre-determined threshold range; (**c**) Acquired 3D OCT volumetric image.

3. Results and Discussion

3.1. Morphological Analysis of Dental Caries along with Quantitative Evaluations

Figure 3a–c show the cross-sectional comparison between healthy, partially demineralized, and completely demineralized (carious) molar tooth samples. Figure 3d,e present the three-dimensional volumetric images of partially demineralized and carious molar tooth samples for a better view. In Figure 3a, the structural layers such as, enamel, dentino-enamel junction, and dentin can be visualized along with the depth ranges of 250 μm, 600 μm, and 800 μm, respectively. The progression of the demineralization can be identified in Figure 3b due to the demineralized enamel region and the formation of pits region in the depth range of 500 μm below the enamel range, and the remaining dentino-junction and dentin layer thickness was about 300 μm. Moreover, a clearly distinguishable demineralized enamel and dentino-junction (in the depth range of 800 μm), which leads to a formation of a carious region including pits and fissures were identified in Figure 3c. In addition, the remaining dentin thickness was about 100 μm. The three-dimensional images (Figure 3d,e) emphasize the top view of the partially demineralized and carious molar teeth samples. The infected microstructures, formation of pits and fissures, as well as the enamel loss, can be clearly visualized through the obtained volumetric images, owing to the high depth penetration. The desired morphological changes owing to demineralization mostly occurred in the enamel and dentin regions, which belong to a depth range that can be sufficiently achieved from the developed OFDI technique, and therefore, the necessity of histological images could be minimized by using the two-dimensional cross-sectional images acquired from the developed non-invasive OCT system [32–35]. Although the customized SD-OCT system implemented in this preliminary study improves the anatomical evaluation of the enamel and dentin, due to the low image acquisition speed and low sensitivity, the image quality has a limitation in SD-OCT compared to optical frequency domain imaging based high-speed swept source OCT (SS-OCT) [36]. Though the implementation of high-speed 1.3 μm SS-OCT can be beneficial, the customized cost effective OFDI system of this preliminary study was capable of obtaining a sufficient depth visibility to confirm the desired morphological results.

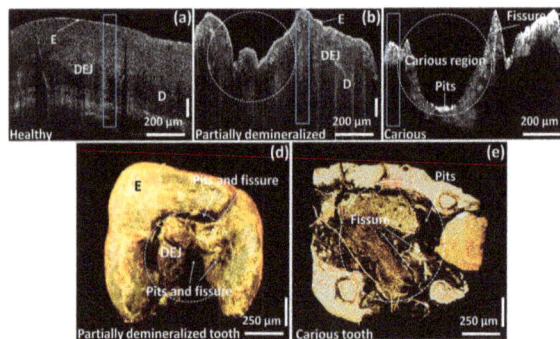

Figure 3. Two-dimensional OCT image comparison between healthy, partially demineralized, and completely demineralized (carious) molar tooth samples along with three-dimensional OCT images. (**a**) 2D OCT image of a healthy molar tooth region; (**b**) 2D OCT image of a partially demineralized molar tooth region; (**c**) 2D OCT image of a completely demineralized (carious) molar tooth region; (**d**) 3D OCT volumetric image of a partially demineralized molar tooth sample; and (**e**) 3D OCT volumetric image of a carious molar tooth sample.

The blue color box regions of Figure 3a–c depict the averaged A-scan depth profile regions. In Figure 4a, the blue solid line, red dotted line, and black dashed line represent the A-scan depth profiles of healthy, partially demineralized, and carious samples, respectively. Owing to the high scattering coefficient of the healthy structure region, a high backscattered signal intensity can be identified compared to partially demineralized and carious samples. In addition, it is difficult to detect dentin enamel junction and dentin regions of the partially demineralized and carious samples (within depth range of 500 μm to 1000 μm) due to low signal intensity from the structure. The demineralization mainly affects the hard calcium based structural surface of the tooth enamel region by decreasing the calcium constitution and simultaneously increase the progression of caries, which contain soft tissues and blood vessels. Owing to the aforementioned increase of the soft tissue region containing blood vessels, light scattering coefficient decreases. Therefore, the degree of demineralization affects the OCT signal in depth direction. As a consequence, low signal intensity could be detected from partially demineralized samples compared to healthy samples.

The aforementioned depth dependent intensity fluctuation according to each sample within each depth range is shown in the Figure 4b graph. The total intensity fluctuation of the healthy sample, partially demineralized sample, and carious sample are illustrated in blue, red, and gray color plots, respectively. Owing to the high optical scattering coefficient, the healthy sample performs the highest total intensity in all depth ranges, and the least intensity values could be identified in the carious sample. Furthermore, the partially demineralized sample performed less total intensity than the healthy sample and a higher intensity than the carious sample, which confirms the progression of dental caries. All the obtained intensity values are shown along with the corresponding graph bars. Furthermore, the enamel thickness was evaluated, and the next bar graph shown in Figure 4c represents the depth direction enamel thickness values of the aforementioned three samples using two-dimensional cross-sectional image based A-scan depth profile analysis. The thickness of the healthy enamel region was measured as 255.45 ± 15.03 µm, a partially demineralized molar specimen was measured as 150.30 ± 10.02 µm (with a reduction of 41.1% compared to the healthy sample), and the enamel residual of the carious region was measured as 100.20 ± 6.68 µm (with a reduction of 60.8% compared to the healthy sample), respectively.

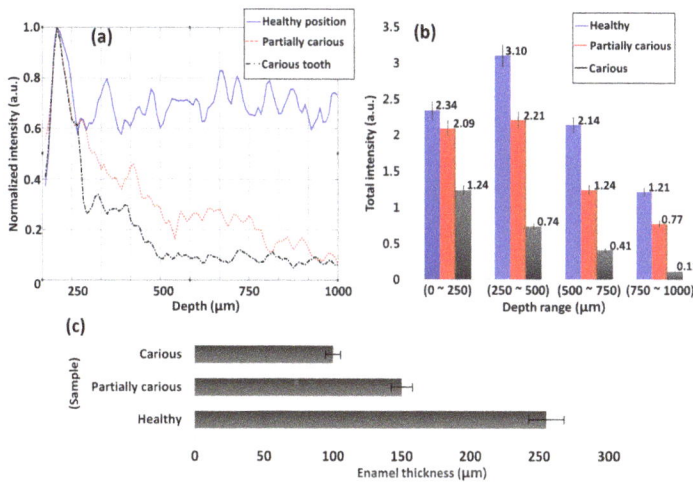

Figure 4. The quantitative evaluation method for healthy, partially demineralized, and completely demineralized (carious) molar tooth samples. (**a**) A-scan depth profiles of healthy, partially demineralized, and carious samples; (**b**) The total intensity fluctuation of healthy, partially demineralized molar, and completely demineralized (carious) molar tooth samples for the entire visible depth range of 1 mm with a gap of 250 µm depth range; (**c**) The depth direction enamel thickness values of the healthy, partially carious, and carious samples.

To gain a better understanding about the enamel demineralization, we repeated the aforementioned similar experimental method using partially demineralized canine and pre-molar tooth samples, which have a healthy appearance externally. Figure 5a,c emphasize the 2D OCT images along with the acquired 3D OCT volumetric images (Figure 5b,d) and sample photographs. The scanned positions of the samples are shown by red dashed lines. Although the samples have a healthy appearance, the formation of the demineralized enamel and root cavity region were identified in cross-sectional images and 3D OCT images of both canine and pre-molar tooth samples. Moreover, the enamel of the pre-molar tooth sample was demineralized towards a 750 µm depth to form the cavity region, which can be quantitatively evaluated using A-scan depth profile analysis. To acquire the most accurate quantification of enamel residual and the demineralized enamel region, we repeated the previous quantitative methods under the same experimental conditions.

The obtained A-scans of partially demineralized canine tooth sample and partially demineralized pre-molar tooth sample were compared with a healthy sample and shown in Figure 6a. In the A-scan profile, the blue solid line, black dashed line, and green dotted line represent the A-scan depth profiles of healthy sample, canine sample, and pre-molar sample, respectively. Similar signal intensity behavior was confirmed as before, owing to the low scattering coefficient of partially demineralized samples, which confirms the changes of the sample composition compared to the healthy sample. Then, we analyzed and compared the total intensity fluctuation of both partially demineralized samples according to each imaging depth range (Figure 6b).

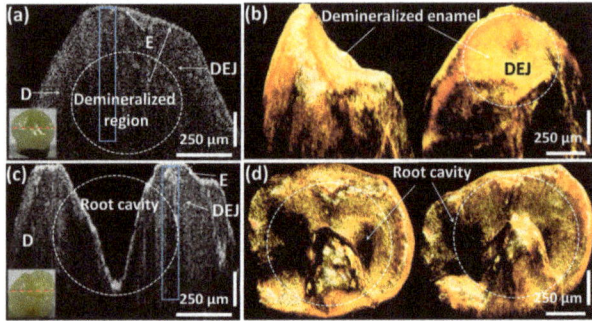

Figure 5. Two-dimensional OCT image comparison between a partially demineralized but healthy appearing canine tooth sample and a partially demineralized but healthy appearing pre-molar tooth sample with three-dimensional OCT images. (**a**) 2D OCT image of a partially demineralized but healthy appearing canine tooth sample; (**b**) 3D OCT volumetric image of a partially demineralized but healthy appearing canine tooth sample; (**c**) 2D OCT image of a partially demineralized but healthy appearing pre-molar tooth sample; (**d**) 3D OCT volumetric image of a partially demineralized but healthy appearing pre-molar tooth sample.

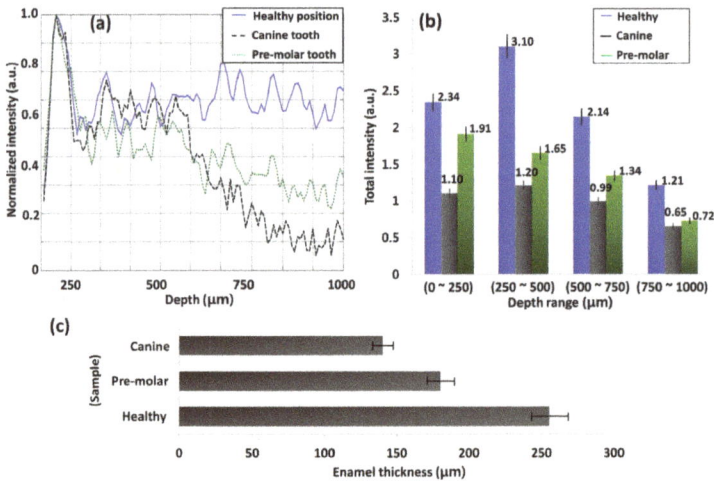

Figure 6. The quantitative evaluation for a healthy sample and partially demineralized but healthy appearing canine and pre-molar tooth samples. (**a**) A-scan depth profiles of healthy and partially demineralized but healthy appearing canine and pre-molar tooth samples; (**b**) the total intensity fluctuation of healthy, canine, and pre-molar tooth samples for the entire visible depth range of 1 mm with a gap of 250 μm depth range; (**c**) the depth direction enamel thickness values of the healthy, partially demineralized but healthy appearing canine and pre-molar tooth samples.

All the obtained intensity values are shown along with the corresponding graph bars. Although a reduction of the total intensity was noticed in partially demineralized samples (compared to the healthy sample), all the intensity levels were comparatively higher than the intensity levels of the carious sample. Therefore, the results confirm that the experimentally tested samples were neither healthy nor carious and verify the progression of demineralization. Next, we analyzed and compared enamel thickness of all three samples, and the bar graph shown in Figure 6c represents the obtained depth direction enamel thickness. The thickness of the healthy enamel region was measured as 255.45 ± 15.03 μm, partially demineralized pre-molar tooth sample was measured as 180.36 ± 12.02 μm (reduction of 29.4% compared to the healthy sample), and partially demineralized canine tooth sample was measured as 140.28 ± 9.35 μm (reduction of 45.1% compared to the healthy sample), respectively. Therefore, the obtained quantitative evaluations confirm the progression of early caries, and, moreover, the obtained quantitative evaluations can be utilized as threshold parameters to detect the progression of early caries. To gain a better understanding about the quantified thickness values and total intensity fluctuations of the experimented tooth specimens, the summarized quantifications are illustrated in Table 3.

Table 3. The quantified enamel thickness and depth direction total intensity fluctuations.

Specimen Category	Enamel Thickness (μm)	Total Intensity Fluctuation in Each Depth Range (a.u.)			
		0–250 μm	250–500 μm	500–750 μm	750–1000 μm
Healthy molar	255.45 ± 15.03	2.34 ± 0.2	3.10 ± 0.2	2.14 ± 0.2	1.21 ± 0.2
Dem. molar	150.30 ± 10.02	2.09 ± 0.2	2.21 ± 0.2	1.24 ± 0.2	0.77 ± 0.1
Carious molar	100.20 ± 6.68	1.24 ± 0.1	0.74 ± 0.05	0.41 ± 0.02	0.11 ± 0.01
Dem. canine	140.28 ± 9.35	1.10 ± 0.1	1.21 ± 0.1	0.99 ± 0.1	0.65 ± 0.1
Dem. premolar	180.36 ± 12.02	1.91 ± 0.1	1.65 ± 0.1	1.34 ± 0.1	0.72 ± 0.05

3.2. Volumetric Evaluation Technique to Identify Initial Caries

We quantified the volume of the enamel residual by applying the described volumetric algorithm in Section 2.4. Thus, we calculated the enamel residual of a selected particular position determined by the expert orthodontist for the healthy tooth specimen, three partially demineralized but healthy appearing tooth specimens, and the carious tooth specimen. All the performed calculations were based on the refractive index of 1.63, and the calculated enamel residual volume evaluations are illustrated along with the parameters in Table 4.

Table 4. The volumetric evaluation results of the enamel residual.

Tooth Specimen	Total Number of 2D OCT Images	Total Number of Enamel Residual Pixels	Enamel Residual Volume (mm³)
Healthy molar tooth	500	2.13×10^7	28.72
Part.dem. molar	500	1.31×10^7	17.70
Carious molar	500	0.91×10^7	12.26
Part.dem. canine	500	1.28×10^7	17.20
Part.dem. pre-molar	500	1.42×10^7	19.15

Hence, the obtained results confirmed that the proposed volumetric evaluation method will be more useful to detect the progression of caries, since the gradual reduction of the enamel volume owing to the gradual growth of caries can be detected quantitatively in advance. Therefore, medical treatments can be initiated immediately in order to obstruct the progression of caries, once the volume reduction of teeth is identified.

3.3. Structural Comparison between OCT and Conventional Methods

Figure 7 shows the structural analysis of a carious molar tooth sample and a comparison between imaging results obtained from various inspection methods. Figure 7a shows the *in vivo* radiographic image of the carious tooth, which was captured before early childhood caries (ECC) surgery performed on a 10-year-old male volunteer. The images were acquired to inspect the dental caries and cavity filling portions using a system that is currently applied in standard clinical practice: ultra speed (D-speed) film (Kodak, Rochester, NY, USA), 150 kVp, 15 mA, and 20 impulses. In this radiographic method, resolving a sub-millimeter tissue structure proves to be difficult, and only the surface structures of the cavity fillings, carious region, partially demineralized regions, pulps, and root canals along with healthy tooth were visualized. Thus, the obtained results were neither quantitative nor sensitive, and the cavity depths could not be imaged as well. Hence, precise radiographic detection of demineralization is a challenging task, since minimally demineralized regions are unable to reach the threshold of resolution. Figure 7b shows the photograph of the carious tooth, which was obtained after early childhood caries (ECC) surgery. Figure 7c,d represent the *ex vivo* 3D OCT images of the same sample and show the top and the side views of the sample. A precise enhancement could be identified, compared to radiographic images. Both 3D OCT figures give a clear view of the distinguishable anatomical structures e.g., dentin tubules, pulp, root canals, and cement owing to the high axial and lateral resolutions. Therefore, the applicability and the reliability of our system were verified because the dental caries, demineralization, and the inner microstructures of dentin were confirmed simultaneously through the obtained results.

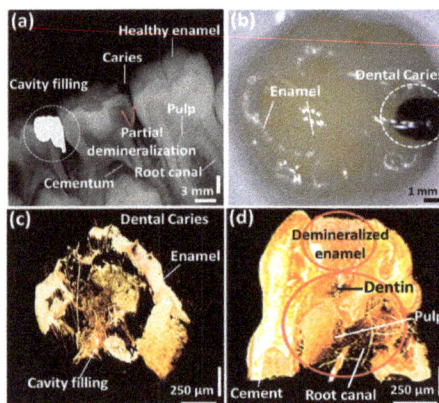

Figure 7. Structural analysis of the carious tooth sample using various inspection methods. (**a**) Radiographic image of the carious tooth sample before the surgery; (**b**) Photograph of the carious tooth sample after the surgery; (**c,d**) top and side views of 3D OCT images of the carious tooth sample.

4. Conclusions

We have demonstrated an optical frequency-domain imaging technique based quantitative evaluation method as an initial *ex vivo* study to detect the progression of dental caries by comparing partially and completely demineralized tooth samples with healthy tooth specimens. The quantification techniques were carried out by evaluating precise volume and thickness of enamel residual. Next, the total intensity fluctuation in each imaging depth range of all the specimens was quantified to confirm the changes that occurred in the internal composition of partially and completely demineralized tooth samples compared to a healthy sample. The performed study was a preliminary descriptive observational study, which was performed to confirm the feasibility of the three developed quantification techniques. The representative *ex vivo* tooth specimens as well as the experimental procedure was conducted according to the guidelines provided by an expert orthodontist. The results obtained using our high-resolution OFDI system revealed anatomic and quantitative information in a relatively nondestructive manner. The threshold parameters to detect the progression of early caries were determined on the basis of the quantitative results obtained from partially demineralized samples. Therefore, the physicians were able to diagnose the tooth volumetric and thickness changes at an initial stage by considering the obtained results as promising threshold parameters, which will be useful to barricade the progression of caries. To enhance the accuracy of the threshold parameters, quantitative (thickness and volumetric) information of multiple *in vivo* specimens will be evaluated, averaged, and normalized along with clinical trials in future studies.

Acknowledgments: This research was supported by the Industrial Strategic Technology Development Program, Grant No. 10047943; the "Development of Micro-Surgical Apparatus Based on 3D Tomographic Operating Microscope" program, funded by the Ministry of Trade, Industry and Energy (MI, Korea, No. 10047943). This study was also supported by the BK21 Plus project funded by the Ministry of Education, Korea (21A20131600011).

Author Contributions: R.E.W. and N.H.C. conducted the experiment, and analyzed and drafted the manuscript. K.P. designed the experimental setup with software and hardware components. M.J. and J.K. designed the study and critically revised and finalized the intellectual contents of manuscript.

Conflicts of Interest: The authors declare no conflict of interest.

References

1. Selwitz, R.H.; Ismail, A.I.; Pitts, N.B. Dental caries. *Lancet* **2007**, *369*, 51–59. [CrossRef]
2. Fejerskov, O. Changing paradigms in concepts on dental caries: Consequences for oral health care. *Caries Res.* **2004**, *38*, 182–191. [CrossRef] [PubMed]
3. Dove, S.B.; McDavid, W. A comparison of conventional intra-oral radiography and computer imaging techniques for the detection of proximal surface dental caries. *Dentomaxillofac. Radiol.* **1992**, *21*, 127–134. [CrossRef] [PubMed]
4. Fercher, A.F. Optical coherence tomography. *J. Biomed. Opt.* **1996**, *1*, 157–173. [CrossRef] [PubMed]
5. Ding, Z.; Ren, H.; Zhao, Y.; Nelson, J.S.; Chen, Z. High-resolution optical coherence tomography over a large depth range with an axicon lens. *Opt. Lett.* **2002**, *27*, 243–245. [CrossRef] [PubMed]
6. Boppart, S.A.; Herrmann, J.; Pitris, C.; Stamper, D.L.; Brezinski, M.E.; Fujimoto, J.G. High-resolution optical coherence tomography-guided laser ablation of surgical tissue. *J. Surg. Res.* **1999**, *82*, 275–284. [CrossRef] [PubMed]
7. Nassif, N.; Cense, B.; Park, B.; Pierce, M.; Yun, S.; Bouma, B.; Tearney, G.; Chen, T.; de Boer, J. In vivo high-resolution video-rate spectral-domain optical coherence tomography of the human retina and optic nerve. *Opt. Express* **2004**, *12*, 367–376. [CrossRef] [PubMed]
8. Wijesinghe, R.E.; Park, K.; Kim, P.; Oh, J.; Kim, S.-W.; Kim, K.; Kim, B.-M.; Jeon, M.; Kim, J. Optically deviated focusing method based high-speed sd-oct for in vivo retinal clinical applications. *Opt. Rev.* **2016**, *23*, 307–315. [CrossRef]
9. Welzel, J. Optical coherence tomography in dermatology: A review. *Skin Res. Technol.* **2001**, *7*, 1–9. [CrossRef] [PubMed]
10. Cho, N.H.; Lee, J.W.; Cho, J.-H.; Kim, J.; Jang, J.H.; Jung, W. Evaluation of the usefulness of three-dimensional optical coherence tomography in a guinea pig model of endolymphatic hydrops induced by surgical obliteration of the endolymphatic duct. *J. Biomed. Opt.* **2015**, *20*, 036009. [CrossRef] [PubMed]
11. Lee, J.; Kim, K.; Wijesinghe, R.E.; Jeon, D.; Lee, S.H.; Jeon, M.; Jang, J.H. Decalcification using ethylenediaminetetraacetic acid for clear microstructure imaging of cochlea through optical coherence tomography. *J. Biomed. Opt.* **2016**, *21*, 081204. [CrossRef] [PubMed]
12. Akkaya, N.; Kansu, Ö.; Kansu, H.; Çağirankaya, L.; Arslan, U. Comparing the accuracy of panoramic and intraoral radiography in the diagnosis of proximal caries. *Dentomaxillofac. Radiol.* 2014. [CrossRef] [PubMed]
13. Seneadza, V.; Koob, A.; Kaltschmitt, J.; Staehle, H.; Duwenhoegger, J.; Eickholz, P. Digital enhancement of radiographs for assessment of interproximal dental caries. *Dentomaxillofac. Radiol.* 2014. [CrossRef] [PubMed]
14. Featherstone, J.; Ten Cate, J.; Shariati, M.; Arends, J. Comparison of artificial caries-like lesions by quantitative microradiography and microhardness profiles. *Caries Res.* **1983**, *17*, 385–391. [CrossRef] [PubMed]
15. Bühler, C.M.; Ngaotheppitak, P.; Fried, D. Imaging of occlusal dental caries (decay) with near-ir light at 1310-nm. *Opt. Express* **2005**, *13*, 573–582. [CrossRef] [PubMed]

16. Cochrane, N.J.; Iijima, Y.; Shen, P.; Yuan, Y.; Walker, G.D.; Reynolds, C.; MacRae, C.M.; Wilson, N.C.; Adams, G.G.; Reynolds, E.C. Comparative study of the measurement of enamel demineralization and remineralization using transverse microradiography and electron probe microanalysis. *Microsc. Microanal.* **2014**, *20*, 937–945. [CrossRef] [PubMed]

17. Fried, D.; Xie, J.; Shafi, S.; Featherstone, J.D.; Breunig, T.M.; Le, C. Imaging caries lesions and lesion progression with polarization sensitive optical coherence tomography. *J. Biomed. Opt.* **2002**, *7*, 618–627. [CrossRef] [PubMed]

18. Ishibashi, K.; Ozawa, N.; Tagami, J.; Sumi, Y. Swept-source optical coherence tomography as a new tool to evaluate defects of resin-based composite restorations. *J. Dent.* **2011**, *39*, 543–548. [CrossRef] [PubMed]

19. Baumgartner, A.; Dichtl, S.; Hitzenberger, C.; Sattmann, H.; Robl, B.; Moritz, A.; Fercher, A.; Sperr, W. Polarization–sensitive optical coherence tomography of dental structures. *Caries Res.* **1999**, *34*, 59–69. [CrossRef]

20. Huynh, G.D.; Darling, C.L.; Fried, D. Changes in the optical properties of dental enamel at 1310 nm after demineralization. In Proceedings of the Biomedical Optics 2004, San Jose, CA, USA, 28 May 2004; pp. 118–124.

21. Cahill, L.; Lee, A.M.; Pahlevaninezhad, H.; Ng, S.; MacAulay, C.E.; Poh, C.; Lane, P. Passive endoscopic polarization sensitive optical coherence tomography with completely fiber based optical components. In Proceedings of the SPIE BiOS, San Francisco, CA, USA, 2 March 2015; p. 930413.

22. Jones, R.S.; Staninec, M.; Fried, D. Imaging artificial caries under composite sealants and restorations. *J. Biomed. Opt.* **2004**, *9*, 1297–1304. [CrossRef] [PubMed]

23. Popescu, D.P.; Sowa, M.G.; Hewko, M.D. Assessment of early demineralization in teeth using the signal attenuation in optical coherence tomography images. *J. Biomed. Opt.* **2008**, *13*, 054053. [CrossRef] [PubMed]

24. Shimada, Y.; Sadr, A.; Burrow, M.F.; Tagami, J.; Ozawa, N.; Sumi, Y. Validation of swept-source optical coherence tomography (ss-oct) for the diagnosis of occlusal caries. *J. Dent.* **2010**, *38*, 655–665. [CrossRef] [PubMed]

25. Cara, A.C.; Zezell, D.M.; Ana, P.A.; Maldonado, E.P.; Freitas, A.Z. Evaluation of two quantitative analysis methods of optical coherence tomography for detection of enamel demineralization and comparison with microhardness. *Lasers Surg. Med.* **2014**, *46*, 666–671. [CrossRef] [PubMed]

26. Hsieh, Y.-S.; Ho, Y.-C.; Lee, S.-Y.; Chuang, C.-C.; Tsai, J.-C.; Lin, K.-F.; Sun, C.-W. Dental optical coherence tomography. *Sensors* **2013**, *13*, 8928–8949. [CrossRef] [PubMed]

27. Keane, P.A.; Ruiz-Garcia, H.; Sadda, S.R. Clinical applications of long-wavelength (1000-nm) optical coherence tomography. *Ophthalmic Surg. Lasers Imaging Retin.* **2011**, *42*, S67–S74. [CrossRef] [PubMed]

28. Jeon, M.; Kim, J.; Jung, U.; Lee, C.; Jung, W.; Boppart, S.A. Full-range k-domain linearization in spectral-domain optical coherence tomography. *Appl. Opt.* **2011**, *50*, 1158–1163. [CrossRef] [PubMed]

29. Jung, U.-S.; Cho, N.-H.; Kim, S.-H.; Jeong, H.-S.; Kim, J.-H.; Ahn, Y.-C. Simple spectral calibration method and its application using an index array for swept source optical coherence tomography. *J. Opt. Soc. Korea* **2011**, *15*, 386–393. [CrossRef]

30. Lee, C.; Lee, S.-Y.; Kim, J.-Y.; Jung, H.-Y.; Kim, J. Optical sensing method for screening disease in melon seeds by using optical coherence tomography. *Sensors* **2011**, *11*, 9467–9477. [CrossRef] [PubMed]

31. Wijesinghe, R.E.; Lee, S.-Y.; Kim, P.; Jung, H.-Y.; Jeon, M.; Kim, J. Optical inspection and morphological analysis of diospyros kaki plant leaves for the detection of circular leaf spot disease. *Sensors* **2016**, *16*, 1282. [CrossRef] [PubMed]

32. Shellis, R. Relationship between human enamel structure and the formation of caries-like lesions in vitro. *Arch. Oral Biol.* **1984**, *29*, 975–981. [CrossRef]

33. Silverstone, L.; Poole, D. The effect of saliva and calcifying solutions upon the histological appearance of enamel caries. *Caries Res.* **1968**, *2*, 87–96. [CrossRef] [PubMed]

34. Ekstrand, K.; Kuzmina, I.; Bjørndal, L.; Thylstrup, A. Relationship between external and histologic features of progressive stages of caries in the occlusal fossa. *Caries Res.* **1995**, *29*, 243–250. [CrossRef] [PubMed]

35. Go, E.-J.; Jung, H.-S.; Kim, E.-S.; Jung, I.-Y.; Lee, S.-J. Histology of dental pulp healing after tooth replantation in rats. *J. Korean Acad. Conserv. Dent.* **2010**, *35*, 273–284. [CrossRef]

36. Yun, S.; Tearney, G.; de Boer, J.; Iftimia, N.; Bouma, B. High-speed optical frequency-domain imaging. *Opt. Express* **2003**, *11*, 2953–2963. [CrossRef] [PubMed]

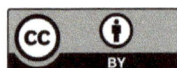

sensors

MDPI

Article

An Objective Balance Error Scoring System for Sideline Concussion Evaluation Using Duplex Kinect Sensors

Mengqi Zhu, Zhonghua Huang, Chao Ma and Yinlin Li *

School of Mechatronical Engineering, Beijing Institute of Technology, Beijing 100081, China;
vivian_zmq@yahoo.com (M.Z.); huangzh@bit.edu.cn (Z.H.); 20081124@bit.edu.cn (C.M.)
* Correspondence: liyinlin@bit.edu.cn; Tel.: +86-10-6891-1081

Received: 10 September 2017; Accepted: 18 October 2017; Published: 20 October 2017

Abstract: Sports-related concussion is a common sports injury that might induce potential long-term consequences without early diagnosis and intervention in the field. However, there are few options of such sensor systems available. The aim of the study is to propose and validate an automated concussion administration and scoring approach, which is objective, affordable and capable of detecting all balance errors required by the balance error scoring system (BESS) protocol in the field condition. Our approach is first to capture human body skeleton positions using two Microsoft Kinect sensors in the proposed configuration and merge the data by a custom-made algorithm to remove the self-occlusion of limbs. The standing balance errors according to BESS protocol were further measured and accessed automatically by the proposed algorithm. Simultaneously, the BESS test was filmed for scoring by an experienced rater. Two results were compared using Pearson coefficient r, obtaining an excellent consistency ($r = 0.93$, $p < 0.05$). In addition, BESS test–retest was performed after seven days and compared using intraclass correlation coefficients (ICC), showing a good test–retest reliability (ICC = 0.81, $p < 0.01$). The proposed approach could be an alternative of objective tools to assess postural stability for sideline sports concussion diagnosis.

Keywords: concussion evaluation; postural stability; balance error scoring system; Kinect sensor

1. Introduction

Sports-related concussion is common in most sports with a higher incidence in American football, hockey, rugby, soccer, and basketball, of which 78% occur during games as opposed to training [1,2]. The Centers for Disease Control estimates that 1.6 to 3.8 million concussions occur in the US per year in competitive sports and recreational activities [3]. Failure of early recognition and removal of the concussed athlete from play may put the individual at risk for potential complications and long-term consequences [4]. This often requires a rapid and accurate sideline assessment in the midst of competition by certified athletic trainers and team physicians [5].

Since 1997, a multidimensional approach consisting of the systematic assessment of cognition, balance and symptoms has been recommended for the diagnosis and management of sports concussion (SC) [2,6,7]. The multidimensional approach emphasizes multiple diagnostic elements including a physical examination, a survey of post-concussion symptoms, performance-based measures of acute mental status and postural stability, and careful consideration of clinical history [5,8]. Unfortunately, this approach is neither time- nor cost-effective, making them difficult to employ at varying levels of sport. A recent survey of certified athletic trainers indicated that only 21% of respondents used the recommended multidimensional approach to assess SC [9]. When used in isolation, each of the aforementioned clinical measures of cognition, balance, and/or symptoms has been demonstrated to have suboptimal reliability and validity [10–12].

As an alternative to the multidimensional approach, the Balance Error Scoring System (BESS) provides an objective measure of balance with the nature of being time- and cost-effective [13]. The BESS relies on the observational skills of trained sports administrator to count the total number of predefined balance errors that a subject makes during three standing stances on firm and foam surfaces. The BESS has been adopted as the current clinical standard of care for balance assessment in concussed athletes on the sideline [14]. However, several studies have addressed the measurement properties of the BESS showing variable inter-rater and test–retest reliability [4,15,16], which are partially based on the raters' subjective interpretations of errors committed throughout the test and different strictness of the scoring criteria.

To overcome the subjective nature of the BESS, technologies have been used to automate the assessment of postural stability. Such efforts can be divided into two main approaches: postural sway and error scoring [14,17]. The first has been evaluated by using force plate [17–19] or wearable devices [14,20,21]. Different from the scores of BESS, the metrics of postural sway are quantified by measured changes in body sway amplitude, velocity, frequency and direction of anterior-posterior, medial-lateral or trunk-rotation movements [20]. The primary clinical balance test for concussion assessment and most often used clinically and described in the literature is the BESS [14]. Therefore, the automated approach of error scoring with increased objectivity and subsequent reliability and validity could have great utility. Brown et al. provided insight into the relationship between inertial sensor-based kinematic outcomes and BESS errors' scores [22]. Potentially being able to track the six balance errors [23] as they are defined in the BESS standard, the Microsoft Kinect®sensor V1 [24] and V2 [23] have been investigated for the purpose. The use of a single Kinect sensor in the previous studies, however, has been called into the problem of self-occlusion happening when some parts of a human body are hidden. In addition, none of the previous studies have accounted for the error of eye-opening. As such, a large level of variability of the counted errors can result, leading to inaccurate BESS scores. Self-occlusion may be addressed by using multiple Kinect sensors instead of one [25–27]. The configuration of two Kinect sensors has been demonstrated to enhance the recognition rate, therefore limiting the issue of self-occlusion [28,29]. Nevertheless, the use of multiple Kinect sensors has not been explored or validated specifically as a way to count the BESS errors.

The aim of the current study is to present and validate a portable, untethered, and affordable solution for sideline sports concussion BESS test using two Kinect sensors. A custom algorithm is developed to automatically score errors committed during each BESS trial from duplex-views. The system is verified by concurrent validity and test–retest reliability in healthy participants. We hypothesized that the use of two Kinect sensors will effectively address the issue of self-occlusion, leading to strong concurrent validity and test–retest reliability when compared to a human rater.

2. Methods

2.1. Balance Error Scoring System (BESS) and Test Protocol

The BESS is a clinical accepted measure of postural stability prior to and following a sport concussion. To complete the BESS test, participants are required to maintain balance in three different stances, as shown in Figure 1. Each stance is performed on firm ground and pad form, respectively. The foam pad is medium density and measured 40 cm × 40 cm × 8 cm in size [30]. All trials are 20 s in length. During the completion of each trial, participants are asked to maintain a double leg, single leg or tandem stance with their hands on their iliac crests and with their eyes closed. The BESS errors consist of removal of hands from hips (balance error a), opening of the eyes (balance error b), stepping, stumbling, or falling (balance error c), abduction or flexion of the hip beyond $30°$ (balance error d), lifting the forefoot or heel off of the firm or foam surface (balance error e), and/or remaining out of the testing position or more than 5 s (balance error f). A maximum of 10 errors could be committed during each trial. If a subject committed multiple errors simultaneously, only one error was recorded. For example, if a subject stumbled, removed his or her hands from their hips and opened their eyes simultaneously, only one error is counted [13]. The balance error is identified by human skeleton data from two Kinect sensors and the final test score is counted. Testing consists of two parts separated by 7 days.

To complete the BESS, subjects are asked to stand at 2.5 m away from the sensors. Each participant is then instructed on how to complete the BESS. Following instruction and assurance of participant understanding, each participant completes the BESS test as previously described. After each trial, a 30 s rest period is employed. An experienced rater (over 60 h of grading experience) simultaneously counts the number of BESS errors for each trial. All trials are video recorded for a follow-up proof counting in order to ensure the accuracy of error numbers. The same testing protocol is administered seven days after the first session.

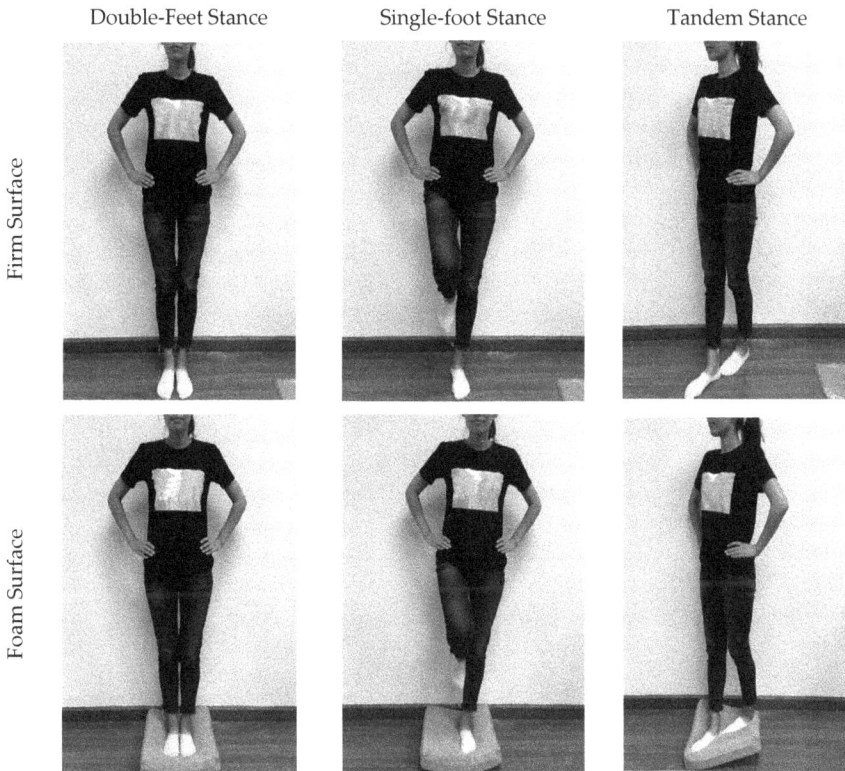

Figure 1. Trials of BESS test in three different stances (double feet, single foot and tandem) on two different surfaces (firm and foam).

2.2. Instrumentation and Configurations

The Kinect V2 sensors (Microsoft Corporation, Redmond, WA, USA) were deployed to measure the 3D coordinates of the skeletons and joints of the human body, which were then being used to judge the aforementioned balance errors a–f using custom-made algorithms. Though the camera is capable of obtaining 25 human skeletal joints through the depth image, only wrists, hips, ankles, spine, shoulder and hip center are used in the method, as denoted by the nine white circles in Figure 2. Experimental equipment includes two Kinect V2 cameras and two laptop computers with Windows 8.1 operating system (Microsoft Corporation, Redmond, WA, USA), Intel Core i5 processor and 4 GB memory. The algorithms were implemented in Visual Studio 2013 (Microsoft Corporation, Redmond, WA, USA) and Kinect SDK 2.0 (Microsoft Corporation, Redmond, WA, USA).

The basic configuration consideration for a Kinect sensor is to put the subject conducting the trial stances in the field of view (FOV), even when the movement of the hip is up to 30° of abduction. Moreover, the nine skeletal joints, as denoted in Figure 2, should not be occluded by body parts in the camera vision, or there should be no self-occlusion, for all three of the stances.

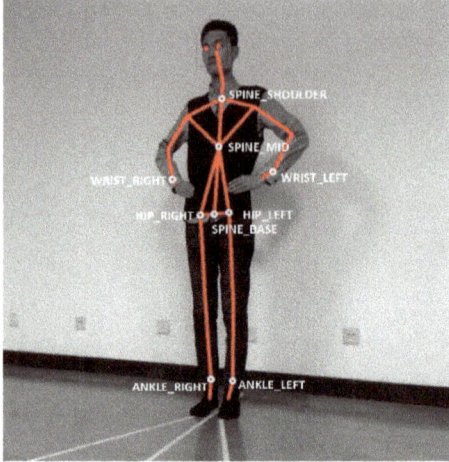

Figure 2. The selected joints used for the BESS test.

The vertical FOV of a single Kinect is up to 60°, illustrated as angle ∠C′K1B′ in Figure 3a; Point K1 represents the Kinect sensor mounted at height of 65 cm, which is regarded as the ideal operating value of Microsoft Xbox One floor mounting stand; Point B is the test position where the subject stands, and line BC denotes the height of subject, herein taking 2 m as the representative value.

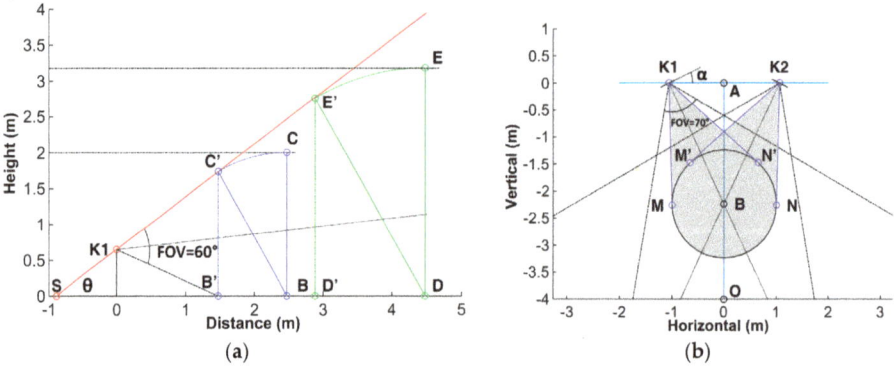

Figure 3. Illustration of duplex Kinect sensor placements. (**a**) the vertical field of view (FOV) of single Kinect sensor and setup for a 2 m high subject; (**b**) the positions, horizontal FOVs and required space (gray color) of the two sensors.

When the subject leans the hip maximally to 30°, the projection height in the vertical axis is under the curve CC′ in math. The point C′ corresponds to the subject's head position at the abduction angle 30°, which determines the upward tilt angle of the Kinect sensor and the minimal camera to subject distance (MCSD) that is able to watch the whole body skeletons. Under the prescribed condition, the distance is computed to be 2.48 m and the radius BB' of the test area is 1 m mathematically. The duplex sensor setup in horizontal view is shown in Figure 3b, in which *K1* and *K2* denote the two Kinect sensors. The distance between the two sensors is 2.12 m and the required test space as illustrated by a gray color in Figure 3b is 5.21 square meters. Since the horizontal FOV of the camera is 70°, the horizontal rotation angle of the camera, α, is allowed to be between 15° and 36°.

Although the above configurations are determined supposing 2 m as the height of participant, the sensor can track the whole body skeletons of shorter subjects as well, without any alteration of the setup parameters. When the subject is taller than 2 m, the mathematical expression between the MCSD value *d* and the subject height h can be described as

$$
\begin{cases}
d = \left(\frac{\sqrt{3}}{2} \cot \theta + 0.5 \right) \times h - H_s \cot \theta \\
\frac{\cot(60° - \theta)}{\cot \theta} = \frac{\frac{\sqrt{3}}{2} H_r - H_s}{H_s}
\end{cases}
\tag{1}
$$

where θ is the angle $\angle C'SB'$ as denoted in the Figure 3a, H_s and H_r are the sensor mounting height of 0.65 m and the reference subject height of 2 m, respectively. Equation (1) is obtained according to the triangular relationships of the sensor setup, as shown in Figure 3a, in which the setup parameters including the tilt angle, horizontal rotation angle and mounting height of the sensors are all the same as the case of the 2 m high subject. Typical numerical solutions of Equation (1) are present in Table 1. In the situation, the subject would simply move a distance referring to Table 1, along line AO toward point O as denoted in Figure 3b. The fixed installation parameters will help to ease the use of the system.

Table 1. The height of the subject and the required minimal camera to subject distance.

Height h (m)	MCSD d (m)
2.1	2.65
2.2	2.82
2.3	2.99
2.4	3.12
2.5	3.32
2.6	3.49
2.7	3.67
2.8	3.83
2.9	3.99

It is noteworthy that the above setup parameters are the worst case values. For example, there is less chance that one can fall like a rigid body without flexing one's hip, and hence the test area diameter should be less than 2 m. Therefore, in a real situation when these values are smaller, the system will have better performance in terms of required installation space and MCSD distance.

2.3. Algorithm Development

Microsoft Kinect SDK 2.0 provides all the methods or functions to acquire the skeletal joints coordinates of recognized users. In the tracking loop, *NuiSkeletonTrackingEnable* method is called to enable the tracking and *NuiSkeletonGetNextFrame* method is to access the members of the *NUI_SKELETON_FRAME* structure to receive information about the users. In the members of the skeleton frame structure, the *NUI_SKELETON_DATA* structure has a *SkeletonPositionTrackingState* array, which contains the tracking state for each joint. A tracking state of a joint can be "tracked" for a clearly visible joint, "inferred" when a joint is not clearly visible and Kinect is inferring its position, or "non-tracked". In addition, the *SkeletonPositions* array in the skeleton frame structure contains the position of each joint.

Once the positions and tracking states of the participants are obtained, the data from two Kinect sensors will be fed into a custom-made algorithm to compute BESS scores. It is mainly composed of two parts: error motion recognition and scoring algorithm.

2.3.1. Error Motion Recognition Algorithm

The error motion recognition algorithm (EMRA) functions to determine whether the balance errors occur during the BESS test. Specifically, the EMRA obtains the coordinates of skeletal joints from the two Kinect sensors and then extracts the feature vectors of the predefined balance errors, which is further processed by comparing the deviation of the joints away from its original position. Subsequently, the EMRA merges the results of two cameras by weighting a fusion coefficient in order to choose the best candidate of the skeletal joints from the two Kinect sensors, especially when one is self-occluded or incurred poor accuracy. Supposing the coordinate of a joint at time t is $p_i^t = (x_i^t, y_i^t, z_i^t)$, the vector between joint i and joint j at time t can be expressed as $p_{i,j}^t = p_i^t - p_j^t$. Then, the error equation $\delta^t(i,j)$ for balance error a, c, e is described as follows:

$$\delta^t(i,j) = \begin{cases} 1, & \|p_i^t - p_j^t\| > H, \|p_i^{t-1} - p_j^{t-1}\| \leq H \\ 0, & otherwise \end{cases} \tag{2}$$

where H is the predefined threshold. When the $\delta^t(i,j)$ is computed to be 1, a balance error is found. In the case of balance error a, the p_i and p_j are the coordinates of the joint wrist and hip, respectively; the term $\|p_i^t - p_j^t\|$ is $\|p_{wrist}^t - p_{hip}^t\|$, and the H equals to $\|p_{wrist}^0 - p_{hip}^0\|$, which means the distance between joint wrist and hip at the initial time. For the balance error c, the p_i is joint spine_mid and p_j is its initial value, and the term $\|p_i^t - p_j^t\|$ is then $\|p_{spine\_mid}^t - p_{spine\_mid}^0\|$. For the balance error e, the p_i is joint ankle and the term $\|p_i^t - p_j^t\|$ becomes $\|p_{ankle}^t - p_{ankle}^0\|$. The threshold H is set to 10 cm in the study for balance error c and e, the amount of which is determined by experiments and set to be large enough to reflect slight balance error motion meanwhile suppressing the jitter caused by the camera vision noise.

The error equation of balance error d is defined by:

$$\delta^t(i,j) = \begin{cases} 1, & \cos(p_{i,j}^{t-1}, v) > H, \cos(p_{i,j}^t, v) \leq H \\ 0, & otherwise \end{cases} \tag{3}$$

where $p_{i,j}$ is the vector from joint spine_base to spine_shoulder, v means a vertical vector, and threshold H is 0.866 corresponding to the cosine 30° of the maximal allowed hip flexion angle.

The error recognition fusion equation is expressed as:

$$\varphi^t = \begin{cases} 1, & \omega_A^t(i,j) \cdot \delta_A^t(i,j) + \omega_B^t(i,j) \cdot \delta_B^t(i,j) \geq 1 \\ 0, & \omega_A^t(i,j) \cdot \delta_A^t(i,j) + \omega_B^t(i,j) \cdot \delta_B^t(i,j) < 1 \end{cases} \tag{4}$$

where $\delta_A^t(i,j)$ and $\delta_B^t(i,j)$ represent the results of error recognition at time t from Kinect sensor A and B, and $\omega_A^t(i,j)$ and $\omega_B^t(i,j)$ are the weight coefficients of sensor A and B at time t, respectively. The values of $\omega_A^t(i,j)$ and $\omega_B^t(i,j)$ are determined according to the capture state of joint (well tracked, inferred and not tracked), which are provided by the Microsoft Kinect SDK. The values of $\omega(i,j)$ are shown in Table 2.

As for the balance error b, it can be achieved directly by calling the *GetFaceProperties* function of the Microsoft Kinect SDK to recognize the states of the eye (open, closed and unknown).

Table 2. The weight coefficient for error recognition fusion.

i	j	$\omega(i,j)$
Not tracked	Not tracked	0
Not tracked	Inferred	0
Not tracked	Well tracked	0
Inferred	Inferred	0.25
Inferred	Well tracked	0.5
Well tracked	Inferred	0.5
Well tracked	Well tracked	1

2.3.2. Scoring Algorithm

In addition to the error motion recognition, the software should also be able to score the BESS trials automatically. As one error might be accompanied by multiple simultaneous or subsequent errors, redundant errors count should be screened out. For the balance errors α and β, $t^{\alpha}_{i,begin}$ is the start time of the i-th occurrence of the balance error α, and the end time is $t^{\alpha}_{i,end}$; $t^{\beta}_{j,begin}$ is the start time of the j-th occurrence of the balance error β, and the end time is $t^{\beta}_{j,end}$. Whether the balance error α and β occur simultaneously is determined by the following equation:

$$\begin{cases} t^{\alpha}_{i,begin} - t^{\beta}_{j,begin} < 0 \\ t^{\alpha}_{i,end} - t^{\beta}_{j,begin} \geq 0 \end{cases} \quad or \quad \begin{cases} t^{\beta}_{j,begin} - t^{\alpha}_{i,begin} < 0 \\ t^{\beta}_{j,end} - t^{\alpha}_{i,begin} \geq 0 \end{cases}. \tag{5}$$

If simultaneous errors are detected, the later one will be ignored.

A total of six stances are performed in sequence (double feet, one foot, tandem) on the firm surface followed by the foam surface. For each stance, there are six types of balance errors a–f. The equation of BESS test score at j-th stance is defined as follows:

$$Score_j = \begin{cases} \sum\limits_{i=1}^{6} \varphi_i - \gamma, & 0 \leq \sum\limits_{i=1}^{6} \varphi_i - \gamma + \varepsilon < 10 \\ 10, & \sum\limits_{i=1}^{6} \varphi_i - \gamma + \varepsilon \geq 10 \end{cases}, \tag{6}$$

where φ_i is the number of occurrences of balance error i, and γ represents the number of simultaneous errors that should be ignored. The constant ε is to indicate whether or not the subject fails to maintain the testing stance less than 5 s or remains out of a proper testing position for longer than 5 s. If so, ε is 0; otherwise, ε is 10. The maximum score of each stance is limited to 10, and the total BESS score is the sum of $Score_j$ counted during all six stances. The total score acquired automatically using the above algorithm is then compared with the rater score to verify the Duplex Kinects System's validity and reliability.

2.4. Subjects

The current study was approved by the institutional academic board. Thirty healthy and physically active subjects (12 female and 18 male) between the 22 and 31 years (yr) of age (25.6 ± 2.56 yr), and who were 158 to 190 cm tall (171.1 ± 6.72 cm) participated in the current study. Exclusion criteria included neurological or musculoskeletal conditions, respiratory or cardiovascular problems, and pregnancy. All subjects were informed of the purpose, methods and instructions to complete the BESS and signed informed consent.

2.5. Analysis

Concurrent validity of scores obtained by the custom-made duplex Kinect BESS software and by the rater were assessed using Pearson correlation coefficients. In addition, intraclass correlation coefficients ICC (2,1) (2-way random effect, single measure model) were used to assess the test–retest reliability of the custom-made duplex Kinect BESS software between days 1 and 8. A modified version of BESS (mBESS) using only three stance conditions on the firm surface, which is currently included in the SCAT3 protocol and the Official NFL Sideline Tool [31], has also been accessed. All analyses were conducted with $p < 0.05$ as the significance level and performed using SPSS Version 20.0 (IBM Corporation, Armonk, NY, USA). For the Pearson coefficient r, it was excellent relationship if r was greater than 0.90, good relationship if r was between 0.8 and 0.89, a fair degree if r was between 0.7 and 0.79, and poor if r was below 0.70 [32]. Regarding the ICC coefficients, it was excellent if ICC was greater than 0.90, good if ICC was between 0.75 and 0.90, moderate if ICC was between 0.50 and 0.75, and poor if ICC was below 0.50 [33].

3. Results

In order to validate the self-occlusion of the proposed sensor configuration, representative images captured by sensors are shown in Figure 4. Direct view indicates the image captured by the sensor placed at position A in Figure 3b, facing directly to the subject; left and right view shows images captured by sensors placed at position K1 and K2 in Figure 3b, respectively, facing to the subject in the same way as depicted in Figure 3b. In Figure 4a, the rear ankle is occluded by the front one during tandem stance in direct view, resulting in a self-occlusion joint denoted as E in the figure. However, the rear ankle joint occluded in direct view is tracked properly in the right view. The same result could be found in the other three stance situations. The red dots overlaid on the eyes were generated by software automatically in case the eyes were tracked by the sensor, as shown in Figure 4.

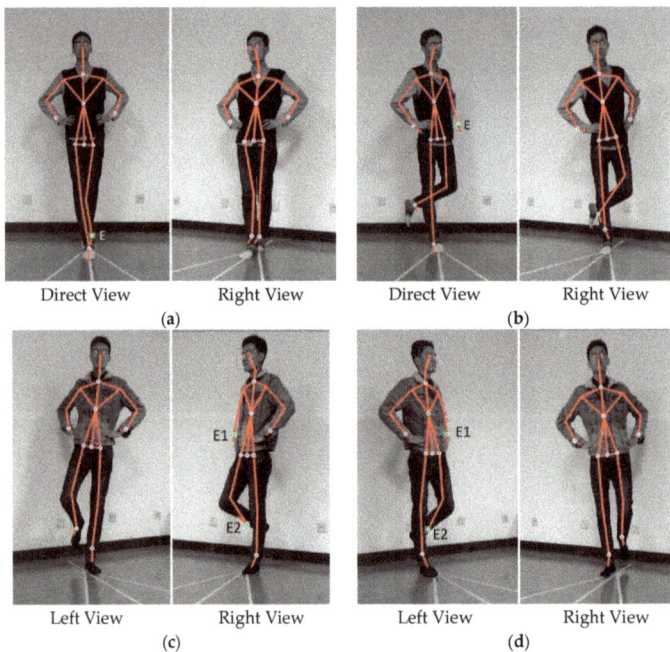

Figure 4. Representative self-occlusion images in direct, left or right view of Kinect sensors. (**a**) in the direct view, the rear ankle joint E is occluded whereas not in the right view; (**b**) in the direct view, the left wrist joint E is occluded when the body twisted, whereas not in the right view; (**c**) in the right view, the joints E1 and E2 are occluded, whereas not in the left view; (**d**) in the left view, joints E1 and E2 are occluded whereas not in the right view.

Further experiments were performed to examine the performance of the system for the purpose gof the BESS test. Table 3 shows the statistical results of the system measurements and the rater counting of the six balance conditions. In each condition, balance errors a–f committed by the subject were counted, including the error b of eye opening. Concurrent validity of the system and the rater counting shows that the system's BESS total score is 11.83 ± 7.62, and the rater's is 11.33 ± 7.89, and the Pearson coefficient r is 0.93 ($p < 0.05$). The total mBESS scores counted by system and rater are 4.67 ± 3.13 and 4.43 ± 3.40, respectively, indicating that the system score accurately fits the rater's ($r = 0.92$, $p < 0.05$) in the subset of balance conditions (firm surface only).

Table 3. The statistical results of the system and rater scores with Pearson coefficient value of each condition ($p < 0.05$).

Balance Condition	System Score	Rater Score	Pearson Coefficient r
Double feet firm	0.10 ± 0.40	0.10 ± 0.40	0.78
Single foot firm	3.37 ± 2.38	3.10 ± 2.34	0.89
Tandem firm	1.20 ± 2.34	1.23 ± 2.50	0.93
Double feet foam	0.33 ± 0.61	0.10 ± 0.30	0.55
Single foot foam	4.43 ± 3.13	4.30 ± 3.19	0.82
Tandem foam	2.37 ± 2.85	2.50 ± 3.08	0.87
BESS total	11.83 ± 7.62	11.33 ± 7.89	0.93
mBESS total (only firm)	4.67 ± 3.13	4.43 ± 3.40	0.92

A scatter plot is also presented in Figure 5, indicating that the system and rater score correlated positively and agreed with each other.

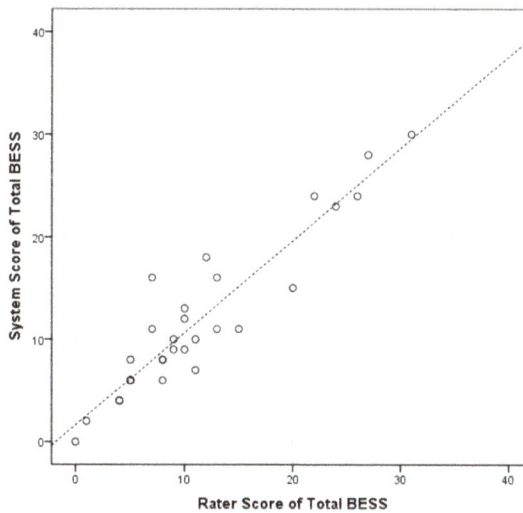

Figure 5. BESS score for rater and system.

Test–retest reliability of the system measurements on the first and eighth day as well as the ICC value in each condition shows that the first day total score of the BESS test is 12.07 ± 7.75, the eighth day total score of the BESS test is 11.47 ± 6.93, and the ICC was 0.81 ($p < 0.001$). The mBESS test score is 4.73 ± 3.17 on day 1 while 4.70 ± 3.76 on day 8, with ICC value of 0.84 ($p < 0.001$). The detail is illustrated in Table 4. The scatter plot of the BESS score for the first day and the eighth day is shown in Figure 6.

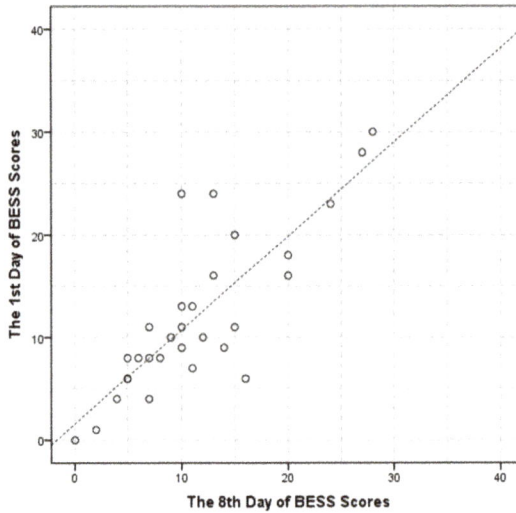

Figure 6. BESS score for day 1 and day 8.

Table 4. The statistical results of system score on the first and eighth day as well as the ICC value of each condition.

Balance Condition	Day 1	Day 8	ICC	p
Double feet firm	0.13 ± 0.30	0.10 ± 0.30	0.83	<0.001
Single foot firm	3.37 ± 2.36	3.67 ± 2.95	0.78	<0.001
Tandem firm	1.23 ± 2.36	0.93 ± 2.18	0.57	0.012
Double feet foam	0.33 ± 0.61	0.23 ± 0.50	0.58	0.010
Single foot foam	4.57 ± 3.21	4.40 ± 3.22	0.68	0.001
Tandem foam	2.40 ± 2.89	2.10 ± 2.93	0.87	<0.001
BESS total	12.07 ± 7.75	11.47 ± 6.93	0.81	<0.001
mBESS total (only firm)	4.73 ± 3.17	4.70 ± 3.76	0.84	<0.001

4. Discussion

The BESS is recognized as the current standard for the evaluation of sports related concussion. However, the intra- and inter-raters reliability of BESS scores has been questioned. In an attempt to overcome the subjective limitations of the BESS, the proposed method used two Kinect sensors along with a custom-made algorithm to track the postural balance errors committed by the participant. The primary findings derived from the results include: (1) the duplex views from two Kinect sensors can compensate for each other and track the key human body skeletal joints without blind spot or self-occlusion, even during the challenging tandem stance; and, (2) due to the constraint of the sensor's field of view, placement parameters including sensor separation distance, tilt angle and mounting height, etc., should be properly determined by taking into consideration the portability, installation space and ease of setup.

Our proposed custom-made algorithm for duplex Kinect BESS yielded excellent correlation coefficients to the human rater's BESS scores ($r = 0.93$, $p < 0.05$) and test–retest reliability (ICC = 0.81, $p < 0.05$) across an eight-day test–retest interval. Our method has greater test–retest reliability compared to that of human rater's BESS scores present by Finnoff et al. (ICC = 0.74) [16] and by Valovich et al. for high school participants (ICC = 0.70) [34]. These results indicate that the suggested duplex Kinect BESS method may be an objective and reliable measure of postural stability.

Brown et al. employed inertial sensors to evaluate the oBESS scores using a custom-made equation in an effort to overcome the subjectivity of the BESS scoring system [22]. Even though their oBESS was able to produce scores with accurate fit to raters in certain conditions, it didn't match well (ICC = 0.68) when using data from the subset of conditions (firm surface only). Contrary to the result of Brown et al., our system's mBESS scores are able to accurately fit the rater's ($r = 0.92$, $p < 0.05$) in the subset of balance conditions (firm surface only) as well. The support for the mBESS test of our method implies a time-saving test of postural stability when required. Moreover, the methodology by Brown et al didn't take into consideration the error of eye opening, which results in further discrepancy relative to the BESS standard.

Dave's study [24] using Kinect sensor V1 can only recognize three balance errors out of a total of six BESS test errors. In our study, we expanded on Dave's work by using a second Kinect sensor which tracked the six total BESS errors, resulting in system-derived scores with accurate fit to raters ($r = 0.93$, $p < 0.05$) compared to Dave's ($r = 0.38$) [24]. Furthermore, in Dave's study, the subject's balance loss may introduce unwanted error detection or may not detect errors during the BESS test, due to the joints' location outside the FOV of the Kinect sensor. In this regard, our work suggested a method to determine the advisable sensor configuration size and hence successfully removed the problem. Moreover, Dave only used a single Kinect sensor V1 and found the camera was limited to detect eye opening during the completion of each balance trial [24]. However, the use of the Kinect V2 improved upon the its predecessors' capability and was able to detect eye-opening, potentially as a result of an improvement of the Kinect V2 camera's resolution from 640×480 to 1920×1080 pixels of color image, and from 320×240 to 512×424 pixels of depth image. These results suggest that the proposed methodology is an improvement over previous attempts at automating error counting while participants complete the BESS.

In addition, Napoli et al. developed an automated assessment of postural stability (AAPS) algorithm based on a single Kinect Sensor V2 to evaluate the BESS errors [23], in which low AAPS performance levels were detected in single-leg and tandem stances on foam. In a separate paper on the same work, they reported the issues detecting the back leg that is hidden behind the other leg during the tandem stance [35]. Their works were only validated by comparing the level of agreement of system's BESS scores with that of rates and a professional camera. In our study, however, the aforementioned limitations have been addressed and verified by concurrent validity and test–retest reliability metrics.

Our study was limited to healthy normal subjects with a mean BESS score of 11.83 ± 7.62 errors. The thresholds used in the error detection algorithm, which influences the sensitivity of the BESS scoring, were determined through experiment and selection of optimal values. Therefore, the threshold values should be further considered when applied to the concussed participants. Our future research will also validate the duplex Kinect system in a clinical setting to assess errors in a large amount of concussed samples.

5. Conclusions

In the current study, we presented a novel Balance Error Scoring System by using duplex Kinect sensors and a custom-made algorithm. Our approach overcomes the self-occlusion problem of a previous solution using the Kinect sensor, realizing the recognition of balance error and the automatic administration of the BESS test, with a stronger test–retest reliability and concurrent validity compared to previous works. The current methodology provides a contactless clinic-based concussion administration and scoring approach that accurately detects all balance errors as per BESS instructions. Our method could be used as an affordable, portable and reliable tool for the concussion assessment in the field.

Acknowledgments: We would like to thank Jacob E. Resch from the Exercise and Sport Injury Laboratory at the University of Virginia for his idea of using Kinect to measure BESS errors, guidance and revision of the current manuscript.

Author Contributions: Mengqi Zhu built the system, designed the algorithm, performed the experiments, and also contributed to the data collection, analysis and writing of the corresponding paragraphs; Zhonghua Huang provided many useful comments and constructive discussions; Cao Ma helped in the experiment and manuscript formatting; Yinlin Li conceived of the technical solution of the study and contributed to the drafting of the manuscript. All authors read and approved the final manuscript.

Conflicts of Interest: The authors declare no conflict of interest.

References

1. Ravdin, L.D.; Barr, W.B.; Jordan, B.; Lathan, W.E.; Relkin, N.R. Assessment of cognitive recovery following sports related head trauma in boxers. *Clin. J. Sport Med.* **2003**, *13*, 21–27. [CrossRef] [PubMed]
2. Harmon, K.G.; Drezner, J.A.; Gammons, M.; Guskiewicz, K.M.; Halstead, M.; Herring, S.A.; Kutcher, J.S.; Pana, A.; Putukian, M.; Roberts, W.O. American Medical Society for Sports Medicine position statement: Concussion in sport. *Br. J. Sports Med.* **2013**, *47*, 15–26. [CrossRef] [PubMed]
3. Langlois, J.A.; Rutland-Brown, W.; Wald, M.M. The epidemiology and impact of traumatic brain injury: A brief overview. *J. Head Trauma Rehabil.* **2006**, *21*, 375–378. [CrossRef] [PubMed]
4. Valovich McLeod, T.C.; Barr, W.B.; McCrea, M.; Guskiewicz, K.M. Psychometric and measurement properties of concussion assessment tools in youth sports. *J. Athl. Train.* **2006**, *41*, 399–408. [PubMed]
5. Putukian, M. Clinical Evaluation of the Concussed Athlete: A View From the Sideline. *J. Athl. Train.* **2017**, *52*, 236–244. [CrossRef] [PubMed]
6. Kelly, J.P.; Rosenberg, J.H. Diagnosis and management of concussion in sports. *Neurology* **1997**, *48*, 575–580. [CrossRef] [PubMed]
7. Broglio, S.P.; Cantu, R.C.; Gioia, G.A.; Guskiewicz, K.M.; Kutcher, J.; Palm, M.; Valovich McLeod, T.C. National Athletic Trainers' Association position statement: management of sport concussion. *J. Athl. Train.* **2014**, *49*, 245–265. [CrossRef] [PubMed]
8. Lovell, M.R.; Iverson, G.L.; Collins, M.W.; Podell, K.; Johnston, K.M.; Pardini, D.; Pardini, J.; Norwig, J.; Maroon, J.C. Measurement of symptoms following sports-related concussion: Reliability and normative data for the post-concussion scale. *Appl. Neuropsychol.* **2006**, *13*, 166–174. [CrossRef] [PubMed]
9. Lynall, R.C.; Laudner, K.G.; Mihalik, J.P.; Stanek, J.M. Concussion-Assessment and -Management Techniques Used by Athletic Trainers. *J. Athl. Train.* **2013**, *48*, 844–850. [CrossRef] [PubMed]
10. Broglio, S.P.; Macciocchi, S.N.; Ferrara, M.S. Sensitivity of the concussion assessment battery. *Neurosurgery* **2007**, *60*, 1050–1057. [CrossRef] [PubMed]
11. Register-Mihalik, J.K.; Guskiewicz, K.M.; Mihalik, J.P.; Schmidt, J.D.; Kerr, Z.Y.; McCrea, M.A. Reliable change, sensitivity, and specificity of a multidimensional concussion assessment battery: Implications for caution in clinical practice. *J. Head Trauma Rehabil.* **2013**, *28*, 274–283. [CrossRef] [PubMed]
12. Resch, J.E.; Brown, C.N.; Schmidt, J.; Macciocchi, S.N.; Blueitt, D.; Cullum, C.M.; Ferrara, M.S. The sensitivity and specificity of clinical measures of sport concussion: Three tests are better than one. *BMJ Open Sport Exerc. Med.* **2016**, *2*, e000012. [CrossRef] [PubMed]
13. Riemann, B.L.; Guskiewicz, K.M. Assessment of mild head injury using measures of balance and cognition: A case study. *J. Sport Rehabil.* **1997**, *6*, 283–289. [CrossRef]
14. Alberts, J.L.; Thota, A.; Hirsch, J.; Ozinga, S.; Dey, T.; Schindler, D.D.; Koop, M.M.; Burke, D.; Linder, S.M. Quantification of the Balance Error Scoring System with Mobile Technology. *Med. Sci. Sports Exerc.* **2015**, *47*, 2233–2240. [CrossRef] [PubMed]
15. Hunt, T.N.; Ferrara, M.S. Age-Related Differences in Neuropsychological Testing Among High School Athletes. *J. Athl. Train.* **2009**, *44*, 405–409. [CrossRef] [PubMed]
16. Finnoff, J.T.; Peterson, V.J.; Hollman, J.H.; Smith, J. Intrarater and Interrater Reliability of the Balance Error Scoring System (BESS). *PM&R* **2009**, *1*, 50–54.
17. Chang, J.O.; Levy, S.S.; Seay, S.W.; Goble, D.J. An Alternative to the Balance Error Scoring System: Using a Low-Cost Balance Board to Improve the Validity/Reliability of Sports-Related Concussion Balance Testing. *Clin. J. Sport Med.* **2014**, *24*, 256–262. [CrossRef] [PubMed]
18. Merchant-Borna, K.; Jones, C.M.; Janigro, M.; Wasserman, E.B.; Clark, R.A.; Bazarian, J.J. Evaluation of Nintendo Wii Balance Board as a Tool for Measuring Postural Stability After Sport-Related Concussion. *J. Athl. Train.* **2017**, *52*, 245–255. [CrossRef] [PubMed]

19. Alsalaheen, B.A.; Haines, J.; Yorke, A.; Stockdale, K.; Broglio, S.P. Reliability and concurrent validity of instrumented balance error scoring system using a portable force plate system. *Physician Sportsmed.* **2015**, *43*, 221–226. [CrossRef] [PubMed]

20. King, L.A.; Mancini, M.; Fino, P.C.; Chesnutt, J.; Swanson, C.W.; Markwardt, S.; Chapman, J.C. Sensor-Based Balance Measures Outperform Modified Balance Error Scoring System in Identifying Acute Concussion. *Ann. Biomed. Eng.* **2017**, *45*, 2135–2145. [CrossRef] [PubMed]

21. King, L.A.; Horak, F.B.; Mancini, M.; Pierce, D.; Priest, K.C.; Chesnutt, J.; Sullivan, P.; Chapman, J.C. Instrumenting the Balance Error Scoring System for Use With Patients Reporting Persistent Balance Problems after Mild Traumatic Brain Injury. *Arch. Phys. Med. Rehabil.* **2014**, *95*, 353–359. [CrossRef] [PubMed]

22. Brown, H.J.; Siegmund, G.P.; Guskiewicz, K.M.; Van Den Doel, K.; Cretu, E.; Blouin, J.S. Development and validation of an objective balance error scoring system. *Med Sci Sports Exerc* **2014**, *46*, 1610–1616. [CrossRef] [PubMed]

23. Napoli, A.; Glass, S.M.; Tucker, C.; Obeid, I. The Automated Assessment of Postural Stability: Balance Detection Algorithm. *Ann. Biomed. Eng.* **2017**. [CrossRef] [PubMed]

24. Dave, P.T. Automated BESS Test for Diagnosis of Post-Concusive Symptoms Using Microsoft Kinect. Master's Thesis, Temple University, Philadelphia, PA, USA, 2014.

25. Asteriadis, S.; Chatzitofis, A.; Zarpalas, D.; Alexiadis, D.S.; Daras, P. Estimating human motion from multiple Kinect sensors. In Proceedings of the 6th International Conference on Computer Vision/Computer Graphics Collaboration Techniques and Applications, Berlin, Germany, 6–7 June 2013.

26. Azis, N.A.; Choi, H.J.; Iraqi, Y. Substitutive Skeleton Fusion for Human Action Recognition. In Proceedings of the International Conference on Big Data and Smart Computing (BigComp), Jeju, Korea, 9–11 February 2015; pp. 170–177.

27. Kaenchan, S.; Mongkolnam, P.; Watanapa, B.; Sathienpong, S. Automatic multiple kinect cameras setting for simple walking posture analysis. In Proceedings of the IEEE International Computer Science and Engineering Conference, Nakorn Pathom, Thailand, 4–6 September 2013; pp. 245–249.

28. Yeung, K.Y.; Kwok, T.H.; Wang, C.C.L. Improved Skeleton Tracking by Duplex Kinects: A Practical Approach for Real-Time Applications. *J. Comput. Inf. Sci. Eng.* **2013**, *13*, 041007. [CrossRef]

29. Gao, Z.; Yu, Y.; Zhou, Y.; Du, S. Leveraging Two Kinect Sensors for Accurate Full-Body Motion Capture. *Sensors* **2015**, *15*, 24297–24317. [CrossRef] [PubMed]

30. Bell, D.R.; Guskiewicz, K.M.; Clark, M.A.; Padua, D.A. Systematic review of the balance error scoring system. *Sports Health* **2011**, *3*, 287–295. [CrossRef] [PubMed]

31. Herring, S.A.; Cantu, R.C.; Guskiewicz, K.M.; Putukian, M.; Kibler, W.B.; Bergfeld, J.A.; Boyajian-O'Neill, L.A.; Franks, R.R.; Indelicato, P.A.; American College of Sports Medicine. Concussion (mild traumatic brain injury) and the team physician: A consensus statement—2011 update. *Med. Sci. Sports Exerc.* **2011**, *43*, 2412–2422. [PubMed]

32. Cicchetti, D.V. The precision of reliability and validity estimates re-visited: distinguishing between clinical and statistical significance of sample size requirements. *J. Clin. Exp. Neuropsychol.* **2001**, *23*, 695–700. [CrossRef] [PubMed]

33. Koo, T.K.; Li, M.Y. A Guideline of Selecting and Reporting Intraclass Correlation Coefficients for Reliability Research. *J. Chiropr. Med.* **2016**, *15*, 155–163. [CrossRef] [PubMed]

34. Valovich, T.C.; Perrin, D.H.; Gansneder, B.M. Repeat Administration Elicits a Practice Effect With the Balance Error Scoring System but Not With the Standardized Assessment of Concussion in High School Athletes. *J. Athl. Train.* **2003**, *38*, 51–56. [PubMed]

35. Napoli, A.; Ward, C.R.; Glass, S.M.; Tucker, C.; Obeid, I. Automated assessment of postural stability system. *Conf. Proc. IEEE Eng. Med. Biol. Soc.* **2016**, *2016*, 6090–6093. [PubMed]

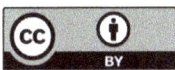

MDPI

St. Alban-Anlage 66

4052 Basel

Switzerland

Tel. +41 61 683 77 34

Fax +41 61 302 89 18

www.mdpi.com

Sensors Editorial Office

E-mail: sensors@mdpi.com

www.mdpi.com/journal/sensors

www.ingramcontent.com/pod-product-compliance
Lightning Source LLC
Chambersburg PA
CBHW051720210326
41597CB00032B/5546